p#53   Postmenopausal estrogen Rx
        + Stroke

p#96   Blepharospasm — review

p#121   Lambert Eaton .
 #125   No assn. ALS c/CA
 #127   Benign mononuclei amyotrophy

#210   PeT Scan in B-Tumors 1990

**YEAR BOOK OF
NEUROLOGY AND
NEUROSURGERY®**

#405   No theended trial of Autologous.
       Adrenal transplant in Parki

The 1990 Year Book® Series

Year Book of Anesthesia®: Drs. Miller, Kirby, Ostheimer, Roizen, and Stoelting

Year Book of Cardiology®: Drs. Schlant, Collins, Engle, Frye, Kaplan, and O'Rourke

Year Book of Critical Care Medicine®: Drs. Rogers and Parrillo

Year Book of Dentistry®: Drs. Meskin, Ackerman, Kennedy, Leinfelder, Matukas, and Rovin

Year Book of Dermatology®: Drs. Sober and Fitzpatrick

Year Book of Diagnostic Radiology®: Drs. Bragg, Hendee, Keats, Kirkpatrick, Miller, Osborn, and Thompson

Year Book of Digestive Diseases®: Drs. Greenberger and Moody

Year Book of Drug Therapy®: Drs. Hollister and Lasagna

Year Book of Emergency Medicine®: Dr. Wagner

Year Book of Endocrinology®: Drs. Bagdade, Braverman, Halter, Horton, Kannan, Korenman, Molitch, Morley, Odell, Rogol, Ryan, and Sherwin

Year Book of Family Practice®: Drs. Rakel, Avant, Driscoll, Prichard, and Smith

Year Book of Geriatrics and Gerontology: Drs. Beck, Abrass, Burton, Cummings, Makinodan, and Small

Year Book of Hand Surgery®: Drs. Dobyns, Chase, and Amadio

Year Book of Hematology®: Drs. Spivak, Bell, Ness, Quesenberry, and Wiernik

Year Book of Infectious Diseases®: Drs. Wolff, Barza, Keusch, Klempner, and Snydman

Year Book of Infertility: Drs. Mishell, Lobo, and Paulsen

Year Book of Medicine®: Drs. Rogers, Des Prez, Cline, Braunwald, Greenberger, Wilson, Epstein, and Malawista

Year Book of Neonatal and Perinatal Medicine: Drs. Klaus and Fanaroff

Year Book of Neurology and Neurosurgery®: Drs. Currier and Crowell

Year Book of Nuclear Medicine®: Drs. Hoffer, Gore, Gottschalk, Sostman, Zaret, and Zubal

Year Book of Obstetrics and Gynecology®: Drs. Mishell, Kirschbaum, and Morrow

Year Book of Occupational and Environmental Medicine: Drs. Emmett, Brooks, Harris, and Schenker:

Year Book of Oncology: Drs. Young, Longo, Ozols, Simone, Steele, and Weichselbaum

Year Book of Ophthalmology®: Dr. Laibson

Year Book of Orthopedics®: Drs. Sledge, Poss, Cofield, Frymoyer, Griffin, Hansen, Johnson, Springfield, and Weiland

Year Book of Otolaryngology–Head and Neck Surgery®: Drs. Bailey and Paparella

Year Book of Pathology and Clinical Pathology®: Drs. Brinkhous, Dalldorf, Grisham, Langdell, and McLendon

Year Book of Pediatrics®: Drs. Oski and Stockman

Year Book of Plastic, Reconstructive, and Aesthetic Surgery®: Drs. Miller, Bennett, Haynes, Hoehn, McKinney, and Whitaker

Year Book of Podiatric Medicine and Surgery®: Dr. Jay

Year Book of Psychiatry and Applied Mental Health®: Drs. Talbott, Frances, Freedman, Meltzer, Schowalter, and Yudofsky

Year Book of Pulmonary Disease®: Drs. Green, Ball, Loughlin, Michael, Mulshine, Peters, Terry, Tockman, and Wise

Year Book of Speech, Language, and Hearing: Drs. Bernthal, Hall, and Tomblin

Year Book of Sports Medicine®: Drs. Shephard, Eichner, Sutton, and Torg, Col. Anderson, and Mr. George

Year Book of Surgery®: Drs. Schwartz, Jonasson, Peacock, Shires, Spencer, and Thompson

Year Book of Urology®: Drs. Gillenwater and Howards

Year Book of Vascular Surgery®: Drs. Bergan and Yao

1990

The Year Book of NEUROLOGY AND NEUROSURGERY®

"Published without interruption since 1902"

Neurology

Editor

Robert D. Currier, M.D.
Professor and Chairman, Department of Neurology, University of Mississippi Medical Center, Jackson

Emeritus Editor

Russell N. DeJong, M.D.
Professor Emeritus of Neurology, The University of Michigan Medical School

Neurosurgery

Editor

Robert M. Crowell, M.D.
Director of Cerebrovascular Surgery, Massachusetts General Hospital and Harvard Medical School, Boston, Mass.

Year Book Medical Publishers, Inc.
Chicago • London • Boca Raton • Littleton, Mass.

Printed in U.S.A.

International Standard Book Number: 0-8151-2467-8

International Standard Serial Number: 0513-5117

Editor-in-Chief, Year Book Publishing: Nancy Gorham
Sponsoring Editor: Judy L. Plazyk
Senior Medical Information Specialist: Terri Strorigl
Assistant Director, Manuscript Services: Frances M. Perveiler
Assistant Managing Editor, Year Book Editing Services: Wayne Larsen
Production Coordinator: Max F. Perez
Proofroom Supervisor: Barbara M. Kelly

Table of Contents

The material in this volume represents literature reviewed through March 1989.

Journals Represented

Year Book Medical Publishers subscribes to and surveys nearly 850 U.S. and foreign medical and allied health journals. From these journals, the Editors select the articles to be abstracted. Journals represented in this YEAR BOOK are listed below.

Acta Cytologica
Acta Neurochirurgica
Acta Neurologica Scandinavica
Acta Oto-Laryngologica
American Journal of Clinical Nutrition
American Journal of Emergency Medicine
American Journal of Epidemiology
American Journal of Neuroradiology
American Journal of Roentgenology
Anesthesiology
Annals of Emergency Medicine
Annals of Internal Medicine
Annals of Neurology
Archives of Neurology
Archives of Orthopedic and Traumatic Surgery
Archives of Otolaryngology – Head and Neck Surgery
Archives of Physical Medicine and Rehabilitation
Biological Psychiatry
Brain—Journal of Neurology
British Journal of Industrial Medicine
British Medical Journal
Canadian Journal of Neurological Sciences
Cancer
Cancer Research
Cleveland Clinic Journal of Medicine
Clinica Chimica Acta
Clinical Orthopaedics and Related Research
Epilepsia
European Neurology
Experimental Neurology
Headache
Intensive Care Medicine
Journal of Bone and Joint Surgery (American volume)
Journal of Clinical Endocrinology and Metabolism
Journal of Clinical Investigation
Journal of Computer Assisted Tomography
Journal of Epidemiology and Community Health
Journal of Gerontology
Journal of Hand Surgery (American)
Journal of Neurological Sciences
Journal of Neurology, Neurosurgery and Psychiatry
Journal of Neuropathology and Experimental Neurology
Journal of Neurophysiology
Journal of Neurosurgery
Journal of Pediatrics
Journal of the American Geriatrics Society
Journal of the American Medical Association
Journal of Thoracic and Cardiovascular Surgery

Journal of Trauma
Klinische Wochenschrift
Laboratory Investigation
Lancet
Laryngoscope
Microsurgery
Mount Sinai Journal of Medicine (New York)
Muscle and Nerve
Nature
Neurochirurgia
Neurochirurgie
Neurology
Neuropediatrics
Neuroradiology
Neurosurgery
New England Journal of Medicine
New York State Journal of Medicine
Otolaryngology–Head and Neck Surgery
Pain
Paraplegia
Pediatric Infectious Disease Journal
Pediatric Neurology
Pediatric Neuroscience
Pediatrics
Postgraduate Medical Journal
Quarterly Journal of Medicine
Radiology
Revue Neurologique
Scandinavian Journal of Infectious Diseases
Scandinavian Journal of Rehabilitation Medicine
Scandinavian Journal of Rheumatology
Science
Spine
Stroke
Surgery
Surgical Neurology
Western Journal of Medicine
Yale Journal of Biology and Medicine

Publisher's Preface

The publication of the 1990 YEAR BOOK OF NEUROLOGY AND NEURO-SURGERY marks the end of an outstanding era of editorship by Russell N. DeJong, M.D. During Dr. DeJong's twenty-one years of editorship of the YEAR BOOK, readers have been treated to perceptive and informative commentary of the highest caliber. We extend our deepest appreciation for the service Dr. DeJong has provided and for his unending support and enthusiasm for this publication. During Dr. DeJong's forthcoming and well-deserved editorial retirement, he has kindly offered to contribute articles to the YEAR BOOK from time to time. We look forward to our continued contact with him in this regard and wish him well in all his other future endeavors.

Robert D. Currier, M.D., co-editor of the Neurology section will continue to select and comment on the neurology literature. He will be assisted by guest editors in the near future.

NEUROLOGY

———

ROBERT D. CURRIER, M.D.

———

RUSSELL N. DeJONG, M.D.

Introduction

The neurology portion of the YEAR BOOK OF NEUROLOGY AND NEU-ROSURGERY has been in existence since 1902. In this 88-year period it has had few editors. The original neurologist, Hugh Patrick, labored from the beginning, 1902, through 1917. Some editors did double duty, covering both nervous and mental diseases, such as Peter Bassoe, who joined the YEAR BOOK in 1910 and served until 1933. For 13 of those years (1918–1930) he was the only editor. In 1934 Hans Reese took over the Neurology portion and passed it to Dr. Roland Mackay in 1948, who went 20 years—until 1968. Dr. DeJong started his tenure then and went another 20 years. That makes five editors in 88 years—an amazing record, really. I am not sure what moral to draw from it, but tolerance on the part of the readers comes readily to mind.

A careful history of the first 40 years of the YEAR BOOK OF NEUROL-OGY, PSYCHIATRY, AND ENDOCRINOLOGY is found in the preface to the YEAR BOOK for 1940. Hans Reese of Wisconsin was the editor of the neurology portion for that YEAR BOOK, but the authorship of the preface is unknown. Appropriate praise was given to Gustavus P. Head, Profes-sor of Laryngology and Rhinology of the Chicago Postgraduate Medical School, as the founder and to his brother, Cloyd James Head, the busi-ness manager of the YEAR BOOK for many years. These two gentlemen were responsible for carrying the YEAR BOOK through its rocky begin-nings.

Nine years ago when Dr. DeJong asked me to help him with the YEAR BOOK, I was, of course, flattered beyond belief. I could remember in my childhood seeing the book on the cigar stand next to my father's evening chair waiting to be read. Indeed, I have some of those volumes annotated in his hand with comments such as *"read"* next to the abstracts.

Dr. DeJong has decided to give it up.

My acquaintance with this man goes back a long way—50 years. I can remember an evening in the winter of 1938 or '39 when after dinner we were ushered from the living room so that my father might talk with a visitor who was coming. We kids, peeping through the glass of the hall door, saw a young, dark-haired man in a winter coat speaking with my father in the hall. Dr. DeJong had come to discuss his own father's ill-ness. Later, in 1949 when Carl Camp retired after more than 40 years of running the Neurology department at Michigan, Dean Furstenburg sent out letters asking for suggestions for the chairmanship of Neurology. My father's comment was, "They couldn't do much better than to give it to that fellow down there"—Dr. DeJong. Over the last 28 years our paths have crossed more than incidentally. My student training, internship and residency, and time as faculty member at the University of Michigan are dominated by his figure. There are two outstanding traits that character-ize him. The first is his ability to work, and the second is his amazing memory. This combination made him an exemplary first editor of the journal *Neurology* and fifth editor of the YEAR BOOK. For a period he did them both, ran the department, and rewrote his textbook on the neu-rologic examination with practically no secretarial help, composing on his own typewriter. I don't know how he found time to run the department, but it is a matter of record that he saw every patient twice a week and definitely knew what was going on.

Dr. DeJong is a man whose shyness and reserve cause those who don't know him to mistake him as possibly aloof or cold. Nothing could be further from the truth. He and his wonderful wife Madge love people and talking with them, and his ability, knowledge, and memory of people make him a fantastic resource in a gossip session.

I am sorry he is retiring but can understand the load of his various physical problems. It's pertinent to point out that his comments, memory, and intelligence are undiminished with age and, if it weren't for physical infirmities such as his recent arm fracture, he would still be editing.

Without ostentatious humility the truth of the matter is I am a poor second. Nevertheless, imperfect though I am, I plan to continue, at least for the foreseeable future. Dr. DeJong has promised to add his comments from time to time, and we will look forward to that input.

In order to cover some areas more equitably, YEAR BOOK has agreed (in fact, encouraged) that we should add subeditors for various fields. Therefore, we have called upon our own Owen Beverly Evans for his comments in the area of pediatric neurology. Bev has recently become our Chairman of Pediatrics here but will, he says, find time to take on this additional task. Beginning with the 1991 edition Dr. Albert Galaburda of Boston will cover the neglected area of behavioral neurology and cortical function. Stanley Appel will cover more than adequately molecular biology and related fields, and Jim Toole has agreed to look over the area of stroke.

Daniel E. Koshland, editor of *Science,* has a delightful editorial in the January 6, 1989, issue that has set me thinking. He has decided that perhaps as an editor he is not automatically excluded from heaven and as a matter of fact has decided to try for it. As his first step he has determined to become humble but "being humble is not easy for ordinary people and it is extraordinarily difficult for editors."

He says there are at least three things militating against humbleness in editors. The first of the conspiracies is "the heroism of the arbitrary decision." He says after the first few arbitrary decisions the editor finally rationalizes that it is part of the job and eventually regards himself as a hero with "brilliance and integrity not given to ordinary mortals" because of his clever selections without consulting too many other people.

The second enemy of humility is "the euphoria of the adoring multitude." All editors have people who assure them they are doing well, and Koshland hypothesizes that "the human brain is designed to amplify such signals and to diminish or completely eliminate the objections of the 'lunatic fringe' who have the effrontery to suggest that one is doing poorly."

Finally, there is "the lure of evangelism" with the "almost imperceptible shift from a person who is puzzled by the cacophony of facts, theories, and opinions in the modern world to one who suddenly believes he or she has seen a clear light and is called to impress this new wisdom on those still benighted. For editors this mission can lead to a little twisting of the facts, all with the noblest of motives, to help the public to come to the 'right' conclusion."

Finally, he notes that his new modesty will "astonish my friends, bewilder my critics, and have a salutary effect on *Science,* as I wend my way to heaven."

From time to time, that is, every day, I worry about an ordinary neurologist like myself selecting articles and then, God forgive me, commenting on the selections when it is perfectly obvious that there are among you readers many, many persons who know more and could do a better job. But frankly, I like what I am doing. I have always had opinions and a big mouth.

The best I can do is to offer some belated New Year's hopes and wishes.

My first hope is that no comment of mine ever harms a patient either directly or indirectly. That has to be the number one editorial cardinal sin. Second is that no comment will ever so discourage an author-investigator that he considers giving up writing and research. Third is that you who do research and write will forgive me for missing an article of yours that is important, well written, and pertinent to select something that is none of those three and that somehow I will achieve the inner strength necessary to put aside the selection that offers a chance for an easy quip to choose those that are possibly hard to comment on but are of permanent worth to neurology and medicine. Fourth, I hope that the comments are helpful and perhaps even reassuring to both reader and patient.

My and, I would guess, your hopes for neurology at this time in our history are not many and fairly straightforward: that the factors causing amyotrophic lateral sclerosis, parkinsonism, and Alzheimer's be identified, that a harmless and effective treatment for multiple sclerosis be found, that the Huntington's disease gene be exactly located, and that some useful treatment be found for dystrophy now that its gene has been located fairly well. General wishes for medicine in the United States now include a wish for universal health coverage of some kind for all citizens. After having waited expectantly for 40 years for health insurance coverage to include all, I have given up and believe that the government will have to fill in the gap, which is a real one here in Mississippi.

Wishes for the world include a desire that each of the medical schools in the United States and Canada adopt a medical school or hospital in a third world country and that in this one-to-one relationship exchanges of students, faculty, knowledge, instruments, and even treatment modalities could be arranged.

The greatest number of comments I have received from you readers per year is perhaps two or three. I would like to hear from more of you about anything.

Looking over old YEAR BOOKS:

In the YEAR BOOK of 1910 edited by Hugh Patrick and Peter Bassoe there is an item taken from the *Journal of Nervous and Mental Diseases* (April 1910) recounting Huntington's comments before the New York

Neurological Society on the disease named for him. He noted that he would have been "unable to describe the clinical picture completely without the facts and observations handed down to him by his grandfather, Dr. Abel Huntington, and his father, Dr. George Lee Huntington, both of whom had practices in East Hampton, Long Island." So the correct perception and description of that disease was dependent on longitudinal knowledge through three generations of physicians. Much of the 1910 YEAR BOOK is taken up with infections of the meninges and the brain. The section on neuroses included epilepsy and migraine. There is no mention of amyotrophic lateral sclerosis, although a case report of progressive muscular atrophy from Germany by Cassirer and Maas is found (*Deutsche Zeitschr. f. Nervenheilk.*, 1910, p. 321).

The 1930 YEAR BOOK is edited by Bassoe who, in his preface, comments that there is "a ray of hope that both the etiology and treatment (of multiple sclerosis) may have been discovered." He probably was referring to the work of Purvis-Stewart and Chevassut (*Br Med J* May 24, 1930) in which the researchers isolated a virus from 200 consecutive cases of disseminated sclerosis. More than 200 patients had been treated with vaccination of this virus, of whom 73 had been treated for 2 years with "encouraging but not brilliant serological and clinical results." I am wondering what became of that virus.

Hans Reese, in a special article in the 1940 YEAR BOOK, gives a history of scalping and its clinical aspects. He had a patient who was scalped at work by a revolving shaft in a creamery, So he researched the history of scalping. Several persons have survived scalping, and it seems that the American Indians did not always take the entire scalp. The Indians were not the only persons active in scalping. During the early French-American-Indian and Canadian wars on this continent, various governments paid bounties for scalps. Governor Penn published on July 7, 1764, a price list that was as follows:

captured Indian more than 10 years old $150
scalp of a killed Indian 134
captured woman or boy under 10 years old 130
scalp of a slain squaw 50

Reese comments that during the American Revolution scalping was practiced on both sides and Hamilton was called "the hair buyer general."

The recent government suggestion that a bounty be paid for the apprehension of a Central American strongman in the amount of 1 or 2 million dollars thus has precedence. Has the value of a captured human really gone up that much, is it simply inflation, or are the difficulties greater?

I can't help but call to your attention the suggestions to authors by Daroff, Rowland, and Scism in *Neurology* (38:1657–1658, 1988). These are really delightful and not at all boring to read. I am guilty of more than one of their prohibitions, particularly the first, which is "keep it short."

Robert D. Currier, M.D.

1 Diagnosis*

Efficacy of MR vs. CT in Epilepsy
Heinz ER, Heinz TR, Radtke R, Darwin R, Drayer BP, Fram E, Djang WT (Duke
Univ, Durham, NC; Mary Hitchcock Clinic, Hanover, NH; St Joseph's Hosp,
Phoenix)
AJNR 9:1123–1128, November–December 1988   1–1

The comparative values of magnetic resonance imaging (MRI) and
computed tomography (CT) were investigated in 72 patients with seizures. Fifty-nine of them underwent both imaging studies as well as electroencephalography (EEG). Computed tomography was done with contrast enhancement.

Magnetic resonance imaging studies were abnormal in 53% of the 59
patients evaluated but never failed to detect a lesion that had been seen
with CT. It was positive also in 5 CT-negative patients. Both MRI and
CT were positive in 7 patients with negative EEGs. Magnetic resonance
imaging studies were positive in 44% of 34 patients with complex partial
seizures (Fig 1–1); CT studies were positive in 29% of these patients,
and EEG studies in 80%. No surgical patient with a tumor causing seizures had negative imaging studies.

Electroencephalography remains the most sensitive means of localizing
an epileptogenic focus; MRI, however, is the most effective imaging
method for defining a potential surgical focus. There is no need for CT
when an MRI study is normal. Because MRI is not always specific, CT
may be helpful in distinguishing neoplasia from thrombosed vascular
malformation and other lesions.

▶ To no one's surprise, MRI is the best way to find an epileptogenic focus. Of
the 3 procedures—CT, MRI, and EEG—EEG was the most sensitive, but MRI,
after all, is a picture. It is hard to persuade a neurosurgeon to operate on a brain
wave focus. No doubt SPECT and PET scans do add something and will add
more in the future, but the beautiful sharpness of the MRI should leave it at the
top of the diagnostic heap in the work-up of an epileptic focus for some time.

Walker and Blumer have given us a nearly 45-year follow-up on World War II
veterans with posttraumatic seizures (Arch Neurol 46:23–26, January 1989).
The seizures in most decreased or disappeared with time, but 25% had mental
deterioration. Why? I wonder what MRI would show in that group.*

---

*Unless otherwise noted, all comments in the Neurology section are those of Dr. Currier.

Idiopathic Intracranial Hypertension (Pseudotumor Cerebri): MR Imaging

Silbergleit R, Junck L, Gebarski SS, Hatfield MK (Univ of Michigan)
Radiology 170:207–209, January 1989   1–2

The central role of brain imaging in idiopathic intracranial hypertension (IIH) is to exclude other disorders that can cause papilledema and intracranial hypertension. Magnetic resonance imaging was performed in 6 patients with diagnoses of IIH. None had risk factors other than obesity. The patients, all women, had a mean age of 27 years. The median opening lumbar pressure was 375 mm of cerebrospinal fluid. Six healthy persons also were examined.

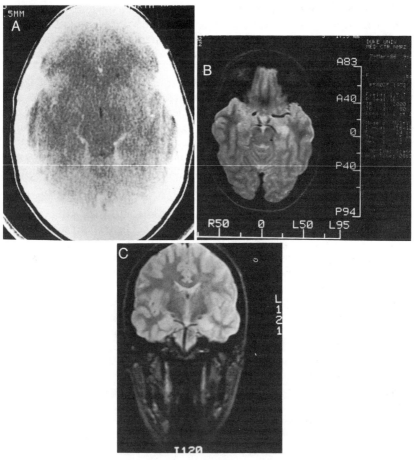

Fig 1–1.—Girl, 17 years, with complex partial seizures for 14 years. Scalp EEG: left spike focus. Depth electrodes: left temporal focus. Computed tomography, negative; magnetic resonance imaging, positive. **A,** contrast-enhanced CT scan is normal. **B,** axial MR image, 2,500/80. Hyperintense focus in medial third of left temporal lobe. **C,** coronal MR image, 2,500/80. Hyperintense focus on fully T_2-weighted sequence is in pes hippocampi. Partial temporal lobectomy was performed by aspiration. (This technique subsequently was changed to partial lobectomy with en bloc removal of specimen.) No tumor was found. (Courtesy of Heinz ER, Heinz TR, Radtke R, et al: *AJNR* 9:1123–1128, November–December 1988.)

Ventricular size and volume did not differ significantly between the patients with IIH and the controls. However, subarachnoid space volume was significantly larger in the patients. Two patients had a partially empty sella. One had signal aberration in the dural venous sinuses, suggesting slow flow. No white-matter signal abnormalities were observed.

These findings fail to support the concept of small or slitlike ventricles in IIH. The subarachnoid spaces are enlarged, but the wide range of normal precludes the clinical use of this parameter in evaluating patients. As is the case with computed tomography, magnetic resonance imaging serves mainly to exclude other diseases.

▶ This is a nice reference on MRI of pseudotumor. The world is waiting for a group of patients with this disorder to be studied carefully with demonstration of the entire venous circulation of the head and neck early in the course of the disorder.

CT, MR, and Pathology in HIV Encephalitis and Meningitis

Post MJD, Tate LG, Quencer RM, Hensley GT, Berger JR, Sheremata WA, Maul G (Univ of Miami; Wistar Inst, Philadelphia)
AJR 151:373–380, August 1988   1–3

Computed tomography (CT) and magnetic resonance imaging (MRI) findings for patients with either autopsy-proved human immunodeficiency virus (HIV) encephalitis or culture-proved HIV meningitis were evaluated. The neurologic and pathologic findings were closely correlated. Atrophy was the most common CT finding; all but 1 of 21 patients with HIV encephalitis had cortical atrophy. Thirteen of these patients had ventricular dilatation on an ex vacuo basis. Seven patients had low-density parenchymal lesions lacking mass effect. Magnetic resonance imaging showed high-intensity parenchymal lesions without mass effect

Location of HIV Infection at Autopsy in 17 Patients*

Site of Involvement	No. of Patients
Cerebral cortical gray matter	16
Cerebral subcortical white matter	15
Centrum semiovale	11
Periventricular white matter	9
Corpus callosum	7
Internal capsule	7
Basal ganglia	11
Thalamus	8
Midbrain	13
Brainstem	14
Cerebellum	9

*Refers to the finding of focal inflammation dominated by microglial nodules containing multinucleated giant cells.

(Courtesy of Post MJD, Tate LG, Quencer RM, et al: *AJR* 151:373–380, August 1988.)

in 5 patients. Detection of demyelinative lesions with MRI was more sensitive than with CT.

Most HIV lesions were not evident on gross study of the brain. They usually were diffuse; no patient had large, focal, mass-producing lesions. The cerebrum was the most frequent site of involvement (table). Sixteen patients had microglial nodules and multinucleated giant cells at multiple sites in both cerebral hemispheres. The CT and MR findings were correlated well both in cortical atrophy and demyelinative white-matter lesions.

Thin-section multiplanar MRI is useful for screening HIV-positive patients with encephalopathy. If findings (e.g., focal mass lesions) are atypical, contrast CT is indicated. Patients with meningeal symptoms should have both studies.

▶ Periventricular changes on MRI and cortical atrophy on CT and MRI seem to be the most important scan findings in HIV encephalitis and meningitis. These findings are not predictive and therefore are probably not helpful in arriving at an early diagnosis.

Diagnosis of Acute Herpes Simplex Encephalitis by Brain Perfusion Single Photon Emission Computed Tomography

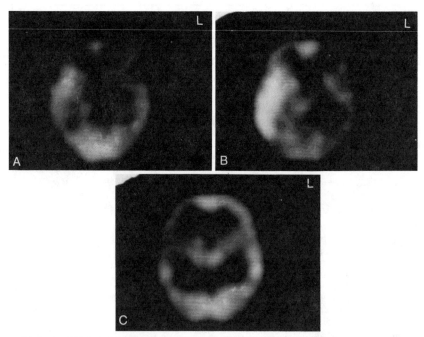

Fig 1–2.—SPECT in HSV encephalitis: case examined with HM-PAO. **A,** a clearly hyperperfused area in the right anterior and middle temporal lobe 4 days after onset of encephalitis. **B,** the rate of hyperperfusion has increased, and the area covers also the posterior temporal aspects 12 days after onset. **C,** an area of hyperperfusion is seen 55 days after onset in the corresponding area where initial hyperperfusion was seen. (Courtesy of Launes J, Nikkinen P, Lindroth L: *Lancet* 1:1188–1191, May 28, 1988.)

Launes J, Nikkinen P, Lindroth L, Brownell A-L, Liewendahl K, Iivanainen M
(Helsinki Univ)
Lancet 1:1188–1191, May 28, 1988   1–4

The clinical picture of herpes simplex virus (HSV) encephalitis may be misleading, and even brain biopsy results may be falsely negative. Because early treatment is important, the potential of brain perfusion scintigraphy using the single photon emission computed tomography (SPECT) technique in 14 patients with viral encephalitis was examined. Either ^{123}I-iodoamphetamine (IMP) or ^{99m}Tc-hexamethylpropyleneamine oxime (HM-PAO) was employed. Seventeen SPECT studies in 6 patients with HSV encephalitis and 10 studies in 8 with non-HSV encephalitis were done. All patients received acyclovir therapy.

Each patient with HSV encephalitis had an area of increased tracer uptake in the affected temporal lobe on initial SPECT study (Fig 1–2). Hyperperfusion increased subsequently in 2 cases, but hypoperfusion followed the hyperperfusion stage, starting 37 days after initial symptoms of encephalitis. No patient with non-HSV encephalitis had focal hyperperfusion during the first 2 weeks. Initial CT scanning results were normal in all patients, and 2 patients with HSV encephalitis had normal results of conventional scintigrams during the time when SPECT results demonstrated hyperperfusion.

Acyclovir therapy should be started when HSV encephalitis is suspected. Using SPECT with IMP or HM-PAO is helpful in distinguishing HSV encephalitis from clinically similar states. However, acyclovir should not be discontinued if SPECT studies fail to show focal abnormality.

▶ It looks as though the MRI scan, good at diagnosing acute herpes encephalitis, may be bettered by the SPECT scan. It would be happy news for those who struggle regularly with acute encephalopathies if it turns out to be true.

MR Imaging Artifacts of the Axial Internal Anatomy of the Cervical Spinal Cord
Curtin AJ, Chakeres DW, Bulas R, Boesel CP, Finneran M, Flint E (Ohio State Univ)
AJNR 10:19–26, January–February 1989   1–5

Transverse magnetic resonance imaging (MRI) studies of the spinal cord regularly show signal variations related to internal cord anatomy that do not coincide with histologic observations and may reflect technical variations. Therefore, a study of MR images of cadaver spinal cords, phantoms, and a normal subject was done. Short repetition-time and echotime (TR/TE) spin-echo studies, cardiac-gated multiecho spin-echo studies, and gradient-refocused-echo studies were carried out, using both 128 × 256 and 256 × 256 matrices with a varying phase-encoded axis.

Significant Fourier truncation and partial-volume imaging artifacts influenced the MRI display of the spinal cord. On short TR/TE images a

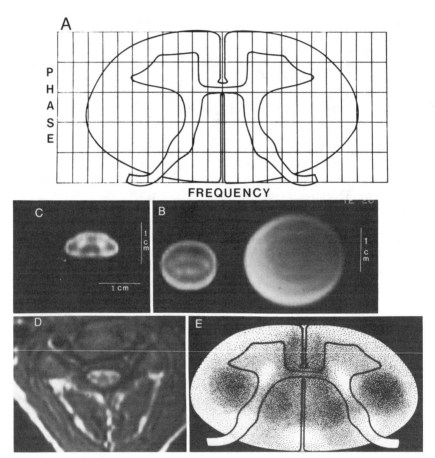

Fig 1–3.—Pixel size and orientation. **A,** grid of rectangular boxes overlying transverse section of cord is drawn to scale approximating the number and size of pixels displaying the human cord when a 128 × 256 matrix and 16-cm field of view is used. Note that when 128 phase-encoded steps run anterior to posterior, only 5 pixels per row span cord. **B,** gel phantom. Axial scan, 800/20, through cylindrical gelatin phantoms in air with 128 × 256 matrix and 128 in phase-encoded direction. Artifactual rings of high and low signal transverse internal structure of homogeneous phantom. Note high signal of periphery, which is thicker in phase-encoded direction. Geometric distortion of circular gel to more oval appearance is due to partial-volume effects. **C,** excised cord. Axial scan of excised human cervical cord in air with parameters identical to those of gelatin phantom (**B**). High-signal rim that is thicker in phase-encoded direction surround 2 lateral circular areas of low signal overlying regions of corticospinal tracts. Butterfly-shaped area of high signal approximates gray matter. Central triangle of low signal approximates anterior and posterior columns. **D,** human volunteer. Axial section of cervical spine, same parameters as **B** and **C**. Note that appearance is similar to that seen in excised cord (**C**). **E,** location of gray-matter tracts with overlay drawing of approximate locations of high and low signal seen on short TR/TE images with 128 × 256 matrix. (Courtesy of Curtin AJ, Chakeres DW, Bulas R, et al: *AJNR* 10:19–26, January–February 1989.)

ring of high signal at the cord periphery represented a truncation artifact (Fig 1–3). The central appearances were affected by partial-volume averaging, depending on matrix size. White matter tracts always were lower in signal than were gray matter tracts, independent of iron deposition or cerebrospinal fluid motion artifact.

A 128 × 256 matrix with 2 averages is suggested when making axial scans of the spinal cord. Truncation artifacts may limit image quality, but with a 256 × 256 matrix longer scan times result in motion artifacts and a lower signal-to-noise ratio.

▶ A similar article by Carvlin and associates (AJNR 10:13–17, January– February, 1989) in the same issue comes to the same conclusion. It is nice to know that the thing on cross-sectional MRI scan that looks like it might relate to the internal anatomy of the spinal cord actually is the internal anatomy of the spinal cord and that the central gray is there and looks white and the white matter is there and looks dark. The rim of white around the periphery of the cord is called a truncation artifact and is not real. It's a real pleasure to be able to see a nice cross section of cord on the MRI scan.

Dizziness in a Community Elderly Population
Sloane P, Blazer D, George LK (Univ of North Carolina at Chapel Hill; Duke Univ)
J Am Geriatr Soc 37:101–108, February 1989   1–6

Dizziness is common among the elderly and often is a perplexing problem. Factors related to dizziness were examined in a series of 1,622 persons aged 60 and older living in 1 community who were interviewed in the course of an epidemiologic catchment area study.

The adjusted lifetime prevalence of dizziness was 34% in this population, and in 18% of patients dizziness prompted a physician visit. After a comparison of approximately 300 patients who had significant dizziness during the previous year with those never experiencing the symptom, dizziness was closely related to overall health status and to perception of self as a nervous person. In addition, dizziness was associated with symptoms of depression and several neurosensory features such as limb numbness, poor vision, and a history of neurologic disease. Furthermore, dizziness was related to several cardiovascular variables. No strong relationships were found between dizziness and smoking or alcohol dependence.

Dizziness may not have high priority in routine systems reviews of elderly patients unless it is a prominent complaint, when it must be pursued vigorously. A significant number of elderly patients experiencing dizziness do have major treatable disorders. In making the medical assessment, particular attention should be given to neurosensory, behavioral, and cardiovascular factors.

▶ The authors come to just about the same conclusion that Drachman and Hart (1) did in their study 15 years ago. Dizziness, of course, is several things, and its etiology in the clinical situation can usually be determined by finding out exactly what the patient means by it, discovering the circumstances in which it occurs, and examining the patient. The advantage of this study, as with Drachman's, is in delineating the group of patients who complain of dizziness but who are depressed or "nervous."

Reference

1. Drachman DA, Hart CW: *Neurology* 22:323–334, 1972.

Sudden Vertigo of Central Origin
Mangabeira-Albernaz PL, Gananca MM (Escola Paulista de Medicina, São Paulo, Brazil)
Acta Otolaryngol (Stockh) 105:564–569, May–June 1988   1–7

The neurotologic literature has described many patients who suddenly have an intense vertiginous attack that lasts for several days and takes weeks or months to disappear completely. Sometimes this attack is accompanied by sudden deafness. The disease is believed to result from the unilateral destruction of the peripheral vestibular end-organ. The vestibular examination typically indicates an intense unilateral peripheral deficit that is permanent. A common name for this disorder is *vestibular neuritis.* A different disorder, intense vertiginous attacks of sudden onset and lasting several months, was observed in 8 patients after viral infection.

The patients were aged 8–46 years. Five were female, and all were white. Complete otolaryngologic examination, audiologic tests, and vestibular assessment were done. Torsion swing tests were performed on 5 patients. For the last 3 patients, auditory brain stem responses were recorded. Different types of signs of involvement of the central vestibular apparatus were found on neurotologic assessment. All of the patients became more dizzy when given vestibular depressor drugs. All obtained symptomatic relief with corticosteroids. Three to 4 months after onset of the disease, all of the patients became asymptomatic. Signs of central vestibular involvement, however, persisted for 6–12 months.

Sudden vertigo of central origin is a vestibular disease characterized by intense vertigo and signs of brain stem involvement. It follows a viral infection, and its symptoms are similar to those of a vestibular neuritis or vestibular paralysis of sudden onset. Patients become asymptomatic after a period of days or months, and a return to normal responses is indicated by neurotologic examination. Although uncommon, this disorder must be considered in the differential diagnosis of sudden vertiginous attacks.

▶ The authors gathered 8 patients with this syndrome over a period of 14 years. They believe it is due to viral involvement of the central vestibular apparatus, is a benign encephalitis, and responds to corticosteroids but not to vestibular depressor drugs.

The Mental Status Evaluation: Application in the Emergency Department
Zun L, Howes DS (Northwestern Univ; Univ of Illinois, Chicago)
Am J Emerg Med 6:165–172, March 1988   1–8

Emergency physicians may have to evaluate mental status in order to detect neuropsychiatric disease, identify a focal lesion, determine mental competence, or distinguish organic from functional illness. Common specific indications for assessment of mental status include head injury, behavioral abnormality, and drug ingestion.

The patient's appearance first is evaluated, and his motor behavior and relation to the environment are noted. Speech is an important characteristic. The way in which the patient thinks, including suicidal or homicidal thought or intent, is also an important consideration. Disorders of perception are considered, and the patient's affect and judgmental ability assessed. Finally the sensorium and intelligence are evaluated. Most often an extensive, formal mental status evaluation is not required. A brief test of cognitive function such as the Cognitive Capacity Screening Examination or Mini-Mental Status Examination often is appropriate.

▶ This is a nice review of the need for and possible methods of obtaining a brief mental status evaluation in the emergency room. There is no question that it should be done, but perhaps unfortunately, the CT scan gets more attention.—R.N. DeJong, M.D., and R.D. Currier, M.D.

Evaluation of Thermography in the Diagnosis of Selected Entrapment Neuropathies
So YT, Olney RK, Aminoff MJ (Univ of California, San Francisco)
Neurology 39:1–5, January 1989   1–9

The diagnostic accuracy of infrared thermography was compared with that of conventional electrodiagnostic studies in 22 patients with carpal tunnel syndrome and 15 with ulnar neuropathy at the elbow. Twenty normal subjects also were studied. A microprocessor-controlled infrared camera was used to obtain skin surface images.

An interside temperature difference exceeding the upper normal limit was found in 9 patients with carpal tunnel syndrome and in 4 with ulnar neuropathy. One or more fingers always were involved. The hand was affected in 6 patients with carpal tunnel syndrome and 2 with ulnar neuropathy. When both increased interside temperature difference and altered thenar-hypothenar temperature gradient were considered, 55% of patients with carpal tunnel syndrome and 47% with ulnar neuropathy had abnormalities. Thermography was considerably less sensitive than electrodiagnosis. In addition, thermographic changes could not be used to reliably identify the side of the lesion nor distinguish between median and ulnar nerve involvement.

Current thermographic methods cannot be substituted for conventional electrophysiologic studies in evaluating carpal tunnel syndrome or ulnar neuropathy.

▶ A friend asked me last year what I thought of thermography. Since then I have tried to find out about it. These authors believe that thermography is not as sensitive as EMG and believe that it sometimes may be misleading, at least in the diagnosis of carpal tunnel syndrome and ulnar neuropathy at the elbow. No doubt this is not the last word. It would be good if a comparable trial of the 2 diagnostic techniques could be arranged somehow, not only for ulnar neuropathy and carpal tunnel syndrome but also for the other syndromes for which thermography is said to be diagnostically helpful, such as lumbosacral root syndromes. Wishful thinking, perhaps?

Tilting Towards a Diagnosis in Recurrent Unexplained Syncope
Fitzpatrick A, Sutton R (Westminster Hosp, London)
Lancet 1:658–660, March 25, 1989   1–10

In about 50% of patients with recurrent syncope, no diagnosis can be established. A group of patients with recurrent syncope that remained unexplained after standard clinical and electrophysiologic investigation underwent a 60-degree head-up tilt test that aided diagnosis.

The 45-minute orthostatic head-up tilt test was used in 71 patients. The procedure reproduced symptoms with vasovagal syncope in 53 patients (74%). Forty of these patients had bradycardia, some with prolonged asystole, during syncope. The remaining 13 had predominant vasodepression with hypotension. After tilt, the mean time to syncope was 25 minutes. Patients with conduction tissue disease had a 14% incidence of tilt syncope, compared with 7% in age-matched controls. Temporary dual-chamber pacing aborted syncope in 85% of the patients, improving cardiac index and systemic blood pressure during tilt. Long-term results suggested that certain patients may benefit from permanent dual-chamber pacing.

Head-up 60-degree tilt for 45 minutes is useful in investigating patients with recurrent unexplained syncope in whom other electrophysiologic studies have been normal.

▶ This is a better way to study unexplained syncope than the usual simple tilt test. The patient is in the tilted state for at least half an hour. Cardiac pacing seemed to be the answer for most of these patients although it is usually difficult to persuade the cardiologists to pace.

Clinical Brain Death With Preserved Cerebral Arterial Circulation
Kosteljanetz M, Øhrstrøm JK, Skjødt S, Teglbjærg PS (Aalborg Sygehus, Denmark)
Acta Neurol Scand 78:418–421, 1988   1–11

The determining factor of brain death is the irreversible cessation of the function of the brain stem. The absolute requirement for the angiographic diagnosis of brain death is nonfilling of all brain vessels in a 4-vessel angiogram. A patient who had preserved cerebral circulation for at least 2 days after a clinical diagnosis of brain stem death later confirmed by autopsy was evaluated.

Man, 44, had a sudden, severe headache. He was previously healthy. Within minutes, his mentation changed. He lapsed into unconsciousness and stopped breathing. His blood pressure increased from 110/90 mm Hg to 200/140 mm Hg. Results of computed tomography scanning showed pronounced subarachnoid hemorrhage and moderate ventricular dilation. Extraventricular drainage was established. The next day, the patient was still comatose. Both pupils were dilated and unreactive to light. All brain stem functions were absent. On the third day, brain stem reflexes and spontaneous respiration were still absent. His condition had not improved on the fourth day. Repeat angiogram revealed no intracranial filling. The ventricular drainage was then opened and functioned with a single drop or 2 in the next 40 minutes. The patient was subsequently disconnected from the respirator, and cardiac arrest occurred within minutes. Autopsy showed a ruptured 3-mm saccular aneurysm on the basilar artery and massive subarachnoid hemorrhage. Histologic examination showed acute infarction of the entire brain stem and the caudal part of the mesencephalon.

In this case, clinical examination on 3 consecutive days fulfilled the criteria for the diagnosis of clinical brain death. However, intracranial filling was seen on cerebral angiograms until the third day after bleeding. Autopsy revealed acute infarction of the brain stem and cerebellum.

▶ The authors conclude that confirmatory angiography is not necessary if the clinical diagnosis of brain death appears certain. Although it may be betraying my ignorance, I have never understood why total cessation of circulation is characteristic of brain death. Cannot the brain die without total closure of the microcirculation? Perhaps not if one assumes that there is always swelling with brain death.

Primary Brainstem Death: A Clinico-Pathological Study
Ogata J, Imakita M, Yutani C, Miyamoto S, Kikuchi H (Natl Cardiovascular Ctr, Osaka, Japan)
J Neurol Neurosurg Psychiatry 51:646–650, May 1988   1–12

Brain stem death is nearly always a secondary phenomenon in clinical practice. The authors encountered a case of primary brain stem death in a patient having surgery for cerebellar hemorrhage.

Man, 47, was found lying on the floor just before becoming unresponsive, with a blood pressure of 270/140 mm Hg. He was deeply comatose when admitted, with flaccid extremities. Computed tomography showed a mass hematoma in the left cerebellar hemisphere and vermis, with ventricular rupture. Hematoma was evacuated at emergency suboccipital craniotomy, and an extensive decompressive craniectomy was carried out. A fifth of the cerebellar tissue was removed. The patient remained deeply comatose, and despite ventricular drainage, cardiac arrest developed 26 days after the onset of stroke. There were no spontaneous facial or limb movements. A monopolar ECG on day 7 showed disorganized irregular theta activity.

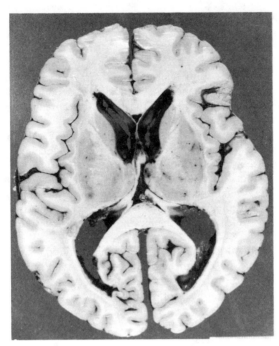

Fig 1–4.—Transverse section of the cerebrum at the level of the splenium of corpus callosum. The lateral ventricles are slightly dilated. (Courtesy of Ogata J, Imakita M, Yutani C, et al: *J Neurol Neurosurg Psychiatry* 51:646–650, May 1988.)

Autopsy within an hour of cardiac arrest showed a necrotic brain stem and cerebellum, but the cerebrum appeared grossly normal (Fig 1–4). The midbrain tegmentum, basis pontis, and medulla were nearly devoid of neurons and replaced by fatty macrophages and proliferating astrocytes. Most cerebellar tissue also was necrotic. The cerebrum exhibited no specific pathologic changes in the cortical or subcortical gray matter; there was some rarefaction of deep white matter.

Among 22 cases of acute infratentorial vascular disease seen during the past 10 years were 4 cases of primary brain stem death lasting longer than 24 hours. Brain stem functions were absent from these cases because of irreversible structural brain stem damage independent of hypothermia and drugs. Acute vascular lesions of the brain stem or cerebellum may lead to irreversible loss of all testable brain stem function despite prolonged somatic survival.

▶ Brain stem death is differentiated from whole-brain death by the presence of persisting EEG activity and the absence of diabetes insipidus. Structural damage to the brain stem may occur with all loss of brain stem functions, but with prolonged somatic survival. This is associated with acute vascular lesions.— R.N. DeJong, M.D.

2 Cerebral Localization and Neurology of Behavior

The Association of Ventral Tegmental Area Histopathology With Adult Dementia
Torack RM, Morris JC (Washington Univ, St Louis)
Arch Neurol 45:497–501, May 1988   2–1

Pathologic changes in the ventral tegmental area (VTA) have been reported infrequently, but this may partly reflect the difficulty in localizing this area. Of 27 adults with clinical dementia who were autopsied within a 1-year period, 6 had mesolimbic pathology. These patients and 1 other had neuronal loss, free pigment, and reactive gliosis in the substantia nigra, associated with neuronal depletion in the VTA.

The core syndrome in these patients consisted of parkinsonism, dementia, and psychiatric disorder—most often depression. Symptoms usually began gradually and progressed, as expected of a neurodegenerative process. The parkinsonism likely was related to severe neuronal depletion in the substantia nigra, but pathologic involvement of the VTA may have contributed to extrapyramidal dysfunction. Four patients became seriously depressed. Dementia eventually developed in all patients who could be evaluated.

These patients had clinical and pathologic findings like those previously described as mesolimbocortical dementia. Nonstriatal dopaminergic pathways, especially the VTA and the hippocampus, are involved. Involvement of the hippocampal and entorhinal cortex distinguishes mesolimbocortical dementia from parkinsonian dementia. The presumed dopaminergic deficit must be confirmed before mesolimbocortical dementia is accepted as a dementing disorder.

▶ How a lesion at this site causes dementia is difficult to understand, so difficult that one tends to doubt it and wonder whether it isn't an epiphenomenon. Such a comment may simply reflect my tendency to disbelieve new ideas. That there could be a connection with thinking that far down the brain is bothersome, but the idea is, to a degree, substantiated by the findings of Katz, Alexander, and Mandell (1), who last year noted slow mentation and poor memory in 6 patients with strokes in the paramedian thalamic-mesencephalic areas. So maybe thinking does go as far down as the red nucleus. We'll see.

Reference

1. Katz, Alexander, Mandell: *Arch Neurol* 44:1127–1133, 1987.

Aphasic Victim as Investigator
Wender D (Wheaton College, Norton, Mass)
Arch Neurol 46:91–92, January 1989   2–2

The author, a classics professor, is a 45-year-old woman who had a cerebrovascular accident (CVA) that produced aphasia. She lost many English words, some syntax, and the ability to read and write. In addition, recall of ancient Greek and Latin, which she had taught for 20 years, was almost totally missing. The patient had computed tomographic findings of left temporal lobe hematoma extending to the level of the internal capsule.

The patient, having been told by speech pathologists that she could benefit much by working hard to relearn words—and by neurologists the opposite—decided to study ancient Greek grammar and vocabulary, leaving Latin alone as a control. After 10 months she was able to teach elementary Greek, and at 2 years taught advanced Greek courses. Her command of Greek was not as it had been before the CVA, but the difference between Greek and Latin abilities was marked. A trial of learning vocabulary suggested that the patient, had she wished, could have relearned Latin rather than Greek.

This experience supports the view that speech therapy can benefit victims of CVA. Other patients with aphasia also have reported that they are able to improve, from work and from long periods of treatment, and have improved beyond the point at which they would have with healing of the injured brain alone.

▶ This contribution is not well named; it should be something like "By All Means, Give Your Aphasic Patients Speech Therapy" or "An Important Contribution to Neurology by a Nonneurologist." There is no question that her Greek came back to the point where she was able to teach even advanced courses and that her Latin stayed elementary. Her conclusion is just and correct: ". . . at least some people may improve from working or from long periods of therapy, not simply from the early healing of the injured brain." This lady, performing a simple experiment on herself, has taught me something.

Impaired Grammar With Normal Fluency and Phonology: Implications for Broca's Aphasia
Nadeau SE (VA Med Ctr; Univ of Florida, Gainesville)
Brain 111:1111–1137, October 1988   2–3

The fundamental nature of Broca's aphasia and the lesion necessary and sufficient to produce it are debated. Broca attributed the linguistic deficit in his famous patient to destruction of the dominant third frontal convolution. Its destruction does not result in lasting linguistic impairment readily evident, but what linguistic function it does fulfill is still not known. The outstanding feature of Broca's aphasia is agrammatism. Two patients with large dominant frontal lobe lesions that included and considerably exceeded the third frontal convolution were studied. One patient had severe generalized impairment in frontal lobe function.

Both patients were fluent and had normal phonologic production. Except for some mild anomia, neither patient had readily evident aphasia on bedside testing. A detailed study of their grammar was done, including tests of inflectional morphology, ability to produce grammatical structures, ability to manipulate word order and function words, grammatical comprehension, and the ability to perceive syntactic relationships. Neither patient was agrammatic, suggesting that even very large frontal lesions do not produce Broca's aphasia and that language cortex proper is confined to the postcentral perisylvian region. Both patients had impaired use of more complex syntactic structures. One patient also had impaired judgment of the use of placement of functors.

This study supports the dissociability of syntactic and morphological aspects of grammar in aphasic patients and links these functions with the frontal lobe and postcentral perisylvian cortex, respectively. Despite a very extensive lesion, 1 patient had a sparing of grammatical judgment, suggesting that very large parts of the frontal lobe are involved in grammatical function. The nature of frontal lobe function in syntax seems consistent with the role of the frontal lobes in other aspects of behavior.

▶ It's instructive what a careful observer can find in examining the same patients that we all see in our daily practice. The observation that the patient with a dominant frontal lobe lesion, although not aphasic by any measure, had erroneous use of language in a "frontal lobe fashion" is of interest.

Evidence for Modality-Specific Meaning Systems in the Brain
McCarthy RA, Warrington EK (Natl Hosp for Nervous Diseases, London)
Nature 334:428–431, August 1988   2–4

Patients with cerebral lesions present an opportunity to study the organization of meaning systems in the brain. Recent observations have suggested that our semantic knowledge base is categorical in organization. A patient was described whose semantic knowledge deficit was not only category-specific but also modality-specific.

Man, 63, said his use of language and comprehension of the spoken word had progressively deteriorated. A relatively well circumscribed abnormality in the left temporal lobe was found. Clinical observation suggested that this deficit was not simply one of word retrieval but that certain names appeared almost totally meaningless to him. This observation contrasted with an excellent ability to derive meaning from a picture. Further observation revealed that he had greater difficulty comprehending the spoken names of animate (dolphin) than inanimate objects (wheelbarrow). These observations were formally tested, which confirmed that this patient had a category-specific impairment affecting his knowledge of the spoken names of living things. The impairment was found to be consistent over time.

These observations raise questions about the widely accepted view that the brain has a single all-purpose meaning store.

► This is a most amazing finding and strikes a blow for the localizers. Zeki and Shipp (1) say that the visual cortex "segregates features of the visual image into separate cortical areas and that communication between them produces a coherent percept." Such a segregation for verbal description in the human brain could explain why a person could not describe a dolphin but could a wheelbarrow.

Reference

1. Zeki, Shipp: *Nature* 335:311–317, September 1988.

The Medical Evaluation of Elderly Patients With Major Depression
Sweer L, Martin DC, Ladd RA, Miller JK, Karpf M (Univ of Pittsburgh)
J Gerontol Med Sci 43:M53–M58, May 1988   2–5

The frequency of new medical problems among 100 depressed geropsychiatric inpatients, who were largely free of cognitive impairment, was determined. All patients fully met criteria of the *Diagnostic and Statistical Manual of Mental Disorders, Third Edition,* for major depression. Their mean age was 72 years.

The most frequent symptoms at presentation were constipation, arthralgia, and headache. Hypertension, osteoarthritis, urinary tract infection, atherosclerotic cardiovascular disease, and diabetes all were frequent. Seven patients had known parkinsonism. Antidepressants were among the many drugs frequently being taken at the time of admission. The EEG result was abnormal for one third of the patients studied. New medical diagnoses included bacteriuria, electrolyte abnormality, thyroid hypofunction, and medication reaction or abuse. About half the population had at least 1 unsuspected medical problem identified. The average patient had 0.77 problems defined.

Undiscovered physical illnesses are frequent among elderly depressed patients. The history, physical examination, and simple laboratory evaluation appear to suffice for work-ups of these patients. More than half these patients had previously unrecognized medical illnesses that affected their health.

► It has long been taught that neurologic examination should be accompanied by a thorough physical examination. This article avers that this should apply also to every psychiatric patient. The brain and the nervous system are only parts of the body as a whole.—R.N. DeJong, M.D.

Acute Pseudobulbar Mutism Due to Discrete Bilateral Capsular Infarction in the Territory of the Anterior Choroidal Artery

Helgason C, Wilbur A, Weiss A, Redmond KJ, Kingsbury NA (Univ of Illinois, Chicago)
Brain 111:507–524, June 1988   2–6

The sudden onset of mutism with pseudobulbar palsy is rarely caused by discrete bilateral infarction of the internal capsule. Eight cases of such destruction were seen in which interruption of the corticobulbar tract caused mutism and facial, oropharyngeal, and glossal paralysis. The patients also had hemisensory and hemiparetic signs.

Computed tomography and magnetic resonance imaging results showed infarcts beginning in the posterior limb of the internal capsule and medial globus pallidus (Fig 2–1). The infarcts were thought but not proved to be in the area supplied by the anterior choroidal artery. The mirror infarctions appeared sequentially, once with a capsular warning syndrome and sometimes with waxing and waning of symptoms. The patients either died within 1 year or remain severely impaired.

The pathogenesis was related to poorly controlled or untreated hypertension and sudden, transient rise in blood pressure. Most patients had cardiac disease, and 1 had arterial atheroma near the anterior choroidal artery.

Early recognition of unilateral capsular infarction and treatment of underlying cardiac or vascular problems may prevent a contralateral lesion. The deterioration associated with bilateral disease may then be avoided.

▶ This is a nice study. Although they couldn't prove it, the authors believe that these infarcts were in the bilateral territories of the anterior choroidal arteries affecting the posterior limb of the internal capsule and sometimes the medial

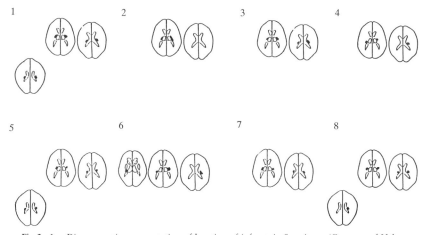

Fig 2–1.—Diagrammatic representation of location of infarcts in 8 patients. (Courtesy of Helgason C, Wilbur A, Weiss A, et al: *Brain* 111:507–524, June 1988.)

globus pallidus and caudate nucleus. Half the patients had pseudobulbar emotionality, and all had hemiparesis or hemisensory loss. The best causal associations found were with hypertension, often uncontrolled, and diabetes. The infarcts were not simultaneous but occurred within a few months of each other. The prognosis was poor. This could turn out to be a landmark paper.

3 Aging and Dementia

Genetic Linkage Studies in Alzheimer's Disease Families
Pericak-Vance MA, Yamaoka LH, Haynes CS, Speer MC, Haines JL, Gaskell PC, Hung W-Y, Clark CM, Heyman AL, Trofatter JA, Eisenmenger JP, Gilbert JR, Lee JE, Alberts MJ, Dawson DV, Bartlett RJ, Earl NL, Siddique T, Vance JM, Conneally PM, Roses AD (Duke Univ; Indiana Univ, Indianapolis)
Exp Neurol 102:271–279, December 1988   3–1

Alzheimer's disease (AD) is a neurodegenerative disease that has no successful treatment or cure. The age of onset varies from the fourth to the ninth decade. Although the etiology of AD is unclear, familial clustering occurs, and autosomal dominant inheritance for AD has been proposed. Recent work linked familial Alzheimer's disease (FAD) in 4 families with early onset AD (mean age of onset, 39.9–52.0 years) to 2 DNA probes on chromosome 21. The DNA from 106 members, including 32 affected members of 13 FAD families was studied for the possibility of linkage of AD to the 2 chromosome 21 probes previously tested (D2 1S1/D2 1S11 and D2 1S16). Ten of the 13 families tested had late onset Alzheimer's disease (mean age of onset, more than 60 years).

Simulation studies using the computer program SIMLINK showed that the data set used would be useful in FAD linkage studies. The results of the linkage studies performed failed to support linkage of autosomal dominant FAD to the regions of chromosome 21 specified by the 2 probes. The family with the highest individual lod score ($\hat{z} = 0.98$) was an early onset family (mean age of onset, 49 years).

These studies failed to demonstrate linkage of autosomal dominant late onset AD with the region of chromosome 21 to which the gene for early onset AD has been localized. This, combined with clinical and neurochemical differences between early and late onset FAD, suggests that multiple etiologies may exist for FAD. More families need to be tested for linkage to probes from both chromosome 21 and other chromosomes.

▶ Ten of these 13 families had disease of the late onset type, and linkage of the disease to chromosome 21 was not found. In the study of Goate and associates (1) 6 families with early onset were localized in the long arm of chromosome 21.

Bird and co-workers (2) report 24 kindreds with 49 neuropathologic specimens and divide the disease neuropathologically and clinically into 6 different types. Five families with early onset, 8 families with late onset, 7 families of Volga German ancestry with early onset, 1 family with tangles but no amyloid plaques and a "schizophrenia-like" onset, 1 family with late onset with anterior horn cell disease, and 1 family with état criblé with marked cortical and meningeal amyloid angiopathy. How many of these should be called Alzheimer's disease? Perhaps Alzheimer's disease is 6 different diseases. Or more.

References

1. Goate et al: *Lancet* 1:352–355, Feb 18, 1989.
2. Bird et al: *Ann Neurol* 25:12–25, 1989.

Diagnosis of Dementia: Clinicopathologic Correlations
Boller F, Lopez OL, Moossy J (Pittsburgh VA Med Ctr; Univ of Pittsburgh)
Neurology 39:76–79, January 1989   3–2

Most studies of the accuracy of diagnosis in demented patients have used clinicopathologic correlation and found diagnostic accuracy to range from 43% to 87%. In several patients with dementia, unexpected neuropathologic findings were noted. It was hypothesized that, in a large series, there would be a significant number of discrepancies between clinical diagnoses and autopsy findings.

Data from 54 demented patients undergoing autopsy consecutively at 1 center were analyzed. Thirty-nine (72.2%) patients had Alzheimer's disease. Other central nervous system diseases represented included multi-infarct dementia, Creutzfeldt-Jakob disease, thalamic and subcortical gliosis, and Parkinson's disease. Two neurologists studied the clinical records of each patient independently without knowing the patient's identity or clinical or pathologic diagnoses. Each neurologist made a clinical diagnosis based on criteria derived from those of the NINCDS/ADRDA. Both clinicians were correct in 63% of the patients, 1 was correct in an additional 17%, and neither was correct in 20%.

In a population of patients with dementias of various types, diagnoses could be correctly inferred by at least 1 of 2 neurologists for about 80% of the patients. The etiology of dementia in patients with a clinical diagnosis of dementia cannot be predicted accurately during life.

▶ Well, I knew we weren't perfect, but I really didn't believe we were that bad and frankly doubt that we are. Alzheimer's disease is becoming a diagnosis and can be made by the checkout lady at the supermarket with a fair degree of accuracy.

Psychotic Symptoms and the Longitudinal Course of Senile Dementia of the Alzheimer Type
Drevets WC, Rubin EH (Washington Univ, St Louis)
Biol Psychiatry 25:39–48, January 1988   3–3

Persons with senile dementia of the Alzheimer type (SDAT) frequently have delusions and hallucinations. The occurrence of psychotic symptoms was studied in 43 patients with SDAT observed since 1979, in 24 in a new longitudinal series, and in 43 patients with clinical dementia ratings of 2 or 3 who were assessed only once.

Rates of psychosis in patients with moderate to severe SDAT ranged from 42% to 84%. At least half of the patients with no past psychiatric history apparently can be expected to be psychotic at some time. Psychotic symptoms were associated with more rapid cognitive deterioration but not with greater mortality.

More than half of the patients with SDAT are psychotic at some time, with symptoms most frequent among moderately demented patients. It is difficult to analyze psychotic symptoms in cognitively impaired persons. Systematized delusions are less frequent than simple persecutory delusions are. Hallucinations are most often visual. Modern imaging methods may lead to a better understanding of the relation between psychiatric symptoms and brain changes in patients with SDAT.

▶ I have difficulty determining what is Alzheimer's dementia and what is psychosis. The authors admit the same problem but believe their analysis was good enough to differentiate the 2 conditions in individual patients and found half or more of the Alzheimer's patients were psychotic some time during the course of the disease. Does this finding have any meaning? Would not a brain that is falling apart cell by cell do such? And thus is it not to be expected? I suppose in some diagnostic situations this knowledge will be helpful.

Age and Simple Reaction Time: Decade Differences for 5,325 Subjects
Wilkinson RT, Allison S (Applied Psychology Unit, Cambridge, England)
J Gerontol 44:P29–P35, March 1989   3–4

A large sample of participants was solicited for reaction time (RT) testing at a booth in a public science exhibition. Representing both sexes and all ages, the participants performed a 1-minute test of simple RT with a preparatory interval of 1–10 seconds. The test used has been employed in assessing clinical drugs for their effects on arousal.

Average RT increased progressively in adults aged in their 20s to age 60 and older, whereas adolescents and young children had progressively shorter reaction times (Fig 3–1). The single fastest RT in each test comprising 10 trials varied much less with age; only participants in their 20s were clearly faster than the others (Fig 3–2). Intrasubject variability in RT was increased only among persons aged less than 10 years and those aged more than 60.

Gross differences in RT with age may reflect the ability to sustain attention during longer preparatory intervals. Better RTs shown in the 20s group, on the other hand, may indicate the presence of some more basic neural property in young persons.

▶ There is a slight rise with age, on the average, in reaction time, but as the graph clearly shows the majority of persons aged more than 69 years have just

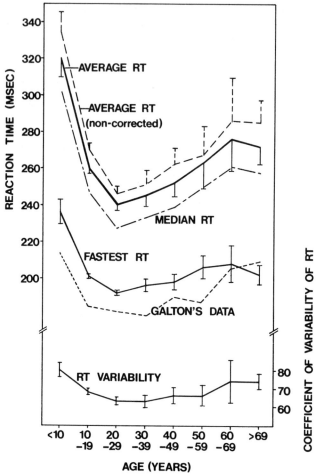

Fig 3-1.—Average reaction time *(RT)*, fastest RT, RT variability, and median RT as a function of age in 8 groups. Confidence limits (95%) are shown for the first 3 scores. The variable breadth of these limits in each group will be a function of the widely varying numbers in each age group as well as the intrinsic variability of subjects within each group. The *dashed curve* gives average RT data derived as for the *full curve* for that score but without removing unduly long RTs more than twice the duration of the average for the test concerned. The *dotted curve* shows, for comparison, Galton's data plotted on the same scale and for approximately the same age. (Courtesy of Wilkinson RT, Allison S: *J Gerontol* 44:P29–P35, March 1989.)

about the reaction time of a 20-year-old. So much for telling grandpa he can't drive anymore because his reaction time is too slow. It's his ability to sustain attention that's poorer.

Nimodipine Facilitates Associative Learning in Aging Rabbits
Deyo RA, Straube KT, Disterhoft JF (Northwestern Univ)
Science 243:809–811, Feb 10, 1989

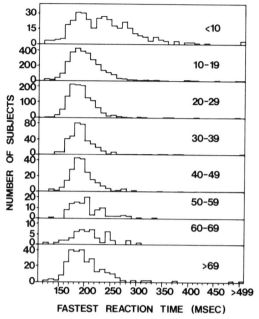

Fig 3–2.—Distribution of fastest reaction time over all subjects and in each age group. (Courtesy of Wilkinson RT, Allison S: *J Gerontol* 44:P29–P35, March 1989.)

Reportedly, when the calcium channel blocker drug nimodipine was given to elderly patients with chronic cerebrovascular disease in an attempt to promote cerebral blood flow, learning was facilitated. Increased intraneuronal calcium can be toxic, and calcium channel blocking agents might be expected to improve learning and memory through lowering the influx of calcium ion.

The effects of nimodipine on eye-blink conditioning were examined in 36 rabbits. A deficiency in acquiring this conditioned response has been found in both aged rabbits and humans. Nimodipine accelerated the acquisition of conditioned eye blink in both young and aging rabbits. It did not alter the amplitude of responses to conditioned or unconditioned stimuli and did not cause nonspecific responding. The drug was given by infusion in a dose of 1 μg/kg/minute.

Nimodipine may facilitate learning by enhancing cerebral blood flow. Alternately, the findings were consistent with evidence of an important role for calcium ion metabolism in age-related dementia. In any event calcium antagonists such as nimodipine could ameliorate learning deficits in aging rabbits, and perhaps in humans as well.

▶ I am wondering whether I might not start on a bit of this stuff. Having pooh-poohed all treatments for the aging brain until now, who do I hope there is something to this one?

4 Stroke

Decline in US Stroke Mortality: Demographic Trends and Antihypertensive Treatment
Klag MJ, Whelton PK, Seidler AJ (Johns Hopkins Med Institutions, Baltimore)
Stroke 20:14–21, January 1989   4–1

Age-adjusted stroke mortality has been declining in the United States since the turn of the century and even more rapidly since 1973. Interrelated effects of age, race, and sex on stroke mortality were examined in a review of vital statistics for 1950–1972 and 1973–1981.

Since 1973 the rapid rate of decline in stroke mortality has resulted in more than 200,000 fewer deaths than would otherwise have occurred. The decline was greater in the later than in the earlier review period and increased with advancing age. Younger black persons had an especially marked fall in stroke mortality, but no consistent gender effects on mortality were observed. The more marked decline among older persons and black persons was related to higher baseline mortality in these groups. Overall stroke mortality declined by about 2% per year in the earlier period and by about 7% per year after 1973. The recent decline did not correspond with changes in the treatment or control of hypertension.

The ongoing decrease in stroke deaths has had markedly beneficial effects on the national health. The reasons for the decrease remain uncertain, but the higher risk for stroke observed among cigarette smokers may be relevant. A relationship with improved antihypertensive treatment remains to be demonstrated.

▶ The considerable decrease in U.S. mortality is now thought to be due to increased control of hypertension, but the decline began before widespread hypertension control. So what was it due to? A great mystery. One wonders about the correlation between the number of neurologists and the decline in mortality. Could not increased diagnostic accuracy related to increased numbers of neurologists be part of the reason? Were death certificates listing stroke as accurate in 1950 as they are now? Perhaps some of the early decline was more apparent than real.

Meta-Analysis of Relation Between Cigarette Smoking and Stroke
Shinton R, Beevers G (Univ of Birmingham, England)
Br Med J 298:789–794, March 25, 1989   4–2

The possible risk for stroke from cigarette smoking remains uncertain. Published data on this association were reviewed to obtain relative risk estimates. Pooled relative risk values were calculated from estimates of the precision of individual risk figures in 32 separate epidemiologic studies that focused on risk factors in people, not populations.

The overall relative risk of stroke associated with smoking was 1.5, with a 95% confidence interval of 1.4–1.6. Risk estimates ranged from 0.7 for cerebral hemorrhage through 1.9 for cerebral infarction to 2.9 for subarachnoid hemorrhage. Risk values declined with advancing age; before age 55 the relative risk was 2.9. Women were at slightly higher risk than men. A dose-response relationship was found between the number of cigarettes smoked and relative risk. Ex-smokers younger than 75 years of age retained an appreciable risk for stroke.

Stroke should definitely be considered as one of the disorders related to cigarette smoking. The excess risk may be modest in epidemiologic terms, but a large potential for preventing strokes, especially in younger persons, is indicated.

▶ Years ago, a fellow neurologist who was interested in stroke commented that all of his patients were smokers. It took several decades for the relationship to be proven, and now we have an analysis of analyses, a meta-analysis of the relationship. The authors point out that "neither publication bias nor the confounding effects of age, obesity, blood pressure, or alcohol seemed to account for the finding" and conclude that smoking produces a structural effect because the risk seems to remain even after smoking ceases. The risk seems to be greater among younger people.

Weekly Alcohol Consumption, Cigarette Smoking, and the Risk of Ischemic Stroke: Results of a Case-Control Study at Three Urban Medical Centers in Chicago, Illinois
Gorelick PB, Rodin MB, Langenberg P, Hier DB, Costigan J (Michael Reese Hosp, Chicago; Univ of Chicago; Univ of Illinois, Chicago)
Neurology 39:339–343, March 1989
4–3

Alcohol consumption is a risk factor for ischemic stroke. A study conducted in a rural community in Japan found that high alcohol intake was a risk factor for cerebral hemorrhage but not for cerebral infarction. Because the relationship between alcohol consumption and ischemic stroke remains unclear, a case-control study was done to assess the role of current weekly alcohol consumption as a risk factor for ischemic stroke.

A questionnaire was administered to 205 middle-aged and elderly patients hospitalized with acute ischemic stroke in Chicago and 410 outpatient controls who were matched for age, sex, race, and method of hospital payment. The stroke index patients had a higher frequency of hypertension and transient ischemic attacks, higher mean weekly alcohol consumption, and a higher number of mean pack-years exposure than the controls. There was a 54-gm-per-week difference in mean alcohol consumption among current drinkers, with index patients consuming 173 gm of alcohol per week, and controls, 120 gm of alcohol per week.

However, when the possibility of mutual confounding effects of independent variables was assessed, hypertension and smoking were found to be independent risk factors for ischemic stroke, whereas alcohol consumption was not. A statistically significant association between alcohol consumption and ischemic stroke was observed only at the 100–299-gm-per-week level of alcohol consumption. Thus, current weekly alcohol consumption may not be an independent risk factor for cerebral infarction in middle-aged and elderly patients.

▶ Alcohol consumption is not an independent risk factor for stroke, at least in Chicago. It may be that the reason alcohol looked like a risk factor in earlier studies is that the effect of eating the potato chips and smoking the cigarettes while drinking were not adequately factored out.

A Prospective Study of Moderate Alcohol Consumption and the Risk of Coronary Disease and Stroke in Women
Stampfer MJ, Colditz GA, Willett WC, Speizer FE, Hennekens CH (Harvard Univ; Brigham and Women's Hosp, Boston)
N Engl J Med 319:267–273, Aug 4, 1988   4–4

In men, moderate consumption of alcohol has been associated with a decreased risk of coronary heart disease. The association between alcohol intake and cardiovascular diseases in women was studied in a 4-year prospective study involving 87,526 female nurses, aged 34 to 59 years, who completed a dietary questionnaire that assessed their consumption of beer, wine, and liquor. Follow-up was 98% complete.

During the 334,382 person-years of follow-up, 200 incident cases of severe coronary heart disease (including 164 nonfatal myocardial infarctions and 36 deaths from coronary disease), 66 ischemic strokes, and 28 subarachnoid hemorrhages were documented. Compared with nondrinkers, drinkers had a lower relative risk of coronary disease. For women consuming 5–14 gm of alcohol per day (equivalent to about 1 drink per day), the risk of coronary heart disease was 0.6; for 15–24 gm per day, the relative risk was 0.6; and for 25 gm or more per day, the relative risk was 0.4, after adjustment for risk factors for coronary disease.

The apparent benefit was strongest among wine drinkers consuming 5 gm or more alcohol per day and among beer drinkers consuming less than 5 gm per day. A moderate inverse association between alcohol intake and the risk of stroke was also noted. Each level of alcohol consumption was associated with a decreased risk of ischemic stroke, the relative risk being 0.3 for women consuming 5–14 gm per day, and 0.5 for those consuming 15 gm per day or more. In contrast, alcohol intake was associated with an increased risk of subarachnoid hemorrhage, with a relative risk of 4.7 for women consuming 5–14 gm per day. This association was strongest among wine drinkers.

Women who consume moderate amounts of alcohol have substantially reduced risks of coronary disease and ischemic stroke but an increased risk of subarachnoid hemorrhage. The increased plasma high-density lipoprotein concentration is the best documented mechanism of the effect of alcohol on the risk of heart disease. Although the net effect of moderate alcohol consumption is beneficial, further studies are needed to compare the benefit of moderate consumption with the risk of subsequent heavy consumption, increased risk of subarachnoid hemorrhage, and the reported increased risk of breast cancer.

▶ Moderate alcohol consumption decreases the risk of both stroke and coronary artery occlusion. This morning's *USA Today* (June 27, 1989) quotes Dr. Klatsky as saying 1 or 2 drinks a day tends to prevent cerebral infarction, possibly partly by raising levels of high-density lipoprotein. More than 2 a day is bad.

Anabolic Androgenic Steroids and a Stroke in an Athlete: Case Report
Frankle MA, Eichberg R, Zachariah SB (Univ of South Florida, Tampa)
Arch Phys Med Rehabil 69:632–633, August 1988   4–5

Athletes continue to use anabolic androgenic steroids despite well-known serious side effects. A stroke occurred in an otherwise healthy young man after he took anabolic steroids to increase his muscle mass.

Man, 34, had been a bodybuilder for 10 years. He had a 4-year history of taking steroids in cycles consisting of drug intake for 10 weeks followed by 10 weeks of drug-free periods. Seventeen days before a body physique contest, the patient experienced an acute right hemiparesis and difficulty in speaking. A computed tomographic scan with contrast revealed an area of decreased attenuation in the left frontoparietal region with mild compression of the lateral ventricle. Liver enzymes were elevated, and high-density lipoprotein was significantly decreased. The patient sustained a simple partial seizure in the emergency room. An electroencephalogram showed abnormal slowing, indicative of left hemispheric structural lesion. The patient also became hypertensive but was well controlled with medication. The patient underwent a course of rehabilitation, after which he was sufficiently recovered to ambulate independently. At discharge, he had mild motor weakness in the upper right extremity and residual mild receptive deficits, as well as severe expressive deficits.

Apparently, stroke can be added to the list of factors for which a person taking steroids is at risk. Physicians who treat athletes should warn them that they might be at risk for stroke should they use steroids to enhance athletic performance or build muscle mass.

▶ It seems as though every new social evil that comes along is capable of causing a stroke, and here is another evil. No doubt I have missed this diagnosis once or twice over the years. I was innocently unaware up until the last Olympics that athletes were using them.

Clustering of Strokes in Association With Meteorologic Factors in the Negev Desert of Israel: 1981–1983

Berginer VM, Goldsmith J, Batz U, Vardi H, Shapiro Y (Ben-Gurion Univ of the Negev, Beer-Sheva, Israel; Israeli Meteorological Service, Beit Dagan, Israel)
Stroke 20:65–69, January 1989   4–6

Stroke admissions in the Negev desert appeared to occur in clusters. Because the usual risk factors for stroke are not likely to change within a short period, factors such as meteorologic changes were considered. Meteorologic data were reviewed for 895 patients admitted with stroke during 1981–1983.

No or only a few stroke admissions were reported on days or groups of days when the atmosphere was unstable and the ambient temperature was less than the monthly mean for the data. In contrast, up to 5 admissions occurred each day that the atmosphere was stable and the temperature was above the historic monthly mean (Fig 4–1).

In this arid region more strokes are found to occur on warm days. This can possibly be ascribed to the presence of more active thromboembolic mechanisms secondary to physiologic responses to heat such as increased blood viscosity and a decrease in blood pressure. Encouraging those at risk to use air conditioning and consume adequate liquids may be helpful in preventing stroke on especially warm days. In addition, antiplatelet aggregation medication might be considered as a preventive treatment.

▶ We should be able to confirm this association here in Mississippi, but the truth is I had never noticed that stroke admissions went up on warmer days

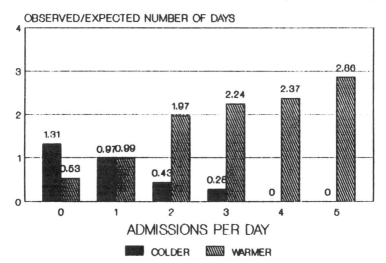

OBSERVED/EXPECTED NUMBER OF DAYS

ADMISSIONS PER DAY

■ COLDER   ▨ WARMER

DEVIATIONS FROM MONTHLY TEMPERATURE

Fig 4–1.—Ratio of observed days with given number of stroke admissions and days expected if there were no meteorologic effects on number of stroke admissions per day. Days warmer than historical mean have relatively more daily admissions. There were never more than 3 stroke admissions on any colder day. (Courtesy of Berginer VM, Goldsmith J, Batz U, et al: *Stroke* 20:65–69, January 1989.)

until today when a patient in his 70s came in to the Veterans' Hospital with a transient ischemic attack that occurred after he had been working in his yard for 3 or 4 hours in what he said was 105 F (40 C) heat. So far, our work-up has shown nothing. As a matter of fact, I had always believed that strokes increased when it began to turn cool in the fall.

Lone Bilateral Blindness: A Transient Ischaemic Attack

Dennis MS, Bamford JM, Sandercock PAG, Warlow CP (Radcliffe Infirmary, Oxford, England)

Lancet 1:185–188, Jan 28, 1989   4–7

Although transient blindness in both eyes may occur after various interventions or in association with epileptic seizures and myocardial infarction and after childbirth, many episodes of transient spontaneous bilateral loss of vision occur without any of these associations. To examine the hypothesis that lone bilateral blindness may be a form of transient focal cerebral ischemia, the general characteristics, vascular risk factors, and subsequent history of affected patients were compared with those of patients with diagnoses of definite transient ischemic attacks (TIAs). Lone bilateral blindness was defined as rapid onset of dimming or loss of vision over all of both visual fields simultaneously that lasts less than 24 hours and is not associated with symptoms of focal cerebral ischemia, epilepsy, or reduction in consciousness.

Among 512 patients with suspected TIAs, 195 were confirmed as having definite TIAs, 184 of whom met the criteria of an incident TIA. Among the other 317 patients were 14 patients, 7 men and 7 women, aged 46 to 82 years, who had episodes of lone bilateral blindness. During a mean follow-up of 2.4 years, 5 of these 14 patients had a first-ever stroke. All cases of stroke were confirmed with computed tomography as being caused by infarction. Based on available age- and sex-specific stroke incidence rates, only 0.31 strokes would have been expected. Thus, patients with lone bilateral blindness had about a 16 times greater risk of stroke than unaffected persons in the general population. Based on these findings, patients with lone bilateral blindness should be included for practical purposes under the diagnostic heading of TIA.

▶ Bilateral blindness, of course, should be considered a TIA and one of more importance than usual if the expected stroke risk in this study is confirmed by others.

Subarachnoid Haemorrhage of Unknown Cause: A Long Term Follow-Up

Hawkins TD, Sims C, Hanka R (Addenbrooke's Hosp, Cambridge; Univ of Cambridge, England)

J Neurol Neurosurg Psychiatry 52:230–235, January 1989   4–8

Some reports have described attempts to identify features that would predict the outcome of subarachnoid hemorrhage of unknown cause, but

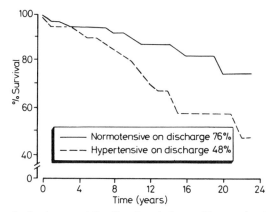

Fig 4–2.—Graphs showing actuarially adjusted survival up to 22 years of patients who were normotensive compared with those who were hypertensive on discharge. (Courtesy of Hawkins TD, Sims C, Hanka R: *J Neurol Neurosurg Psychiatry* 52:230–235, January 1989.)

studies have been small. The survival rates for and the certified causes of death among a larger group of patients followed over a long period were reviewed.

A total of 306 patients who suffered subarachnoid hemorrhage of unknown origin were followed up by questionnaire from 2 to 23 years later, with an average of 10 years. Angiographic studies and medical records were also reviewed. Follow-up angiographic studies were conducted in 23 patients who had no improvement; 9 patients had further subarachnoid hemorrhage. Thirty-four percent of the patients were hypertensive on admission, and 14% were hypertensive at discharge. At the time of the study, 79.5% of patients were known to be alive, 15.5% had died, and 5% were unavailable for follow-up. After 22 years, the cumulative survival for the group was 69%, in contrast to expected survival of 89%. Thirty patients died of diseases of the circulatory system, principally myocardial infarction and cerebrovascular disease, whereas the predicted number of deaths from these causes was 21.8. Evaluation of angiograms showed that 68% of patients had no arterial spasm, 21% had localized spasm, and 11% had more widespread changes. Five of 9 patients with further subarachnoid hemorrhage were hypertensive at discharge, but all were living at the end of the survery. Cumulative proportional survival of normotensive patients was 76%, compared with 48% of patients who were hypertensive at discharge (Fig 4–2). Whether patients died of circulatory disorders or other causes, both men and women in the study group had a reduced life expectancy.

These findings suggest that the long-term outcome for patients who suffer subarachnoid hemorrhage of unknown origin is more guarded than had been previously thought. There appears to be an excess of deaths from circulatory disorders.

▶ The authors are cautious in commenting on this excellent and large follow-up study (only 5% were untraceable). They point out that a large part of the decreased life expectancy might be explained by the hypertension, but even those who were not hypertensive on discharge tended to die at a greater rate. However, the outlook is as much as has been long taught and not nearly that of patients with known aneurysms. No doubt a few of these patients did have aneurysms because some had spasm on their angiograms.

Prostaglandins and Vasoactive Amines in Cerebral Vasospasm After Aneurysmal Subarachnoid Hemorrhage

Chehrazi BB, Giri S, Joy RM (Univ of California, Davis)
Stroke 20:217–224, February 1989   4–9

Delayed cerebral vasospasm is a significant cause of complications after subarachnoid hemorrhage. The cause of vasospasm remains uncertain. Cerebrospinal fluid (CSF) levels of vasoactive amines and prostaglandins in 5 consecutive patients with aneurysmal subarachnoid hemorrhage were determined on a daily basis. The values were correlated with the neurologic course and with the computed tomographic and angiographic findings.

All patients had increased CSF serotonin levels; levels were highest early in the course of vasospasm. The CSF tryptophan content increased markedly in association with vasospasm, and the same was the case for prostaglandin $F_{2\alpha}$. Most of the patients with subarachnoid hemorrhage had reduced levels of prostaglandin E in the CSF.

Levels of CSF prostaglandin $F_{2\alpha}$ are helpful in predicting clinical vasospasm after subarachnoid hemorrhage. It is possible that increased CSF tryptophan indicates disruption of CSF homeostasis, which allows accumulation of prostaglandin $F_{2\alpha}$. In the presence of elevated serotonin, accumulation of prostaglandin $F_{2\alpha}$ may participate in delayed cerebral vasospasm.

▶ This is another small step in the continued attempt to understanding the serious business of vasospasm in ruptured cerebral aneurysms. If prostaglandin F_2 is the culprit, we must look for some effective blocking agent.

Reversible Cerebral Segmental Vasoconstriction

Call GK, Fleming MC, Sealfon S, Levine H, Kistler JP, Fisher CM (Massachusetts Gen Hosp; St Elizabeth's Hosp, Boston)
Stroke 19:1159–1170, September 1988   4–10

Transient, completely reversible vasoconstriction and dilatation that chiefly involved arteries about the circle of Willis developed in 4 patients. No cause of the clinical features or angiographic abnormalities was found.

Woman, 37, had had a severe left-sided headache the night before and soon lost consciousness. Left hemicranial headaches with a visual prodrome had occurred about twice a year for 10 years. After regaining consciousness the patient

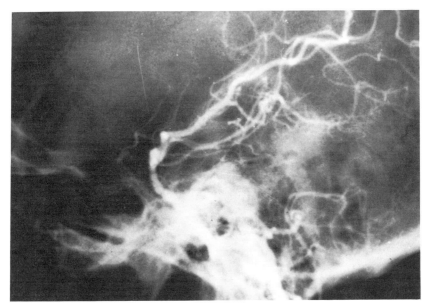

Fig 4–3.—Lateral left vertebral angiogram on day 12 showing multiple constrictions of basilar artery *(white arrow)*. (Courtesy of Call GK, Fleming MC, Sealfon S, et al: *Stroke* 19:1159–1170, September 1988.)

reported headache, tingling in the left fingers, a blurred right visual field, and difficulty in swallowing. The left face, arm, and leg were moderately weak, and there was a left Babinski sign. Headache resolved slowly during treatment with nadolol, dexamethasone, aspirin, dipyridamole, and nifedipine. A similar episode occurred on day 8, and computed tomographic scanning showed a low-density lesion in the right basis pontis. Angiography on day 12 showed irregular arteries near the circle of Willis (Fig 4–3). The basilar artery was normal 2 months later, and the patient has been well for the past 3 years.

All 4 patients had severe headaches and fluctuating or recurring motor or sensory deficits. Narrowing of arteries contributing to and arising from the circle of Willis often was marked, and segmental dilation also was observed. Narrowing was bilateral in all patients.

These patients appear to have physiologic narrowing of arteries with no structural correlate. A similar picture is seen after subarachnoid hemorrhage, surgery, closed head injury, and sympathomimetic drug abuse. Migraine syndrome may be a variant of the disorder, and the study patients may have a severe "cluster" form of migraine.

▶ Well, my father used to talk about vasospasm when he was describing what we now call TIAs. It looks as though it does truly occur in some people with headaches. An exact pharmacologic history on these patients might tell us something.

Prevalence of Patent Foramen Ovale in Patients With Stroke

Lechat P, Mas JL, Lascault G, Loron P, Theard M, Klimczac M, Drobinski G, Thomas D, Grosgogeat Y (Hôpital Pitié-Salpétrière, Paris)
N Engl J Med 318:1148–1152, May 5, 1988   4–11

The cause of ischemic stroke in about one third of young adult patients remains uncertain. Paradoxic embolism through a patent foramen ovale is responsible for some cases, but its prevalence is not known. Two-dimensional contrast echocardiography was used to determine the presence of patent foramen ovale in 60 adults aged younger than 55 years with ischemic stroke and normal cardiac findings and in 100 control patients who were candidates for posterior fossa surgery in the seated position. The method is based on the injection of isotonic saline containing air microbubbles.

The prevalence of patent foramen ovale was 40% in the stroke patients and 10% in the control group, a significant difference. Patent foramen ovale was found in 21% of 19 patients with identifiable causes of stroke and in 40% of 15 patients with risk factors for stroke. Of 26 patients with no identifiable cause or risk factor, 54% had a patent foramen ovale.

Patients with cerebral embolism should have contrast echocardiography if routine ultrasonography and cerebral angiography fail to demonstrate a source. If venous thrombosis is found, anticoagulant therapy is indicated for as long as the thrombosis persists. If this is ineffective, caval interruption or closure of the foramen ovale should be considered.

▶ Armin F. Haerer, M.D., Professor of Neurology, Department of Neurology, University of Mississippi Medical Center, Jackson, comments on this study.

▶ The causes of ischemic strokes in young adults are still often elusive. The present study suggests that paradoxical emboli through a clinically silent patent foramen ovale may be responsible for strokes more often than previously thought because patent foramina were significantly more common among young (aged less than 55) stroke patients than among a control group. Two questions that remain are: When is a stroke "embolic" and therefore to be investigated by contrast echocardiography and what about older persons with "embolic" strokes; do they also have patent foramina more often than controls? Confirmatory studies will help.—A.F. Haerer, M.D.

Patent Foramen Ovale in Young Stroke Patients

Webster MWI, Chancellor AM, Smith HJ, Swift DL, Sharpe DN, Bass NM, Glasgow GL (Auckland Hosp, Auckland, New Zealand)
Lancet 2:11–12, July 2, 1988   4–12

Despite thorough evaluation, no clear underlying cause can be found for about half of cerebral infarcts in patients younger than 40 years. Paradoxical embolism through a patent foramen ovale has been suggested as the origin for some of these strokes. A group of young stroke patients was assessed to determine the prevalence of patent foramen ovale.

Forty patients with a diagnosis of nonhemorrhagic cerebral infarction or transient ischemic attacks underwent contrast echocardiography. These patients were compared with age- and sex-matched normal controls. Echocardiography studies were performed at rest and with a Valsalva maneuver. Results were considered abnormal if microbubbles were visible in the left atrium or left ventricle within 3 cardiac cycles of their appearance in the right atrium.

Among stroke patients, a patent foramen ovale was revealed in 12 (30%) at rest and in 20 (50%) with a Valsalva maneuver. Among controls, the rates were 7.5% at rest and 15% with a Valsalva maneuver. Right-to-left shunting, assessed by the number of bubbles shown in the left side of the heart, occurred to a greater degree in stroke patients.

Though the high incidence of patent foramen ovale among stroke patients does not prove cause and effect, it does suggest a stronger link between paradoxical embolism and stroke than was previously known. Patients younger than 40 with an unexplained stroke or transient ischemic attack should undergo contrast echocardiography. The presence of a patent foramen ovale suggests a right-sided embolic source.

▶ This certainly is food for thought. Should every stroke patient aged less than 40 have this procedure? None had a clinically detectable intracardiac shunt at rest or a deep vein thrombosis at the time of their stroke. The authors comment, "Since recurrent episodes were uncommon, we cannot yet say how these patients should be managed subsequently." They draw attention to the publication of Lechat and co-workers in the *New England Journal of Medicine* (1), which reported closely similar results in patients aged less than 55. It seems to be a real finding. Perhaps this should be added to our list of diagnostic procedures in young stroke patients for whom there is no more obvious explanation.

Reference

1. Lechat et al: *N Engl J Med* 318:1148–1152, 1988.

Asymptomatic Cerebral Infarction in Patients With Chronic Atrial Fibrillation
Kempster PA, Gerraty RP, Gates PC (St Vincent's Hosp, Melbourne)
Stroke 19:955–957, August 1988   4–13

Chronic atrial fibrillation is a risk factor for cerebral infarction. Data on 54 patients who were seen in 1980–1985 with atrial fibrillation and symptoms of cerebral ischemia were reviewed. The control group included 168 persons in sinus rhythm who had symptoms of cerebral ischemia.

Seven (13%) patients with chronic atrial fibrillation had cranial computed tomographic evidence of previous, unsuspected cerebral infarction;

3 of these 7 patients had no cardiac disorder. Four patients sustained severe strokes, and 2, mild strokes; 1 had dementia. In the control group, 7 patients had computed tomographic evidence of clinically silent cerebral infarction; 3 of the 7 patients had small deep lacunar infarcts. The prevalence of asymptomatic cerebral infarction was significantly greater in the patients with atrial fibrillation.

Some patients with atrial fibrillation seen with symptomatic cerebral ischemia have had asymptomatic infarction in the past. Asymptomatic cerebral infarction is more common among such patients than among persons in sinus rhythm.

▶ There is no question that fibrillation is associated with embolization to the brain and that the scan pattern of embolization is different from that of lacunae but questions remain. Is this stroke really due to an embolus from the heart, and if so, does this patient need anticoagulation? Or is aspirin just as good? Halperin and Hart (1) in an editorial on atrial fibrillation and stroke note that we should have some answers soon because 5 studies are under way.

Reference

1. Halperin, Hart: *Stroke* 19:937–941, 1988.

Basilar Artery Blood Flow in Subclavian Steal

Bornstein NM, Krajewski A, Norris JW (Univ of Toronto)
Can J Neurol Sci 15:417–419, November 1988   4–14

To investigate whether subclavian steal is a benign hemodynamic phenomenon or is a cause of brain stem ischemia and stroke, transcranial Doppler studies were performed at rest and on arm exercise in 41 patients with severe subclavian stenosis, 33 of whom had reversed vertebral blood flow. The subclavian steal test (inflating a cuff to greater than the systolic pressure for 3 minutes on the ipsilateral arm) was performed when there was a 20-mm Hg blood pressure between the arms and a monophasic waveform from the subclavian artery, indicating severe stenosis.

No patient had reversed or bidirectional flow in the basilar artery during or after the steal test, and none experienced symptoms. No patient had cerebral ischemia during a 3-year follow-up period. The mean peak basilar blood flow was the same in 22 patients with reversed vertebral flow at rest and 11 with bidirectional vertebral flow. Of the 33 study patients, 8 had severe carotid stenosis.

Reversed blood flow in the vertebral artery appears to be a benign finding that rarely is associated with symptomatic brain stem ischemia. These findings do not support the view that neurologic symptoms occur only when subclavian steal coexists with hemodynamic incompetence elsewhere in the cerebral circulation.

▶ The basilar artery flow is not only in the right direction but even speeded up so the authors feel the syndrome is harmless and of no significance. But what about the patient who has cerebrovascular symptoms and a subclavian steal? A Doppler study of such a group would be interesting.

Stroke Following Coronary-Artery Bypass Surgery: A Case-Control Estimate of the Risk From Carotid Bruits

Reed GL III, Singer DE, Picard EH, DeSanctis RW (Harvard Univ)
N Engl J Med 319:1246–1250, Nov 10, 1988   4–15

Stroke after coronary-artery bypass surgery can be disabling. The causes of stroke after such surgery are largely unknown. This study was done to determine whether carotid bruits increase the risk of these events.

Fifty-four patients with postoperative stroke or transient ischemic attacks (TIAs) were compared with 54 randomly selected control patients. Both groups were taken from 5,915 consecutive patients who had coronary bypass surgery at 1 hospital between 1970 and 1984. Carotid bruits were found preoperatively in 13 patients with postoperative stroke and in 4 control patients. Case-control analysis revealed that the presence of carotid bruits increased the risk of stroke or TIAs by 3.9-fold. This elevated risk was essentially unchanged after adjustment for potentially confounding variables in a multiple logistic regression analysis. Other risk factors associated with a significantly elevated risk of these neurologic deficits were a history of stroke or TIA, a history of congestive heart failure, mitral regurgitation, postoperative atrial fibrillation, a cardiopulmonary-bypass pump time of more than 2 hours, and a previous myocardial infarction.

▶ This study clears up some of the fog surrounding the question of whether the carotid bruit in a preoperative cardiac patient needs to be investigated. The authors point out that although the risk of intraoperative TIA or stroke is increased nearly fourfold it is still, in an absolute sense, small (2.9%) and "comparable to the reported risk of stroke from carotid endarterectomy." Here is a situation into which the clinician can step and make a decision based on the totality of possible risk factors, rather than simply accepting the dictum that, if there is a bruit, an arteriogram needs to be done, and if a lesion is found, it needs to be removed before the cardiac surgery.

The Course of Transient Ischemic Attacks

Werdelin L, Juhler M (Rigshospitalet Copenhagen)
Neurology 38:677–680, May 1988   4–16

Short-term longitudinal studies are necessary to precisely distinguish between transient ischemic attack (TIA) and stroke. The authors followed, over the first 24 hours, 78 patients admitted with a first cerebrovascular episode of presumed ischemic origin. Only patients with specific symptoms of good focal diagnostic value and of presumed ischemic origin were included. The scoring system used (table) was coarse enough

---

Neurologic Grading of Cerebrovascular Symptoms

Gr. 0   Neurologically intact with anamnestic TIA.

Gr. 1   Objective signs of cerebrovascular insult without
        subjective functional limitation. (eg, hyperreflexia
        without paresis)

Gr. 2   Minor deficit: paresis < 50% in one extremity or facial
        palsy. Slight sensory impairment, dyscoordination, or
        aphasia.

Gr. 3   Moderate deficit: paresis > 50% in one extremity or
        hemiparesis < 50%. Severe aphasia, apraxia,
        dyscoordination, or sensory impairment. Hemianopia.

Gr. 4   Severe deficit: hemiparesis > 50%—hemiparalysis.
        Abolished sensory functions. Deviation of gaze.

Note: Inclusion in a given category was based on 1 or more of the listed findings.
Any patient exhibiting findings in more than 1 category was classified according to
the highest score.
(Courtesy of Werdelin L, Juhler M: Neurology 38:677–680, May 1988.)

---

to minimize interobserver differences in evaluation while allowing registration of significant changes in degree of deficit.

Fifty-eight patients had a final diagnosis of stroke, whereas 20 had TIA. Most TIA patients had slight symptoms at the outset, but 70% of stroke patients were in grade 3 or 4. Nearly all stroke patients but only 70% of TIA patients had hemiparesis. Only 7 patients with stroke had hemianopia. About half of each group were aphasic. Half the 20 patients with TIA had remission within 1 hour, and 18 of the 20, within 4 hours. Seven stroke patients had some remission, and 1 remitted completely. Angiography showed occlusion or stenosis in 3 of 8 TIA patients.

Transient ischemic attack and stroke may be distinguished clinically within 24 hours of the onset of an acute cerebrovascular event. Persistence of symptoms beyond a few hours suggests stroke. The severity of symptoms at onset or at admission also is a clue. The distinction may be especially important in clinical trials of intervention in acute ischemic brain disease.

▶ These careful observers have shown that a neurologic examination combined with a 4-hour wait can give good predictive information about whether the patient has suffered a stroke or a TIA. Most of the TIAs cleared within 4 hours, and the presenting symptoms were less dense. So by the time you decide on treatment after having looked at the CT scan, using these criteria you have a 90% chance of being right.—R.N. DeJong, M.D., and R.D. Currier, M.D.

Granulomatous Angiitis of the Central Nervous System: Protean Manifestations and Response to Treatment
Koo EH, Massey EW (Univ of California, San Francisco; Duke Univ)
J Neurol Neurosurg Psychiatry 51:1126–1133, September 1988   4–17

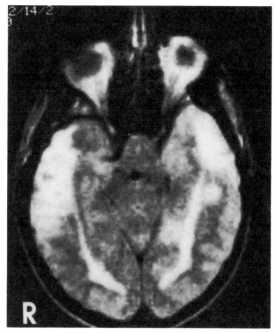

Fig 4–4.—Magnetic resonance imaging of first patient demonstrates multifocal areas of increased signal intensity in T_2-weighted spin-echo image, most marked in both temporal lobes. (Courtesy of Koo EH, Massey EW: *J Neurol Neurosurg Psychiatry* 51:1126–1133, September 1988.)

Granulomatous angiitis of the central nervous system is an uncommon necrotizing vasculitis with an unknown cause. About 30 tissue-proven cases unassociated with Hodgkin's disease or herpes zoster infections have been described. The outcome is generally fatal. Five tissue-proven cases unassociated with systemic illnesses are reported. The cases illustrate the varied manifestations of granulomatous angiitis.

The first patient, a 69-year-old man, had a left temporoparietal mass (Fig 4–4). The second patient, a 65-year-old man, had progressive confusion and memory loss. The third patient, a 44-year-old man, had signs and symptoms suggesting herpes simplex encephalitis. The fourth patient, a 78-year-old man, had a condition that mimicked the multi-infarct state. The last patient, a 60-year-old diabetic man, presented with a cerebellar mass lesion.

In 4 patients who underwent cerebral spinal fluid examination, protein was elevated (81 to 193 gm/L), and 3 patients had mononuclear pleocytosis (12 to 800 white blood cells/mm³). Cerebral arteriogram suggested vasculitis in 1 of 4 patients. Diagnosis was made by brain biopsy in 3 patients, all of whom were successfully treated. In the other 2 cases, the diagnosis was made at postmortem examination.

These cases illustrate the protean manifestations of the disease and the difficulties encountered in making a diagnosis.

▶ This disease is still nearly impossible to diagnose without a brain biopsy.

Younger and associates (1) agree that a biopsy "is the only way to ascertain the diagnosis in living patients." The happy thought in this analysis is that 3 of their cases were treated successfully with high-dose steroids, which may be combined with an immunosuppressive agent such as cyclophosphamide. Therapy may be prolonged.

Reference

1. Younger et al: *Arch Neurol* 45:514–518, 1988.

Diagnosis and Management of Isolated Angiitis of the Central Nervous System
Moore PM (Wayne State Univ, Detroit)
Neurology 39:167–173, February 1989   4–18

Isolated angiitis of the central nervous system (CNS) is an idiopathic, recurrent disorder involving chiefly small and medium-sized blood vessels. Patients generally die after sustaining recurrent cerebral infarction,

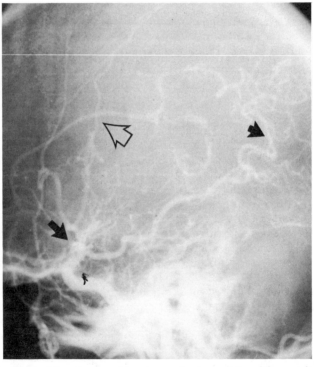

Fig 4–5.—Selective left common carotid angiogram showing occlusion of the supraclinoid segment of the carotid artery associated with neovascularization *(shaded arrow)*. There are extensive collaterals from the external carotid circulation *(open arrow)* and collaterals with the posterior circulation *(arrowhead)* (via retrograde flow). The vertebral injection (not shown) confirms the posterior circulation collaterals to anterior and middle cerebral arteries. (Courtesy of Moore PM: *Neurology* 39:167–173, February 1989.)

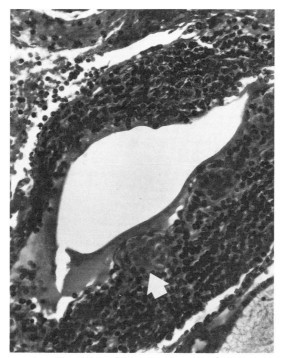

Fig 4–6.—Leptomeningeal biopsy. There is a mononuclear cell infiltrate in the vessel with areas of focal necrosis *(arrow)*. (Courtesy of Moore PM: *Neurology* 39:167–173, February 1989.)

but aggressive immunosuppression with prednisone and cyclophosphamide can alter the outcome.

Five new incidents of isolated angiitis of the CNS were reported. The most frequently seen features were severe headache, focal neurologic abnormalities, and mild encephalopathy. Systemic symptoms and serologic evidence of inflammation are usually absent. All patients had segmental stenotic narrowing of medium-sized arteries (Fig 4–5). In addition, some blood vessels ended abruptly and arterial walls were poorly delineated. The preferred biopsy site (Fig 4–6) is the nondominant hemisphere, usually at the temporal tip.

All 5 patients have done well. Initial treatment should include prednisone, 40–60 mg, and cyclophosphamide, 100 mg, daily, but dosage should be individually adjusted as indicated by weekly monitoring of the leukocyte count. This treatment should not begin until the diagnosis of isolated angiitis is established. The cause of isolated angiitis of the CNS remains unknown.

▶ This author recommends a 4-step diagnostic approach to include the typical symptom complex of headache, mental changes and focal symptoms, a CSF examination, and cerebral angiography, with the last step being leptomeningeal/parenchymal biopsy. She also has had good luck with the suggested treatment.

The Value of Carotid Doppler Ultrasound in Asymptomatic Extracranial Arterial Disease

Bornstein NM, Chadwick LG, Norris JW (Univ of Toronto)
Can J Neurol Sci 15:378–383, November 1988   4–19

Continuous-wave Doppler ultrasonography is 90% accurate in detecting carotid lesions producing more than 50% stenosis. Close correlation is found between the Doppler frequency shift and the degree of stenosis on angiography (Fig 4–7). Periorbital directional flow is reversed only in high-grade stenoses. High-resolution real-time B-mode imaging is a better means of demonstrating plaque and its surface than is angiography, and it has high predictive value in detecting large plaque hemorrhages. B-mode imaging also serves to assess plaque ulceration, but angiography is more sensitive for this purpose.

The asymptomatic cervical bruit is a marker of extracranial carotid disease and a risk factor for stroke. Carotid Doppler study can identify underlying arterial disease in patients with bruits. The finding of stenosis in the internal carotid artery indicates a definite risk for stroke (table). Patients found to have internal carotid stenosis should be instructed as to warning symptoms and in the need to report them immediately.

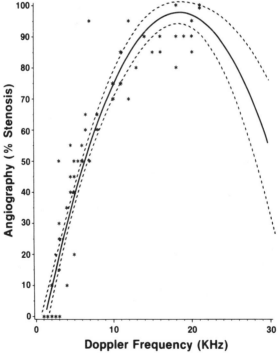

Fig 4–7.—Correlation between the Doppler shift in kilohertz and the percentage of stenosis on angiography using quadratic regression model. (Courtesy of Bornstein NM, Chadwick LG, Norris JW: *Can J Neurol Sci* 15:378–383, November 1988.)

Annual Stroke Rate (%) in All Vascular Territories in 498 Patients (996 Carotid Arteries) With Asymptomatic Cervical Bruits

	Patients	Arteries
Carotid Stenosis (Doppler)	**% Stroke**	**% Stroke**
< 35%	0.9	0.3
35-50%	0.0	0.0
50-75%	0.9	0.6
>75%	6.0	3.0
Overall	1.7	0.6

Note: Kaplan-Meier method.
(Courtesy of Bornstein NM, Chadwick LG, Norris JW: *Can J Neurol Sci* 15:378–383, November 1988.)

Progressive carotid stenosis on a follow-up Doppler study (Fig 4–8) probably indicates "plaque instability."

It is necessary to distinguish between carotid occlusion and severe stenosis because occluded vessels are inoperable. Carotid Doppler ultrasonography has proved to be imperfect in making the distinction; even infrequent errors are unacceptable in this setting. All candidates for surgery who appear to have severe stenosis should undergo angiography if the internal carotid artery is not clearly seen on duplex study. Transcranial Doppler recordings can show the adequacy of hemispheric collateral circulation.

▶ The authors have followed a large number of patients with modern Doppler techniques and find it to be more useful as the machines have improved. They point out that differentiating occlusion from severe stenosis is still a problem, but by combining carotid with transcranial Doppler a good guess can be made.

What is the proper place and use of modern Doppler techniques? Hennerici and associates (1) may have found it. Doppler carotid techniques were carried

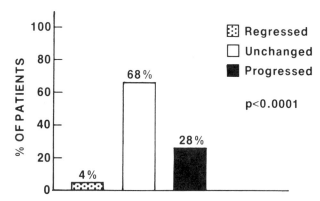

Fig 4–8.—Percentage of arteries that have progressed (28%), regressed (4%), and remained unchanged (68%) over 2 years' follow-up with continuous-wave Doppler. (Courtesy of Bornstein NM, Chadwick LG, Norris JW: *Can J Neurol Sci* 15:378–383, November 1988.)

out in 3,225 patients admitted to the hospital with coronary or peripheral vascular disease and without stroke. Of these, 339 had abnormal results and were studied serially. Progression of the arterial abnormality by Doppler study or transient ischemic attacks (TIA) were the only valid prognostic factors for stroke. So perhaps if there has been no sign or symptom of stroke, following with Doppler and noting TIA symptoms is the best way to determine who should have carotid surgery.

The American Neurological Association's Committee on Health Care Issues (Jack Whisnant) has a position paper on whether or not carotid surgery is useful at all (2) that is worth rereading. Its usefulness is regarded as unproved.

References

1. Hennerici et al: *Brain* 110:777–791, 1987.
2. Whisnant J: *Ann Neurol* 22:72–76, July 1987.

Fatal Ischaemic Brain Oedema After Early Thrombolysis With Tissue Plasminogen Activator in Acute Stroke
Koudstaal PJ, Stibbe J, Vermeulen M (Academic Hosp Dijkzigt, Rotterdam, The Netherlands)
Br Med J 297:1571–1574, Dec 17, 1988   4–20

A pilot study of thrombolysis with tissue plasminogen activator was planned in 10 patients with acute cerebrovascular accident and symptoms of ischemia in the carotid territory. The first 2 patients, with presumed middle cerebral artery occlusion, were treated about 3.5 hours after the onset of symptoms. A bolus of 10 mg of tissue plasminogen

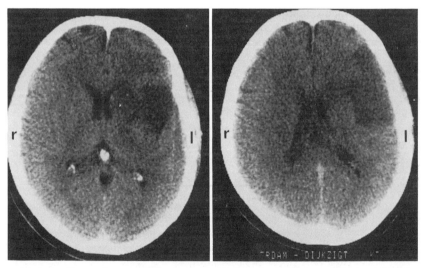

Fig 4–9.—Computed tomographic appearances of brain on day 3. (Courtesy of Koudstaal PJ, Stibbe J, Vermeulen M: *Br Med J* 297:1571–1574, Dec 17, 1988.)

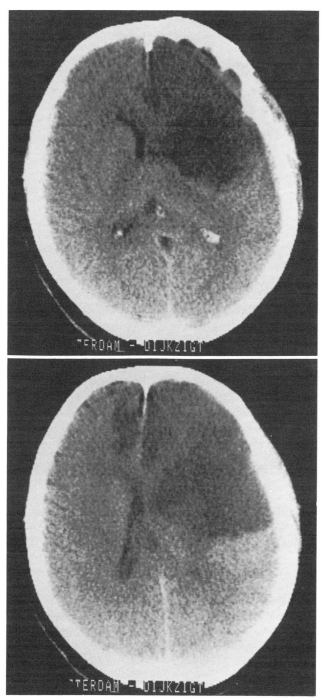

Fig 4–10.—Computed tomographic appearances of brain on day 5. (Courtesy of Koudstaal PJ, Stibbe J, Vermeulen M: *Br Med J* 297:1571–1574, Dec 17, 1988.)

activator was followed by an infusion of 50 mg in the first hour and 40 mg in the second and third hours, for a total dose of 100 mg.

Initial computed tomographic (CT) scans were normal, and there were no significant systemic bleeding complications. Marked fibrinogenolysis was documented. Both patients had extensive infarction, with massive edema on repeat CT scanning (Figs 4–9 and 4–10). The conditions of both patients deteriorated, and the patients died of transtentorial herniation. Autopsy in 1 patient showed bleeding into the subarachnoid space from a microscopic angioma.

Early treatment of ischemic stroke with tissue plasminogen activator can lead to excessive ischemic edema and fatal brain herniation. It is possible that ischemia for 2 to 5 hours damages vessels and results in leakage, with hemorrhage occurring only after a longer period of ischemia.

▶ These workers found just 2 of 59 stroke patients acceptable for the study of tissue plasminogen activator. Both patients died after treatment, and at autopsy their vessels were open. Massive cerebral edema, not hemorrhage, caused their deaths, and the assumption is that the treatment in some way caused massive cerebral infarction. Well, the brain is not the heart. Nature continues to point that out.

Placebo-Controlled, Randomised Trial of Warfarin and Aspirin for Prevention of Thromboembolic Complications in Chronic Atrial Fibrillation
Petersen P, Boysen G, Godtfredsen J, Andersen ED, Andersen B (Univ Hosp, Rigshospitalet, Copenhagen)
Lancet 1:175–179, Jan 28, 1989   4–21

Atrial fibrillation is associated with a high risk of thromboembolic complications. However, paroxysmal atrial fibrillation is associated with a lower risk of stroke. The question of whether to use prophylaxis with anticoagulants or aspirin in patients with chronic nonrheumatic atrial fibrillation has been debated for years. A randomized trial was done to compare the effects of warfarin anticoagulation, low-dose aspirin therapy, and placebo on the incidence of thromboembolic complications in patients with chronic nonrheumatic atrial fibrillation.

Of 1,007 outpatients studied, 335 received warfarin openly and, in a double-blind trial, 336 received 75 mg of aspirin daily and 336 received placebo. Patients were followed up for 2 years or until termination of the study. The primary end point was a thromboembolic complication, and the secondary end point was death. The incidences of thromboembolic complications and vascular death were found to be significantly lower in the warfarin group than in the other 2 groups. The aspirin and placebo groups did not differ significantly. Five patients taking warfarin had thromboembolic complications, compared with 20 taking aspirin and 21 taking placebo. Twenty-one patients on warfarin were withdrawn from the study because of nonfatal bleeding complications, compared with 2 receiving aspirin and none receiving placebo.

These findings suggest that warfarin should be recommended to prevent thromboembolic complications in patients with chronic nonrheumatic atrial fibrillation. The incidence of thromboembolic complications and vascular mortality in this series were significantly lower among patients on warfarin than those on aspirin or placebo.

▶ Bless the Danes. They may be the best-organized nation for studying their population, and the world benefits from it. The patients on warfarin were carried at a therapeutic range of 4.2–2.4 international normalized ratio (INR) and had their blood checked every month. Five patients on warfarin had strokes, and of these 5 strokes, only 1 occurred during sufficient anticoagulation. There was 1 fatal stroke in the warfarin group, 3 in the aspirin group, and 4 in the placebo group. Their complications were minimal. It does look as though careful use of warfarin is the right treatment for chronic atrial fibrillation.

Postmenopausal Oestrogen Treatment and Stroke: A Prospective Study
Paganini-Hill A, Ross RK, Henderson BE (Univ of Southern California, Los Angeles)
Br Med J 297:519–522, Aug 20–27, 1988   4–22

Stroke continues to be the third leading cause of death in the United States. Because stroke is frequently fatal and the impact of treatment on prognosis is limited, control of this disease must be achieved through primary prevention. To determine whether use of postmenopausal estrogen affects the risk of dying of stroke questionnaires eliciting details of estrogen replacement therapy and potential risk modifiers were sent to all 22,781 residents of a California retirement community. Sixty-one percent, with a median age of 73 years, responded. This cohort was followed up, using health department death certificates. Rates of death from stroke among women who did and did not receive estrogen replacement therapy were compared. By the end of the study, there had been 1,019 deaths in the cohort. Twenty of the 4,962 women who used estrogen replacement treatment died ,from stroke, compared with 43 of the 3,845 women who did not use such therapy, yielding a relative risk of 0.53. The protective effect was found in all age groups except the youngest and was unaffected by adjustment for the possible confounding variables of hypertension, smoking, alcohol use, body mass index, and exercise.

Postmenopausal estrogen replacement therapy may protect against death from stroke. A reduction in mortality from stroke was found both in women with and those without a history of hypertension.

▶ This splendid study shows clearly that postmenopausal estrogen replacement does protect against death due to stroke. The reduced risk in this study was found in both hypertensive and nonhypertensive women. The authors also suggest, interestingly enough, that, because adipose tissue is a source of estrogen, obesity in postmenopausal women may not be bad.

I have asked my knowledgeable friends to explain to me why estrogen taken as a method of contraception may lead to stroke, whereas estrogen taken postmenopausally prevents stroke. So far I have not had a clear explanation, but I am sure someone out there knows. Is it a difference in dosage? Probably. For a nice review of the neurology of sex steroids and oral contraceptives see Schipper HM (1).

Reference

1. Schipper HM: *Neurol Clin* 4:721–751, November 1986.

Deep Vein Thrombosis After Ischemic Stroke: Rationale for a Therapeutic Trial
Bornstein NM, Norris JW (Univ of Toronto)
Arch Phys Med Rehabil 69:955–958, November 1988   4–23

Deep venous thrombosis is a major threat to all immobilized patients, including those with ischemic stroke. The feasibility of anticoagulant prophylaxis was studied in a prospective series of stroke patients seen within a 16-month period. Forty-nine of 250 consecutive patients (mean age, 74 years) were studied. They had no contraindications to anticoagulant or antiplatelet therapy.

Deep venous thrombosis was detected in 22.5% of the 49 study patients. All 11 affected patients had marked leg weakness. Six patients required chronic care for their neurologic deficits, and in the other 5 patients, anticoagulant therapy could be justified. Two patients had symptoms of pulmonary embolism. Two patients had proximal vein thrombosis. In 4 patients fibrinogen scanning was positive but deep venous thrombosis was not clinically apparent.

Prophylactic low-molecular-weight heparin may be warranted for some stroke patients but not those with minimal deficits or those who are ambulatory. Treatment should begin as soon as possible after neurologic assessment. Prophylaxis also has a role in the management of patients who make significant recovery in the first few days.

▶ After the first week or 2 with deaths due first to increased pressure and massive infarction and then to pneumonia, the most likely cause of death is pulmonary embolism originating in occluded veins in the paralyzed and often insensitive leg. Some years ago without a proper trial we began requesting that the nurses or the family or both milk both legs, particularly the paralyzed leg, every 8 hours (once each shift), with a deep and strong stroking of the leg as though they were milking blood clots out of the veins.

Since then we have had no deaths of acute stroke patients who had been under our care from the beginning and for whom this had been done. The family doesn't mind doing it; in fact, they appreciate having a part in the care of the patient.

Central Post-Stroke Pain: A Controlled Trial of Amitriptyline and Carbamazepine

Leijon G, Boivie J (Univ of Linköping, Sweden)
Pain 36:27–36, January 1989   4–24

The only common feature in patients with central poststroke pain (CPSP) is disordered cutaneous sensibility, usually of the hyperpathic type. Fifteen patients with a definite stroke and subsequent constant or intermittent pain participated in a trial to evaluate the effects of amitriptyline and carbamazepine. Patients received treatment for 4 weeks with amitriptyline or carbamazepine in final doses of 75 mg and 800 mg daily, respectively.

Both amitriptyline and carbamazepine reduced pain. In the fourth week of treatment, pain intensity scores were about 20% lower than in patients receiving treatment with placebo. Most patients had side effects from active treatment but these usually were mild. Although the pain-relieving effect of amitriptyline was correlated with the total plasma level, no such relationship was seen for carbamazepine.

An antidepressant agent such as amitriptyline should be tried first in patients with CPSP, but controlled studies of the long-term effects of these drugs are needed. Some patients with CPSP may receive pain-relieving benefit from carbamazepine.

▶ Central poststroke pain is more common than realized. It often includes (causes?) the shoulder-hand syndrome on the affected side. Amitriptyline, often used in treatment of CPSP, is now shown by this double-blind study to work but not through the relief of depression per se. How it works is still open to question, although it may be related to serotonin or other central nervous system neurotransmitters. For those interested, the authors characterized the symptoms and pain characteristics of this group is an article just preceding this one in *Pain* (1).

Reference

1. Leijon G, Boivie J: *Pain* 36:13–25, January 1989.

5 Pediatric Neurology

Intraventricular Hemorrhage in the Premature Infant—Current Concepts: Part I
Volpe JJ (Washington Univ, St Louis)
Ann Neurol 25:3–11, January 1989   5–1

The incidence of intraventricular hemorrhage (IVH) has decreased at most neonatal centers in recent years. Hemorrhage generally begins in the subependymal germinal matrix and spreads to the lateral ventricles and throughout the ventricular system. The germinal matrix is destroyed, and the hematoma often is replaced by a cyst. About 15% of infants with IVH also have an area of hemorrhagic necrosis in the periventricular white matter dorsolateral to the external angle of the lateral ventricle. The lesion appears to represent hemorrhagic infarction. Posthemorrhagic ventricular dilation is another sequel to IVH.

Intravascular factors relating to blood flow and pressure regulation in the microvascular bed of the germinal matrix have a role in the pathogenesis of IVH. Fluctuating cerebral blood flow likely is a major factor. Intraventricular hemorrhage has been related temporally to abrupt increases in arterial pressure. Elevated cerebral venous pressure also may contribute to IVH. A fall in cerebral blood flow occurring either before or after birth can be an important factor in IVH in some infants. Disordered platelet-capillary function or coagulation also may contribute. Some studies have proposed that a postnatal decrease in tissue pressure increases the intravascular-extravascular gradient and provokes hemorrhage.

▶ Owen B. Evans, M.D., Professor and Chairman, Department of Pediatrics, University of Mississippi Medical Center, Jackson, comments.

▶ This article is the clinical companion to the second article in a series that discusses diagnoses, prognosis, and prevention (1). The 2 together are remarkable for their clarity of style, scope of the discussion, and the correlation of pathogenesis to diagnosis, management, and prognosis. The concept of fluctuating cerebral blood flow in the pathogenesis of IVH and the role of venous hemorrhagic parenchymal infarction as a major factor that determines subsequent neurologic sequelae are typical examples.

Dr. Volpe has contributed considerable knowledge to the field of neonatal neurology, and these two papers are further evidence of his leadership.—O.B. Evans, M.D.

Reference

1. Volpe JJ: *Ann Neurol* 26, 1989.

Natural History of Fetal Ventriculomegaly

Hudgins RJ, Edwards MSB, Goldstein R, Callen PW, Harrison MR, Filly RA, Golbus MS (Univ of California, San Francisco)
Pediatrics 82:692–697, November 1988
5–2

The efficacy of a treatment can be determined only if the natural history of the disease being treated is known. The natural history of ventriculomegaly is not well understood. Extrapolating the natural history of neonatal hydrocephalus to fetal ventriculomegaly is not valid because of significant selection differences between these groups; fetuses with severe anomalies rarely survive the neonatal period. A retrospective review was done to investigate the natural history of in utero ventriculomegaly.

The outcome of 47 fetuses assessed within a 5-year period was analyzed. In 20 cases, ventriculomegaly associated with other severe abnormalities was diagnosed early in pregnancy; 19 pregnancies were terminated, and the remaining fetus did not survive. In 5 cases, ventriculomegaly associated with severe abnormalities was diagnosed late in pregnancy. None of these features, managed in a routine obstetric fashion, survived. Of the other 22 fetuses, 19 had stable and 2 had progressive ventriculomegaly. In 1 of these, ventriculomegaly resolved in utero. Nineteen of these fetuses survived, 13 with normal intellectual development and 6 with moderately delayed to severely delayed development. In

Patient Population	
Characteristics	No. of Infants or Fetuses
Detected early in pregnancy, all with severe associated abnormalities, no survivors	20
Detected late in pregnancy, all with severe associated abnormalities, no survivors	5
No severe anomalies detected on prenatal ultrasonogram	22
Stable ventriculomegaly	19
Increased intracranial pressure, all shunted	9
Developmentally normal (1 died of sepsis)	6
Moderately delayed	2
Severely delayed	1
Intracranial pressure normal	10
No abnormalities, developmentally normal with stable, mild ventriculomegaly	5
Multiple abnormalities, all developmentally abnormal (2 have died)	5
Progressive ventriculomegaly, both shunted and developmentally normal	2
Resolved ventriculomegaly, developmentally normal	1

(Courtesy of Hudgins RJ, Edwards MSB, Goldstein R, et al: *Pediatrics* 82:692–697, November 1988.)

74% of fetuses, associated abnormalities were found with ultrasonography. There was a 20% false negative detection rate. In 2 cases in which ventriculomegaly was isolated and progressive, the fetuses were delivered at term and a postnatal shunting procedure was performed. Both infants are now neurologically normal (table).

The prognosis for the fetus with in utero ventriculomegaly is poor. In this series, mortality was 70%, and only 50% of the survivors had normal intellectual development. Severe central nervous system and systemic anomalies, associated with fetal ventriculomegaly in 81% of the fetuses, may not be detected in 20% to 39% of the cases. Those fetuses with in utero ventriculomegaly who may benefit from in utero shunting could not be identified.

▶ Technologic advances often exceed clinical applications. This study shows that in utero ventriculomegaly is usually associated with other severe anomalies or is nonprogressive. One fetus had spontaneous resolution, and 2 had progressive ventriculomegaly that did well with traditional postpartum shunting. Demonstrating intrauterine ventriculomegaly is not a reason for premature intervention.—O.B. Evans, M.D.

Cluster of Perinatal Events Identifying Infants at High Risk for Death or Disability

Ellenberg JH, Nelson KB (Natl Inst of Neurological and Communicative Disorders and Stroke, Bethesda, Md)
J Pediatr 113:546–552, September 1988   5–3

The syndrome of hypoxic-ischemic encephalopathy implies a series of events with risks related to the evolution of clinical signs and to the severity of those signs. To determine the prognostic importance of neonatal seizures according to the presence or absence of certain other postnatal characteristics, a population of 39,000 infants with birth weights greater than 2,500 gm was studied.

Babies with clinically recognized neonatal seizures and 5-minute Apgar scores of 5 or less and who had at least 1 of 5 signs compatible with neonatal encephalopathy had a 33% risk of first-year death. Those who survived this cluster of events—low Apgar score, abnormal signs, and seizures—had a risk for motor disability of 55%. Survivors of neonatal seizures who did not have poor Apgar scores or other abnormal signs had a risk for motor disability of only 0.13% (Fig 5–1).

In this series, infants with neonatal seizures had a risk for cerebral palsy 420 times greater if they also had a low 5-minute Apgar score and other neonatal signs.

▶ The prognosis for an infant with neonatal encephalopathy from any cause is worsened if there are associated seizures. This study indicates that seizures, in and of themselves, were not the major determinant. Rather, if an insult to the

A

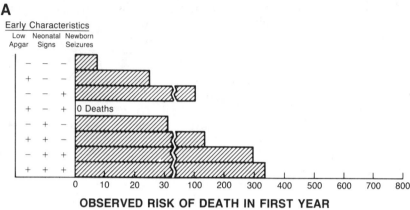

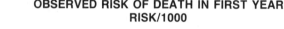

OBSERVED RISK OF DEATH IN FIRST YEAR
RISK/1000

B

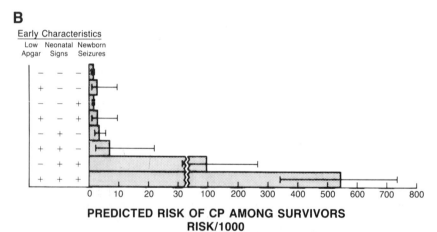

PREDICTED RISK OF CP AMONG SURVIVORS
RISK/1000

Fig 5–1.—Observed risk of death in first year (**A**) by presence or absence of early characteristics, and predicted risk of cerebral palsy (**B**). Ninety-five percent confidence limits for predicted risk of cerebral palsy are indicated by *brackets* superimposed on histogram bars. (Courtesy of Ellenberg JH, Nelson KB: *J Pediatr* 113:546–552, September 1988.)

brain is sufficient enough to cause altered consciousness, abnormal neurologic signs, and seizures, the insult is likely to be significant and cause permanent neurologic deficits or death.—O.B. Evans, M.D.

EEG Diagnoses of Neonatal Seizures: Clinical Correlations and Outcome
Scher MS, Painter MJ, Bergman I, Barmada MA, Brunberg J (Magee-Women's Hosp, Pittsburgh; Children's Hosp of Pittsburgh)
Pediatr Neurol 5:17–24, January–February 1989   5–4

Neonatal seizures are associated with high death rates and incidences of neurodevelopmental delay. Recognizing seizures is difficult because of the nature of neonatal convulsive activity. However, prompt intervention may be important. Abnormal neonatal movements were correlated with the absence or presence of EEG seizure activity to determine the frequency of seizures as a cause of abnormal movements in neonates.

The EEG seizures were assessed in 112 infants (table). The first part of the study included 80 neonates with clinically identified abnormal movements. Eight (10%) of these infants had EEG evidence of seizures coincident with these movements. In the second half of the study, 40 neonates who had electrical seizures were examined, 8 of whom were identified in the first half of the study. Two thirds of the infants were premature. Sixteen (40%) died. Ninety percent had brain lesions documented with computed tomography or autopsy. The most common lesions were cerebral infarction and intraventricular hemorrhage. One third of the surviving infants were normal at a mean age of 3 years, and two thirds had significant neurologic and developmental anomalies.

Suspected Seizure Diagnosis		
Suspicious Movements	**Number of Records**	**EEGs with Electrical Seizures**
Subtle clinical signs		
Bicycling	5	0
Buccolingual	5	2
Eye deviation	2	1
Apnea	2	1
Autonomic*	4	0
Irritability	5	0
Clonic	18	8
Tonic	12	1
Myoclonic	15	1
Tremor (jitteriness)	17	0
Total:	85	14

*Includes sudden heart rate or blood pressure changes.
(Courtesy of Scher MS, Painter MJ, Bergman I, et al: *Pediatr Neurol* 5:17–24, January–February 1989.)

Neonatal seizures are frequently subtle, unassociated with notable clinical expression, and associated with adverse outcomes. Confirmation by EEG is important in assessing seizures in the neonate.

▶ The most interesting findings in this study were that only 10% of the 80 infants with abnormal movements had EEG-documented seizures and 23% of the 40 infants with documented EEG seizures had no abnormal movements noted clinically. With the data, it is an understatement to say that neonatal seizures may be difficult to clinically diagnose. This study suggests that neonatal seizures may be important to diagnose for prognostic reasons but does not answer the question as to whether they are important to treat.—O.B. Evans, M.D.

Oligoantigenic Diet Treatment of Children With Epilepsy and Migraine
Egger J, Carter CM, Soothill JF, Wilson J (The Hosp for Sick Children; Inst of Child Health, London)
J Pediatr 114:51–58, January 1989   5–5

In recent double-blind controlled trials of oligoantigenic diet therapy in children with migraine and hyperactive behavior disorders, 27 children also had epileptic seizures that usually ceased during diet therapy. The efficacy of diet therapy in 45 children with drug-resistant seizures, migraine, and hyperkinetic behavior was compared with that in 18 children with epilepsy but no migraine or conventional allergic symptoms. The 63 children ranged in age from 2 to 16 years and had several types of epilepsy.

After a 4-week oligoantigenic diet, patients who did not improve were offered a second oligoantigenic diet consisting of foods not included in the first diet. Patients who responded entered the reintroduction phase during which foods that caused the reappearance of symptoms were subsequently avoided. In addition, 16 children who had reached an acceptable diet participated in a double-blind, placebo-controlled provocation study.

After 7 months to 3 years on the oligoantigenic diet, 25 of the 45 children with epilepsy, recurrent headaches, abdominal symptoms, or hyperkinetic behavior had achieved complete control of seizures and 11 children had fewer seizures than before diet therapy was initiated. Furthermore, headaches, abdominal pains, and hyperkinetic behavior ceased in all children whose seizures ceased and in some of the children who still had seizures. However, none of the 18 patients with epilepsy alone had improvement from the oligoantigenic diet. Symptoms recurred with the reintroduction of 42 different foods, and seizures recurred with 31 foods. Cow milk was the most common provoking substance among the 10 most frequently incriminated foods (table). Fifteen of the 16 patients who participated in the double-blind, placebo-controlled provocation studies of food reintroduction had recurrence of symptoms, of whom 8 had recurrence of seizures.

Reactions to Foods Reintroduced in More Than 10
Patients and Frequently Incriminated

Food	Tested	Seizures (%)	Other symptoms* (%)
Cow milk	35	37	63
Cow cheese	11	36	55
Citrus fruits	24	29	50
Wheat	35	29	49
Food additives†	12	25	58
Hen eggs	27	19	35
Tomato	20	15	25
Pork	23	13	22
Chocolate	19	11	47
Corn	21	10	19
Grapes	12	8	17
Tea	13	8	15
Beef	31	7	19
Cane sugar	19	5	21
Yeast	21	5	18
Oats	29	3	21
Potato	31	3	10
Rice	31	3	6
Banana	33	3	9
Apple	39	3	6

*Headaches, gastrointestinal symptoms, behavior problems.
†Tartrazine and benzoic acid.
(Courtesy of Egger J, Carter CM, Soothill JF, et al: *J Pediatr* 114:51–58, January 1989.)

Oligoantigenic diet therapy may benefit carefully selected children who have both drug-resistant epilepsy and migraine and whose disease is severe enough to warrant such a socially disruptive and expensive treatment.

▶ Is one to conclude from this article that both seizures and headache in children are precipitated by certain foods or that food precipitates one, which causes the other? The children with epilepsy only did not have improvement with the diet. Gibbs used diet to treat epilepsy decades ago, but I don't recall whether his epileptic patients had a mixture of headache and epilepsy or epilepsy alone.

Low Morbidity and Mortality of Status Epilepticus in Children
Maytal J, Shinnar S, Moshé SL, Alvarez LA (Montefiore Med Ctr–Albert Einstein College of Medicine, Bronx, NY)
Pediatrics 83:323–331, March 1989   5–6

A study was undertaken to establish the current mortality and morbidity of status epilepticus in children. A total of 193 children aged 1 month to 18 years (mean, 5.0 years) with status epilepticus of varying causes were followed up for a mean period of 13.2 months. Of these, 97 were recruited prospectively.

The causes of status epilepticus were classified as idiopathic in 46 children, remote symptomatic in 45, febrile in 46, acute symptomatic in 45, and progressive neurologic in 11. The peak incidence was during the first few years of life, with 64% of cases occurring in the first 5 years of life. Age distribution was significantly correlated with etiology of status epilepticus. Febrile status epilepticus and status epilepticus due to other acute symptomatic illnesses were more prevalent in the first few years of life, whereas unprovoked status epilepticus occurred throughout childhood and adolescence.

Seven children (3.6%) died within 3 months of the episode of status epilepticus. New neurologic deficits occurred in 17 (9.1%) of the 186 survivors. All of the deaths and 15 of the 17 sequelae occurred among children with acute or progressive neurologic insults, whereas only 2 of the 137 children with other causes sustained any new deficits. Duration of the status epilepticus affected outcome only within the acute symptomatic group. The incidence of significant sequelae was a function of age. It declined from 29% among infants aged less than 1 year to 11% among children aged 1 to 3 years and 6% among children aged more than 3 years. This relationship reflected the greater incidence of acute neurologic disease in the younger age groups. For each cause, however, age did not affect outcome. Of the 125 children with no history of prior unprovoked seizures, 37 (30%) had subsequent unprovoked seizures. Recurrence risk was significantly higher in the retrospective group than in the prospective group (Fig 5–2).

In the absence of an acute or progressive neurologic insult, status epi-

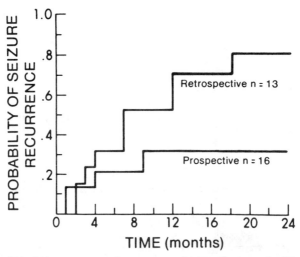

Fig 5–2.—Risk of seizure recurrence after occurrence of status epilepticus as first idiopathic seizure. Data are shown as Kaplan-Meier curves for prospective and retrospective groups. (Courtesy of Maytal J, Shinnar S, Moshé SL, et al: *Pediatrics* 83:323–331, March 1989.)

lepticus has low morbidity and mortality. It appears that the outcome of status epilepticus is primarily a function of the underlying etiology.

▶ The trend in the treatment of seizure disorders has been one of retrenchment. This has been accomplished by a number of studies, such as this one, documenting the natural history of seizures, the cognitive effects of anticonvulsant drugs, and the limitations of anticonvulsants in the treatment of some epileptic disorders. We have been shown the wisdom of withholding treatment after a single seizure and the value of monotherapy. This study also indicates that therapy isn't always necessary after an unprovoked prolonged seizure, and should it recur, the risk of status epilepticus is low.— O.B. Evans, M.D.

Rett Syndrome: Natural History and Management
Moeschler JB, Charman CE, Berg SZ, Graham JM Jr (Dartmouth Med School; Dartmouth-Hitchcock Med Ctr, Hanover, NH)
Pediatrics 82:1–10, July 1988   5–7

Rett syndrome is a newly described developmental disorder affecting girls only. More than 600 patients have been studied, but pediatricians are still learning to recognize the syndrome and to care for the patients. Seven girls and 1 woman with Rett syndrome were evaluated.

The patients ranged in age from 2 to 25 years. Rett syndrome was first diagnosed after psychomotor regression and stereotypic hand movements were noted in a girl aged 2 years. At birth, this patient had aspirated meconium and received ventilatory support because of respiratory dis-

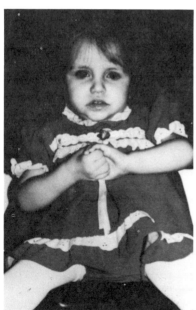

Fig 5–3.— Note hand posture and normal physical features. (Courtesy of Moeschler JB, Charman CE, Berg SZ, et al: *Pediatrics* 82:1–10, July 1988.)

tress. Developmental delays were first recognized at age 11 months, when she was not yet sitting. By age 15 months, she had learned to speak 1 to 2 words but had ceased saying them. At age 18 to 24 months, she lost interest in objects and people. She no longer reached and grasped toys. She held her hands constantly in the midline and wrung them (Fig 5–3). She did not interact with her parents and had bruxism and episodes of inconsolable screaming. She stopped rolling around for locomotion, preferring to sit and wring her hands over any other activity.

In another case, the mother of a 24-year-old woman recognized her daughter's syndrome while reading about Rett syndrome in the newspaper. The affected woman was a dizygotic twin, born at term after a normal gestation, who developed slowly compared with her twin brother. At age 18 months, she began to regress and started prolonged, inconsolable screaming. At age 18 to 24 months, she began the characteristic hand wringing. At age 3 years 8 months, truncal ataxia was observed. By age 4 years 7 months, she had spasticity in the upper and lower extremities. She had gross tremors of her hands and legs when excited. She also had sustained ankle clonus. Menses began at 12 years of age and continued regularly until she was 20 years old, when it became erratic. At age 25 years, she was nonambulatory and had no speech. Hand wringing was prominent, and severe kyphoscoliosis was present. She had thin, cool, mottled extremities and a tremor in 1 foot at rest. Chromosomes were 46,XX, with 1 cell of 30 being 47,XXX (table).

Rett syndrome has a recognizable neurodevelopmental phenotype without a specific biologic marker, making diagnosis difficult sometimes. Treatment is largely supportive. An active parents' association can be helpful.

Neurodevelopmental Phenotypic Features*			
Feature	This Report (N = 8)	Naidu et al[26] (N = 70)	Hagberg et al[3] (N = 35)
Hand wringing or clapping	8	70	35
Loss of hand function	8	70	35
Hyperventilation	5	NR	23
Bruxism	5	NR	NR
Irritability or self-injury	7	38	NR
Sleep disturbance	4	40	NR
Strabismus	5	20	NR
Seizures	6	59	25
Scoliosis	4	25	11
Walking	1	61	13
Gait apraxia	1	45	13
Vasomotor instability	6	22	7
Trunk ataxia	6	NR	34
Hypotonia in infancy	7	NR	NR

*Results are numbers of patients with feature. NR, not reported.
(Courtesy of Moeschler JB, Charman CE, Berg SZ, et al: *Pediatrics* 82:1–10, July 1988.)

▶ Rett syndrome is one of the most common degenerative neurologic diseases in female children. This review is one of several that have emerged in the literature over the past several years. Neurologists are now recognizing the syndrome during its emerging stages because of the stereotyped syndrome. The outer limits of the spectrum have not been fully defined. One should carefully review the histories of adolescent and young adult females with apparent chronic encephalopathies. Many with diagnoses of severe mental retardation, autism, or cerebral palsy in fact have Rett syndrome. The diagnosis can often be made retrospectively with documentation of the typical progression of the disease. Old photographs can be particularly helpful.—O.B. Evans, M.D.

Intramuscular Ceftriaxone Versus Ampicillin-Chloramphenicol in Childhood Bacterial Meningitis
Girgis NI, Abu El Ella AH, Farid Z, Haberberger RL, Galal FS, Woody JN (US Naval Med Research Unit No 3; Abbassia Fever Hosp, Cairo)
Scand J Infect Dis 20:613–617, 1988   5–8

The treatment of bacterial meningitis has been complicated by the emergence of *Streptococcus pneumoniae* strains resistant to penicillin or chloramphenicol or both, of *Haemophilus influenzae* resistant to ampicillin or chloramphenicol or both, and of *Neisseria meningitidis* resistant to penicillin. The search for alternative antimicrobial drugs remains a priority. A randomized controlled study was done to compare the efficacy, safety, and tolerability of ceftriaxone given intramuscularly daily with that of ampicillin plus chloramphenicol given intramuscularly every 6 hours in the treatment of bacterial meningitis in children.

Seventy children aged 4 months to 12 years were treated. Each treatment group consisted of 35 patients. Both groups were comparable in age, sex, duration of illness, and state of consciousness. Twenty-nine children given ceftriaxone and 26 given ampicillin plus chloramphenicol recovered without permanent complications or sequelae. Fifteen children died, 10 of whom were in deep coma when treatment was begun. Three of these children had been given ceftriaxone, and 7, ampicillin plus chloramphenicol.

Ceftriaxone given intramuscularly once a day was much easier to administer. It was as effective as the combination of ampicillin and chloramphenicol in this series. This treatment would be most appropriate for use during epidemics in developing countries, where medical facilities are usually limited. The single intramuscular dose facilitates nursing care and is cost-effective.

▶ Intramuscular and even oral administration of antibiotics for the treatment of meningitis has been used in situations in which the intravenous route is difficult to maintain. Certainly the costs are much reduced by these routes. Along similar lines, reducing the treatment to 7 days instead of the recommended 10–14 days has also been explored.

One must interpret data from these studies carefully. In this study, the age range was skewed toward older children and the causative bacteria reflected this. Only 16 of the 70 patients had *H. influenzae* meningitis, which is much lower than the incidence in the United States. The mortality in this group was 44%, which is higher than expected. Although the numbers were small, intramuscular antibiotic administration for the treatment of meningitis in infants and those with *H. influenzae* meningitis may not be appropriate.—O.B. Evans, M.D.

The Effects of Physical Therapy on Cerebral Palsy: A Controlled Trial in Infants With Spastic Diplegia

Palmer FB, Shapiro BK, Wachtel RC, Allen MC, Hiller JE, Harryman SE, Mosher BS, Meinert CL, Capute AJ (Kennedy Inst for Handicapped Children; Johns Hopkins Univ, Baltimore)
N Engl J Med 318:803–808, Mar 31, 1988   5–9

Physical therapy is a major component of treatment of cerebral palsy, the goal of which is to improve motor development and prevent musculoskeletal complications. To evaluate the effects of physical therapy, 48 infants aged 12 to 19 months with mild to severe spastic diplegia fulfilling the enrollment criteria, were randomly assigned to 2 treatment groups: group A underwent 12 months of physical therapy and group B had 6 months of physical therapy preceded by 6 months of infant stimulation, which included motor, sensory, language, and cognitive activities of increasing developmental complexity. Masked outcome assessment was performed after 6 and 12 months of therapy to evaluate motor quotient, motor ability, and mental quotient.

After 6 months of treatment, infants receiving physical therapy demonstrated no motor, cognitive, or social advantage over infants who received infant stimulation. In fact, the data favored the infants who received infant stimulation. The difference in motor outcome, particularly in walking independently, continued to favor group B 12 months after therapy. There were no significant differences between the groups in the incidence of contractures or the need for bracing or orthopedic surgery. Stepwise multiple regression analysis showed that the motor and mental abilities at the time of enrollment were the most powerful determinants of motor or mental outcome, strongly outweighing any effect of treatment.

The routine use of physical therapy in infants with spastic diplegia offers no short-term advantage over infant stimulation. Because of the small sample size, the data favoring infant stimulation are still preliminary. These findings underscore a fundamental issue in developmental pediatrics and public policy affecting developmentally disabled children: the inclusion of physical therapy as a major component of treatment for cerebral palsy should be examined critically.

▶ This study compares regulation physical therapy with a treatment modality called infant stimulation. Infant stimulation, although sounding complex, is more effective in getting the patient to walk and speeding his mental development. The question is whether this persists or is simply a rapid acceleration that will be equaled by the physical therapy group sometime in the future.

6 Headache and Pain

Treatment of Migraine
Wilkinson M (City of London Migraine Clinic, London)
Headache 28:659–661, November 1988   6–1

Most migraine victims know what can bring on attacks. Stress, whether emotional or physical, is a significant precipitating factor. Hormonal changes may be important in women, although true menstrual migraine is not frequent. Trigger factors cannot always be avoided. Nonpharmacologic approaches to migraine include relaxation exercises, acupuncture, and biofeedback. These measures may not suffice but may reduce the amount of medication needed.

The author's regimen for symptomatic treatment of migraine incorporates sleep, an antinausea agent, simple analgesics, and in about one third of patients, ergotamine tartrate by inhalation or suppository. Most patients' symptoms are relieved in 3 to 4 hours. Metoclopramide and domperidone are the preferred antinausea drugs because they do not suppress normal gastrointestinal activity. Caffeine should be avoided. Symptoms do not become worse with this regimen.

Prophylaxis is warranted if there are more than two migraine attacks a month. Amitriptyline can be effective in patients who are depressed. Other prophylactic medications include β-blockers, antiserotoninergic drugs, and antihistaminergic medications. Methysergide is effective but has many side effects. Recently, calcium channel blockers have been used to prevent migraine headaches.

▶ An abstract can't properly reflect the good sense Dr. Wilkinson shows in her comments. I particularly like sleep as part of the treatment. But something else has lately come to my attention. Relief of the pain of the migraine is not equal to treatment of the headache. The headache tendency will return and perhaps recur for days if rest and sleep are not available at the beginning of the pain. In other words, when the pain decreases and becomes tolerable, discourage the patient from continuing to work or going back to work without a period of good rest or sleep. Do you agree?

Analgesic Rebound Headache
Rapoport AM (Yale Univ)
Headache 28:662–665, November 1988   6–2

When chronic headache sufferers use analgesics frequently and excessively, head pain may be prolonged and worse. A cycle of increased analgesic consumption and more intense headache can ensue. Most patients are in their 30s or 40s and have a history of mild subacute or chronic muscle-contraction headache. Pain occurs 2 to 4 times a week before overusing analgesics; the headaches last 6 to 24 hours. Patients often take analgesics before getting out of bed in the morning; they may take up to 20 tablets a day. The results of Minnesota Multiphasic Personality Inventory profiles suggest "masked depression." In most patients the symptoms improve after discontinuation of analgesics. With abrupt withdrawal from mixed analgesics, withdrawal symptoms may occur.

If the pain of chronic muscle-contraction headache is central in origin and associated with tolerance and rebound pain, it may be secondary to suppression of a central antinociceptive system, such as the serotoninergic system. Aspirin acts centrally to increase serotonin levels, but increased pain occurs as a paradoxic effect. There may be downregulation of serotonin receptors and a reduction of receptor sites in the brain. Augmenting serotonin by giving 5-hydroxy tryptamine or by blocking presynaptic serotonin uptake with tricyclics increases the pain threshold in conjunction with the enkephalin system.

▶ The author is, in my opinion, pointing out a true phenomenon, and Marcia Wilkinson probably would agree, although Miller Fisher (1) in a following discussion points out that patients regularly taking large amounts of aspirin for arthritis do not experience any rebound effect. Fisher's comments end with a note that endears him to me. He has been "against the existence of muscle contraction headache for at least 25 years." The withdrawal of true analgesics may produce a state of heightened sensitivity to pain, which may explain the patient who seemingly can't stop taking analgesics without constant headaches (or other pain) day in and day out. Knowledge of such a heightened pain period after withdrawal of analgesics is helpful in explaining to the patient what he must go through to reduce both the pain and the pain medications.

Reference

1. Fisher M: *Headache* 28:666, 1988.

Randomized Double-Blind Trial of Intravenous Prochlorperazine for the Treatment of Acute Headache
Jones J, Sklar D, Dougherty J, White W (Butterworth Hosp, Grand Rapids, Mich; Akron Gen Med Ctr, Akron, Ohio; Timken Mercy Hosp, Canton, Ohio; Univ of New Mexico Hosp, Albuquerque)
JAMA 261:1174–1176, Feb 24, 1989   6–3

Prochlorperazine, a phenothiazine that does not pose a substantial risk for orthostatic hypotension, was evaluated in 82 adults with severe vascular or tension-type cephalalgia. Elderly patients and those receiving phenothiazines were excluded from the study, as were pregnant women. An intravenous injection of prochlorperazine, 10 mg, or saline was given to participants.

Headache was totally relieved within 1 hour of prochlorperazine injection in 74% of patients and another 14% had partial relief. Forty-five percent of placebo recipients had some degree of pain relief. The difference was significant and remained so after adjusting for age, sex, and headache type and duration. Accompanying nausea and vomiting also responded to prochlorperazine injection. Drowsiness was the most frequently experienced side effect. Only 1 patient had orthostatic hypotension, and none had an extrapyramidal reaction.

In patients with acute vascular or tension headaches, intravenous prochlorperazine is appropriate treatment when medications taken orally have failed and there are no contraindications to phenothiazine therapy. If pain persists, dihydroergotamine or a narcotic analgesic may be given intravenously.

▶ Well, chlorpromazine was reported several years ago to be similarly effective in the emergency room for the relief of severe headache, and later studies did not confirm it. However, see the next abstract.

Comparative Efficacy of Chlorpromazine and Meperidine With Dimenhydrinate in Migraine Headache

Lane PL, McLellan BA, Baggoley CJ (Univ of Toronto)
Ann Emerg Med 18:360–365, April 1989   6–4

Migraine headache affects approximately 20% of the population. Many patients have "fixed" migraines that are refractory to oral medications. These patients often become addicted to narcotics. Because an earlier preliminary study of intravenous (IV) chlorpromazine showed promising results, a double-blind, controlled study was conducted to compare IV chlorpromazine against IV meperidine with dimenhydrinate in providing pain relief to patients who go to an emergency department for treatment of fixed migraine.

The study population consisted of 46 patients of whom 22 were randomly assigned to IV meperidine with dimenhydrinate and 24 were assigned to IV chlorpromazine. The chlorpromazine-treated patients were given a bolus injection of 5 ml of normal saline placebo followed by 0.04 ml/kg of chlorpromazine solution at a dose of 0.1 mg/kg. The others were given a bolus injection of a 5-ml solution containing 25 mg of dimenhydrinate, followed by 0.04 ml/kg of meperidine at a dose of 0.4 mg/kg. Drug administration was repeated in the same dosage every 15 minutes as needed, up to a total of 3 doses. Pain, blood pressure, and adverse effects were assessed at 15, 30, and 45 minutes after drug administration. Pain was assessed by visual and verbal analogue scales.

Two of the 24 chlorpromazine-treated patients and 11 of the 22 meperidine plus dimenhydrinate-treated patients experienced inadequate relief and required other medications. In addition, patients in the chlorpromazine group showed significantly better changes in both the visual and verbal analogue scales. The incidence of minor side effects was acceptable.

The IV chlorpromazine appears to offer effective relief in the treatment of fixed migraine headache while avoiding the potential for narcotic abuse and addiction

▶ Here is a recent study again showing chlorpromazine to be better than the usual emergency room treatment of headaches. It looks as though the day is approaching when narcotics will not be used in the emergency room treatment of migraine.

Possible Benefit of GR43175, A Novel 5-HT₁-Like Receptor Agonist, for the Acute Treatment of Severe Migraine
Doenicke A, Brand J, Perrin VL (Ludwig-Maximilians Univ, Munich; Migraine Clinic, Koenigstein, West Germany; Glaxo Group Research Ltd, Greenford, England)
Lancet 1:1309–1311, June 11, 1988   6–5

GR43175 is a 5-HT₁-like receptor agonist with a short, selective vasoconstrictor effect on the arteriovenous anastomoses of the carotid arterial bed in animals. The pathogenesis of migraine might involve the opening of arteriovenous anastomoses in the carotid circulation. GR43175 is being investigated as a potential antimigraine agent, and the first clinical experience using the intravenous form to treat acute attacks was described.

GR43175 was used to treat 46 attacks of severe migraine in 34 patients. The highest dose given—2 mg infused over 10 minutes in 24 severe attacks—resulted in rapid and complete relief of symptoms in 17 (71%) attacks, and in improvement to a nonmigrainous residual headache in 7 attacks (Fig 6–1). Treatment was judged to be well tolerated. The only adverse effects were transient feelings of heaviness and pressure, mostly in the head, but they were mild and short-lived and stopped when infusion was completed.

It was concluded that GR43175 may be an important advance in the treatment of acute migraine. In this initial clinical trial, GR43175 given intravenously relieved all symptoms without affecting heart rate, blood pressure, or electrocardiogram results.

▶ This paper came across my desk at the same time as one entitled "Induction of Migrainelike Headaches by the Serotonin Agonist m-chlorophenylpiperazine" by Brewerton and associates (1). I was curious as to how a 5-HT₁ agonist could both cause and cure migraine. These are not the same drugs, but both are 5-HT₁ agonists. The intravenous administration of 2 mg of GR43175 over a 10-minute period partially or completely eliminated severe migraine headaches in all subjects. No delayed aftereffects were noted. The other drug, m-chlorophenylpiperazine, caused headaches 4–12 hours after administration by which time approximately 90% of the drug had been cleared from the plasma so the synapses were in a depleted condition relative to 5-HTP₁. The patients were given it for treatment of eating disorders; the headache occurrence was unexpected. On questioning those (28 of 52 subjects) who had the

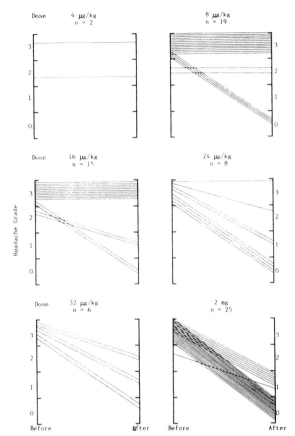

Fig 6–1.—Severity of migraine headache before and after GR43175C. n = number of attacks. Each *line* refers to an attack. Some attacks were treated with more than 1 dose of GR43175C. (Courtesy of Doenicke A, Brand J, Perrin VL: *Lancet* 1:1309–1311, June 11, 1988.)

delayed headache, 90% had a history of severe or migraine headaches. So this apparent contradiction is just that: apparent. The 2 findings are not opposed.

Recently Lance (2) has given us his summary of "50 years of migraine research." He thinks that serotonin is involved in the headache pathway as an intermediate or perhaps final link or both in a chain that starts with the cerebral cortex or hypothalmus, goes to the raphe nuclei and locus ceruleus, and then down the brain stem to eventually influence the cortical microcirculation.

Raskin (3) is of a similar mind and comments that "the only unitary concept thus far put forth regarding the mode of action of the drugs effective in migraine proposes that enhancement of serotonergic neurotransmission is common to them through a variety of mechanisms."

As you know, serotonin is also currently held to be the chief neurotransmitter involved in depression and its therapy. How can this be? Are patients with migraine depressed? Does migraine cause depression or do both result from a common origin? Merikangas and co-workers (4) find a significant association between migraine and depression in families. They conclude that both are strongly familial but that "depression may either be a sequela of migraine or the diathesis which results in both migraine and depression."

The August 1988 issue of *The Journal of Clinical Psychiatry* (vol 49) is devoted to a symposium report of an analysis of serotonin in behavioral disorders and attempts to acquaint the audience with a new serotonin uptake blocker. Can a low serotonin level be responsible for both migraine and depression? Possibly so. I certainly am depressed with a migraine and sometimes high without one. But it must be of a different degree and with a different periodicity in the 2 disorders.

References

1. Brewerton et al: *Clin Pharmacol Ther* 43:605−609, 1988.
2. Lance: *Aust NZ J Med* 18:311−317, 1988.
3. Raskin: *Headache* 28:254−257, 1988.
4. Merikangas et al: *J Psychiatr Res* 22:119−129, 1988.

Plasma Serotonin in Patients With Chronic Tension Headaches
Anthony M, Lance JW (Univ of New South Wales, Sydney, Australia)
J Neurol Neurosurg Psychiatry 52:182−184, February 1989   6−6

Tension headache occasionally has migrainous features, and in some patients evidence of vasodilatation is seen. Because low platelet serotonin levels have been reported in tension headache, the level of platelet serotonin was estimated in 95 patients with chronic tension headache (CTH), 166 with migraine, and 35 normal controls. Analgesia was discontinued for a week before blood was sampled.

The mean plasma serotonin level in patients with CTH was significantly lower than in normal persons and headache-free migraine patients (Fig 6−2). The difference between CTH patients and those with active migraine was not significant.

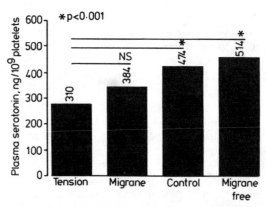

Fig 6−2.—Plasma serotonin in tension headache (statistical comparison between groups). (Courtesy of Anthony M, Lance JW: *J Neurol Neurosurg Psychiatry* 52:182−184, February 1989.)

Chronic tension headache, like migraine, may be a low-serotonin syndrome. In migraine the low platelet serotonin concentration probably reflects reduced levels in other body tissues including the brain stem. Chronic tension headache may reside at 1 end of a spectrum of idiopathic headache, whereas the symptom complex known as migraine may be at the other end.

▶ This is a report of the authors' work over a period of several years in their Sydney headache clinic. Evidently, serotonin levels go below control levels during active migraine, and tension headache patients have even lower levels. The tension headache group had daily headaches, which is a bit peculiar in my experience. Most patients with tension headaches not on medications probably do not have daily headaches. At any rate we wish the authors continued success in their research into this biochemical abnormality and applaud their placing of tension headache and migraine headache on the same spectrum. The world still needs a descriptive term for tension headaches that does not include the word *tension.*

Just yesterday in *U.S.A. Today* (1) there was a note of a deficiency of suppressor T cells in headache patients: headaches may be associated with a dysimmune state, which would not be too surprising. Last, Edmeads has given us a gem on migraine (2). Copies to all the trainees.

References

1. *USA Today* p 1A, May 31, 1989.
2. Edmeads: *Postgrad Med* 85:121–134, 1989.

Headache as a Risk Factor in Atherosclerosis-Related Diseases
Couch JR, Hassanein RS (Southern Illinois Univ, Springfield; Kansas Univ, Kansas City)
Headache 29:49–54, January 1989   6–7

Several previous studies suggested a relationship between migraine and vascular disease. This study was done to further investigate this association.

Data were collected from 87 men and 263 women with migraine and from 104 men and 196 women without migraine who served as controls. All study participants were questioned about the occurrence of atherosclerosis-related disease, diabetes mellitus (DM), hypertension, myocardial infarction, stroke, and recurrent severe headache (RSHA) in their parents. The parents' age was recorded as age at the time of the survey or age at the time of death.

There was no significant difference between the incidence of myocardial infarction, DM, and hypertension among parents of migraine patients and among parents of controls. The data indicated that the presence of migraine in a child was not associated with any increased risk of vascular disease in the parent. After the parents were pooled and resegregated as to the occurrence of RSHA, migraine parents and control parents within the RSHA or no-RSHA groups were compared as to the occurrence of each vascular condition.

For mothers, there was an increased occurrence of stroke and DM in the RSHA group, but the differences were not significant. For fathers, there was an increased incidence of myocardial infarction and hypertension in the RSHA group that was statistically significant. Atherosclerosis-related disease occurred more often in RSHA than in no-RSHA parents. For men, the increase occurred at all ages, but for women, the difference was significant only among women younger than 60 years. These findings suggest that the presence of RSHA may be associated with an increased risk of 1 or more atherosclerosis-related conditions, including stroke, myocardial infarction, DM, or hypertension.

▶ Yes, migraine is a vascular disease and somehow related to hypertension, but is it a predictor?

Treatment of a Cluster Headache Patient in a Hyperbaric Chamber

Weiss LD, Ramasastry SS, Eidelman BH (Univ of Pittsburgh)
Headache 29:109–110, February 1989   6–8

Administration of oxygen effectively relieves the symptoms of refractory cluster headaches. A patient with severe cluster headaches who was treated in a hyperbaric chamber is described.

Woman, 49, had a 26-year history of cluster headaches. At presentation, she had been suffering for 2.5 months from debilitating right-sided retro-orbital headaches that occurred 3 to 5 times per week. Most of her headaches lasted 1 to 4 hours. She had previously undergone arterial embolization, microvascular decompression of the V nerve, and local nerve blocks to relieve the pain. Oxygen therapy by nasal cannula at varying flow rates had also been unsuccessful.

When the patient next presented with a typical headache and nasal congestion, she was placed in a hyperbaric chamber where the oxygen pressure was gradually increased to 2 atmospheres-absolute (ATA) over a 15-minute period. Her pain and congestion completely resolved within 5 minutes after reaching 2 ATA. She was not treated with any analgesics after exiting the hyperbaric chamber and returned to the emergency department 2.5 hours later with a rebound cluster headache that required parenteral narcotic administration. Three days later, she had another typical cluster headache and was given a second hyperbaric oxygen treatment that again promptly relieved her pain. After the second hyperbaric oxygen treatment, the patient did not have a rebound headache and her cluster seemed to have been broken, as she had no other cluster headaches during the next 7 months.

Because the efficacy of 100% oxygen therapy delivered by conventional means in the treatment of cluster headaches has already been confirmed, the efficacy of hyperbaric oxygen therapy should be tested in a prospective trial.

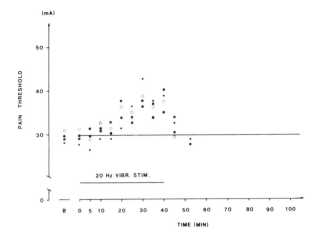

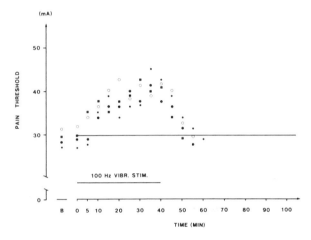

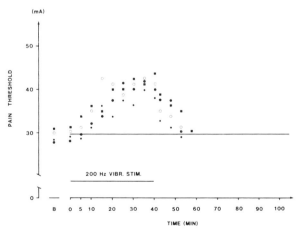

Fig 6–3.—Effects of vibratory stimulation at 20 Hz, 100 Hz, and 200 Hz, respectively, on muscle pain threshold in 4 controls. The duration and frequency of the vibratory stimulation *(VIBR. STIM.)* is indicated by the *horizontal bar*. The pain thresholds are expressed in (mA). The *horizontal line* represents the unconditioned mean value (mA) of the controls. (Courtesy of Lundeberg T, Abrahamsson P, Bondesson L, et al: *Scand J Rehab Med* 20:149–159, 1988.)

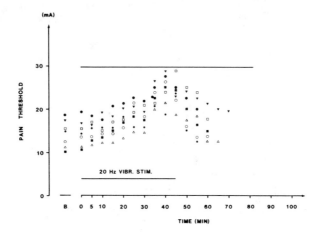

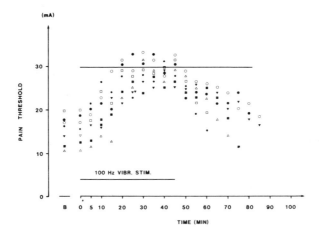

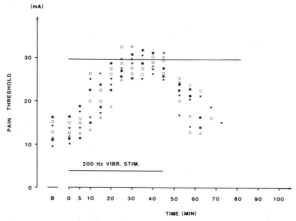

Fig 6–4.—Effects of vibratory stimulation at 20 Hz, 100 Hz, and 200 Hz, respectively, on muscle pain threshold in 7 patients with epicondylalgia. The duration and frequency of the vibratory stimulation *(VIBR. STIM.)* is indicated by the *lower horizontal bar.* The pain thresholds are expressed in (mA). The *upper horizontal line* represents the unconditioned mean value (mA) of the controls. (Courtesy of Lundeberg T, Abrahamsson P, Bondesson L, et al: *Scand J Rehab Med* 20:149–159, 1988.)

% PAIN ALLEVIATION

INDUCTION TIME FOR

MAXIMAL PAIN ALLEVIATION

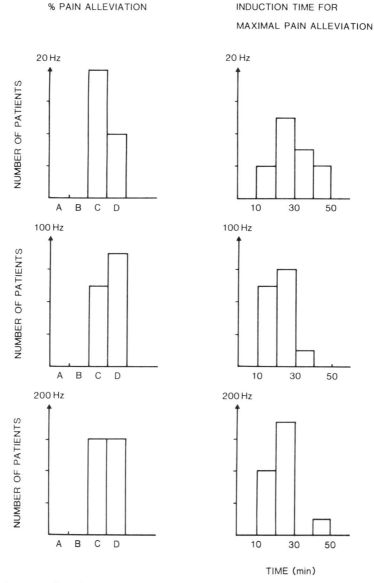

Fig 6–5.—Effect of vibratory stimulation at 20 Hz, 100 Hz, and 200 Hz, respectively, on general subjective pain and induction time for maximal pain alleviation. *A,* pain increase; *B,* no change in pain intensity; *C,* pain alleviation 50% or less; *D,* pain alleviation 51% to 100%. (Courtesy of Lundeberg T, Abrahamsson P, Bondesson L, et al: *Scand J Rehab Med* 20:149–159, 1988.)

▶ This is a nice trick if you happen to have a chamber handy when your patient is having a cluster headache. But what does it tell us about the etiology of cluster headaches? Anything? Is the improvement caused by the production of vasoconstriction?

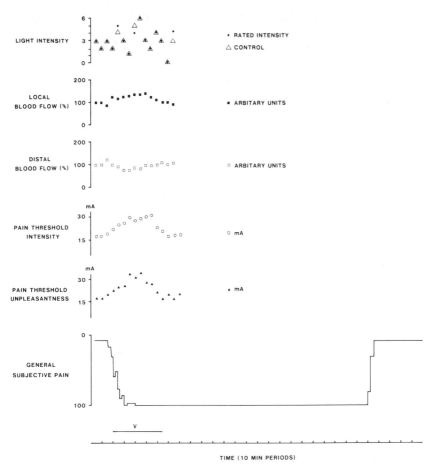

Fig 6–6.—Effect of vibratory stimulation on general subjective pain, pain thresholds, peripheral blood flow, and visual discrimination ability as recorded from a patient. (Courtesy of Lundeberg T, Abrahamsson P, Bondesson L, et al: *Scand J Rehab Med* 20:149–159, 1988.)

Effect of Vibratory Stimulation on Experimental and Clinical Pain

Lundeberg T, Abrahamsson P, Bondesson L, Haker E (Karolinska Inst, Stockholm)

Scand J Rehab Med 20:149–159, 1988   6–9

There is evidence that vibratory stimulation can alter pain thresholds and relieve pain of varying origin. Pain thresholds in skin overlying the extensor carpi radialis longus muscle were measured before and after electrical vibratory stimulation of both healthy persons and patients with epicondylalgia. Eight of the 18 patients had worked with vibrating tools. Pain had been present for 6–14 months and reportedly was relieved by a trial of vibratory stimulation. Sinusoidal mechanical vibration was delivered using an electromechanical vibrator at frequencies of 20, 100, or 200 Hz.

In patients, the experimental pain threshold was lower over the painful muscle than that on the same side in healthy controls. Pain thresholds increased with vibratory stimulation both in healthy persons (Fig 6–3) and in patients with pain (Fig 6–4). The mean duration of pain relief was 4 hours (Fig 6–5). Local blood flow increased with the pain threshold (Fig 6–6). The time course of pain thresholds was not correlated closely with clinical pain relief.

Activation of low-threshold mechanoreceptors by vibratory stimulation may reflect an action at the segmental level in the dorsal horn of the spinal cord. Changes in both pain threshold and peripheral blood flow may result from spinal reflexes, and subjective pain relief results from cognitive changes.

▶ This phenomenon is interesting and probably true. Vibratory stimulation changes pain threshold and relieves pain to a degree. Although the threshold change lasts less than an hour, the pain relief may last for 1 to 7 hours. It looks as though a frequency of 100 Hz is the most effective. A vibrator should certainly be cheaper than a TENS unit and possibly is as effective and not nearly as addicting as narcotics.

7 Degenerative and Genetic Diseases

Localization of an Ataxia-Telangiectasia Gene to Chromosome 11q22-23
Gatti RA, Berkel I, Boder E, Braedt G, Charmley P, Concannon P, Ersoy F, Foroud T, Jaspers NGJ, Lange K, Lathrop GM, Leppert M, Nakamura Y, O'Connell P, Paterson M, Salser W, Sanal O, Silver J, Sparkes RS, Susi E, Weeks DE, Wei S, White R, Yoder F (Univ of California, Los Angeles; Children's Med Ctr, Tulsa, Okla; Virginia Mason Research Ctr, Seattle; Hacettepe Univ, Ankara, Turkey; Erasmus Univ, Rotterdam, The Netherlands; et al)
Nature 336:577–580, Dec 8, 1988   7–1

Ataxia-telangiectasia (AT) is associated with nonrandom chromosomal rearrangements in lymphocytes. A DNA processing or repair protein is suspected to underlie the disparate features of AT. As many as one in five women with breast cancer may carry the AT gene. Cells from heterozygotes are more sensitive than normal to ionizing radiation.

The authors undertook a genetic linkage analysis of 31 families having AT-affected members. A gene for AT was localized in chromosomal region 11q22-23. Because there are at least 4 clinically indistinguishable complementation groups of persons affected by AT, an Amish pedigree was used to screen 171 genetic markers. The highest lod scores were attained when complementation group assignments were disregarded and all families were analyzed.

Reliable genetic markers for identifying AT carriers will permit genetic counseling of families and help elucidate the role of AT gene carriage in cancer.

▶ John F. Jackson, M.D., Professor and Chairman, Department of Preventive Medicine, University of Mississippi Medical Center, Jackson, comments.

▶ A gene for ataxia-telangiectasia has been localized to the distal long arm of chromosome 11 by demonstration of linkage to restriction-fragment length polymorphic markers. The marker THY1 has a likelihood of linkage greater than 2,000 to 1 (lod 4.34) at a recombination frequency of 0.10, and the apparently even closer marker pYNB3.12 has odds of linkage greater than 380,000 to 1 (lod 5.58) at 0.08 recombination frequency. Gene marker studies should allow identification of AT carriers and insight into the contribution of the AT gene(s) to cancer, breast cancer especially, and to associated Purkinje cell degeneration, immunodeficiency, and radiosensitivity.—J.F. Jackson, M.D.

Neurofibrillary Tangles and Senile Plaques in Aged Bears

Cork LC, Powers RE, Selkoe DJ, Davies P, Geyer JJ, Price DL (Johns Hopkins Univ; Harvard Univ; Albert Einstein College of Medicine, New York)
J Neuropathol Exp Neurol 47:629–641, November 1988   7–2

In aged persons and in those with age-associated degenerative disorders, particularly Alzheimer's disease, neurons develop cytoskeletal abnormalities, such as neurofibrillary tangles and senile plaques. Senile plaques occur in several nonhuman species, but neurofibrillary tangles have not been identified in other mammals. A study was done to investigate neurofibrillary tangles and senile plaques in aged bears.

Five bears aged 20–30 years were studied within 1–12 hours after death. Cytoskeletal abnormalities similar to those occurring in humans were found. An aged Asiatic brown bear had neurofibrillary tangles, composed of straight 10–16 cm filaments, that were immunoreactive with antibodies directed against phosphorylated epitopes of neurofilaments; tau; A68; and an antigen associated with paired helical filaments. An aged polar bear was found to have numerous senile plaques; neurites of these plaques were immunoreactive with antibodies against phosphorylated epitopes of neurofilaments, but neurofibrillary tangles were not detected (Fig 7–1).

Nonprimate species have age-related cytoskeletal abnormalities similar to those occurring in humans. Studies of the comparative pathology of aged mammals may be useful in determining the pathogeneses of these anomalies.

► That neurofibrillary tangles and senile plaques can develop in bears and other mammals, monkeys and dogs, is of interest. Behavioral information, available

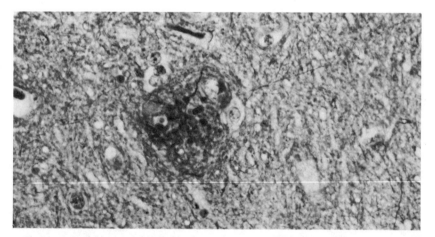

Fig 7–1.—Cerebral cortex of aged polar bear contained numerous senile plaques with argyrophilic neurites that were immunoreactive with antibodies against phosphorylated epitopes of neurofilaments. (Original magnification, ×400.) (Courtesy of Cork LC, Powers RE, Selkoe DJ, et al: *J Neuropathol Exp Neurol* 47:629–641, November 1988.)

for only 1 of the 5 bears was consistent with dementia. It makes one consider the proposed aluminum etiology of Alzheimer's disease in a different light. Of course the bears, monkeys, and dogs in question may have been eating from aluminum dishes, and in the case of zoo animals their food also may have been prepared in aluminum pots and pans. Who knows? On the other hand it would seem likely that, even so, their exposure to aluminum would be less than that of humans. The aluminum-brain relationship is reviewed by Birchall and Chappel (1).

In a nice hypothesis entitled "Brain Evolution and Alzheimer's Disease" (2), Rapoport states that the higher cortex of the human brain may have evolved too rapidly. This rapid evolution may have produced a genomic weakness of the rapidly evolved and added areas, and such a weakness causes a vulnerability to degenerative diseases. This explanation must confront the fact that senile plaques and presumably dementia also occur in dogs. Perhaps dog brains are also considered highly evolved.

In a review of risk factors (3), Henderson concludes that those relating to the activity of free oxygen radicals may be real. These include late age, family history of Down's syndrome, vascular dementia, head injury, exposure to some organic solvents and phenacetin, and vibrating tools.

Finally, a strange note by Manuelidis and associates (4) is intriguing and takes us back to consideration of infectious agents. The authors took blood from 11 first-degree relatives of Alzheimer's patients (2 of whom actually later had Alzheimer's) and injected it intracerebrally into hamsters. In 5 cases a spongiform encephalopathy resulted, and in 3 of the 5 a second passage showed the same alterations. I am resistant to the notion that Alzheimer's disease is a communicable form of spongiform encephalopathy, but I can't throw it out. Nor can we throw out the aluminum theory about the bear evidence.

References

1. Birchall, Chappel: *Lancet* 2:1008–1010, Oct 29, 1988.
2. Rapoport: *Rev Neurol [Paris]* 144:79–90, 1988.
3. Henderson: *Acta Psychiatr Scand* 78:257–275, 1988.
4. Manuelidis et al: *Proc Natl Acad Sci USA* 85:4898–4901, July 1988.

Novel Precursor of Alzheimer's Disease Amyloid Protein Shows Protease Inhibitory Activity
Kitaguchi N, Takahashi Y, Tokushima Y, Shiojiri S, Ito H (Asahi Chemical Industry Co Ltd, Shizuoka, Japan)
Nature 331:530–532, Feb 11, 1988   7–3

In Alzheimer's disease there are cerebral deposits of amyloid β-protein (AP) in the form of senile plaque core and vascular amyloid. A complementary DNA encoding a precursor of this protein (APP) has been cloned from human brain. A cDNA identical to that reported, as well as a new cDNA containing a 225-nucleotide insert, has been isolated from a complementary DNA (cDNA) library of a human glioblastoma cell line. The sequence of amino acids at the N-terminal of the protein deduced from this insert is highly homologous with the basic trypsin inhibitor family.

A lysate of COS-1 cells transfected with the longer APP cDNA showed increased inhibition of trypsin activity. Partial sequencing of the genomic DNA encoding APP showed the 225 nucleotides to be located in 2 exons. Analysis of human brain showed at least 3 messenger RNA species, apparently transcribed from a single APP gene by alternative splicing. Protease inhibition by the longer APP could be related to abnormal APP catabolism.

The new species of APP cDNA could be helpful in studying the pathogenesis of Alzheimer's disease and Down's syndrome.

▶ I am told this is hot news. Accepting my informant's (Arnold Koeppen) word for it, I also admit the article is nearly impossible to understand. Evidently this protein could function as a trypsin inhibitor and thus lead to the formation of amyloid. Simultaneously, Abraham, Selkoe, and Potter (1) report the finding of the serine protease inhibitor α-antichymotrypsin in the brain amyloid deposits of Alzheimer's disease, in an article easier to comprehend. The findings support each other. Perhaps it is too much to hope for, but one wonders whether the answer to Alzheimer's is closer than we think.

Reference

1. Abraham, Selkoe, Potter: *Cell* 52:487–501, February 1988.

Mapping of Mutation Causing Friedreich's Ataxia to Human Chromosome 9
Chamberlain S, Shaw J, Rowland A, Wallis J, South S, Nakamura Y, von Gabain A, Farrall M, Williamson R (Univ of London; Univ of Utah; Karolinska Institutet, Stockholm)
Nature 334:248–250, July 21, 1988   7–4

Friedreich's ataxia is an autosomal recessive disorder characterized by progressive degeneration of the central and peripheral nervous systems. Molecular genetic linkage studies have been done to determine the chromosomal site of the mutation, as a first step in isolating and characterizing the defective gene. The biochemical abnormality underlying Friedreich's ataxia is unknown. The incidence is about 1 in 50,000.

Analysis of 22 families having 3 or more affected siblings had led to assignment of the gene mutation to chromosome 9p22-CEN, through genetic linkage to an anonymous DNA marker MCT112 and an interferon-β gene probe. Interferon-β, MCT112, and Friedreich's ataxia comprise a linkage group spanning about 10 centimorgans. Despite the observed clinical variation in this disorder, there was no evidence of genetic heterogeneity.

There now is strong evidence favoring a single gene locus for classical Friedreich's ataxia. Analysis of large inbred families may allow homozygosity mapping to be used with other strategies to move from linkage to gene, assuming that the region surrounding the disease locus remains homozygous by descent in affected children of consanguineous marriages.

▶ I had to be told the article on Alzheimer's (Abstract 7–3) was blockbusting, but this one is obviously hot news even to me. This group has localized Friedreich's ataxia to the ninth chromosome. We all hope that the characterization of the abnormality will soon follow. One of the really special things about this study is that it included workers from 2 continents, at least 3 countries, and many laboratories in a cooperative effort. The authors are to be congratulated. Of slightly more than incidental interest is that the apparent clinical heterogeneity of Friedreich's is just that—apparent—because clinically dissimilar cases seem to localize to the same chromosome. Of course there could be a slightly different biochemical abnormality at the same genetic locus, as is the case with other genetic diseases, explaining the apparent differences.

Chronic Progressive Spinobulbar Spasticity: A Rare Form of Primary Lateral Sclerosis
Gastaut JL, Michel B, Figarella-Branger D, Somma-Mauvais H (Hôpital Ste Marguerite, Marseilles, France)
Arch Neurol 45:509–513, May 1988   7–5

Most agree that primary lateral sclerosis (PLS), though rare, exists as a form of degenerative disease. Either an isolated spasmodic paraplegia or tetraplegia, or spasmodic tetraplegia associated with a pseudobulbar syndrome, may be observed. The authors encountered 5 cases of chronic progressive spinobulbar spasticity, a subtype of PLS.

Woman, 53, had severe paralytic dysarthria at age 25 years, followed by difficulty chewing and moderate disability in all extremities. Movements became rigid, and the facies, fixed. Median facial reflexes were pronounced. A diffuse upper motor neuron syndrome developed, with bilateral Babinski and Hoffmann signs, but there was no motor deficiency; only very complex movements were impaired. No muscle atrophy or sensory disorder was present, and intellect was normal. Spontaneous electromyographic activity was absent at rest; readings during contraction were normal. A computed tomographic study showed moderate diffuse atrophy. Magnetic resonance imaging showed no abnormality at the brain stem or spinal cord levels.

Primary lateral sclerosis exists in 2 forms, 1 paraplegic or tetraplegic and the other chronic progressive spinobulbar. It is a difficult diagnosis in cases of isolated paraplegia or tetraplegia, but it is appropriate where there is bilateral spinobulbar spasticity, especially if long-term. Primary lateral sclerosis is distinct from the other 2 degenerative disorders involving principal motor pathways, amyotrophic lateral sclerosis, and spinal amyotrophy. Amyotrophic lateral sclerosis involves both central and peripheral neurons, whereas spinal amyotrophy involves only peripheral neurons and PLS involves only central motor neurons.

▶ How did the authors find 5 cases of the very rare chronic progressive spino-bulbar spasticity? If I hadn't seen a case myself, I wouldn't have believed it existed. When the patient comes in, one does all the known tests and finds nothing other than the very gradual progression of spinobulbar symptoms. One might expect some thinning of the midbrain on MRI scanning; our single case showed it, but the authors found none in their 5.

The existence of this rare subtype of primary lateral sclerosis does not seem to be in doubt.

Posterior Cortical Atrophy
Benson DF, Davis RJ, Snyder BD (Univ of California, Los Angeles; West Los Angeles VA Med Ctr; St Paul-Ramsey Med Ctr, St Paul)
Arch Neurol 45:789–793, July 1988   7–6

Some patients with dementia exhibit early visual dysfunction, but retain visual acuity and visual fields until late in the course. Five such patients were studied for this report. Alexia, agraphia, visual agnosia, and components of Balint's, Gerstmann's, and transcortical aphosia syndromes eventually developed in all of these patients.

Causes for the dementia were not known. Primary motor and sensory modalities, including visual fields, were intact. Patients underwent a blood cell count; liver, thyroid, and renal function tests; determinations of glucose, serum calcium, and phosphorus levels; and evaluations of sedimentation rate and folate and vitamin B_{12} levels. Urine samples were

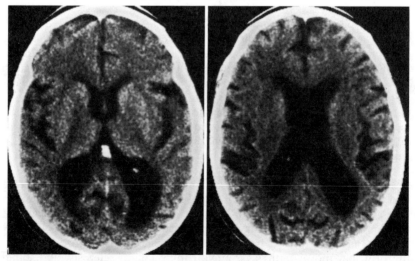

Fig 7–2.—Computed tomographic scan demonstrating striking enlargement of occipital horns bilaterally. (Courtesy of Benson DF, Davis RJ, Snyder BD: *Arch Neurol* 45:789–793, July 1988.)

evaluated for the levels of heavy metals and other toxic substances. All patients also underwent lumbar punctures, electroencephalography, computed tomography, and magnetic resonance imaging, and 3 also underwent angiography. Neuropsychologic tests were administered to the 3 patients who could be tested. Computed tomography and magnetic resonance imaging demonstrated predominant and parieto-occipital atrophy in 2 patients (Fig 7–2). Posterior circulation was normal in the 3 patients studied with angiography.

No pathologic specimens were available for study, but possible underlying pathology includes an atypical variant of Alzheimer's disease, a lobar atrophy similar to Pick's disease, or some previously undiscovered condition. Whatever the pathology, it seems likely that all the persons studied had the same disorder.

▶ This is another one of those lobar atrophies of unknown cause that are being reported. Three of the 5 were angiographically normal, and no pathology is available. The authors consider a localized vascular syndrome of a peculiar progressive nature among the possible causes but a focal progressive dementia similar to Alzheimer's or Pick's diseases is also possible.

A Cohort Study of Amyotrophic Lateral Sclerosis and Parkinsonism-Dementia on Guam and Rota
Reed D, Labarthe D, Chen KM, Stallones R (Natl Heart, Lung, and Blood Inst, Honolulu; Univ of Texas, Houston; Natl Inst of Neurologic and Communicative Disorders and Stroke Research Ctr, Agana, Guam)
Am J Epidemiol 125:92–100, January 1987   7–7

A 15-year prospective study of the incidence of new cases of amyotrophic lateral sclerosis (ALS) and parkinsonism-dementia was conducted by follow-up of 899 Chamorros on Guam and Rota in the Mariana Islands who were examined at baseline in 1968. The study persons initially were aged 20 years and older. At baseline the prevalence of ALS was 130/100,000 on Guam and 324/100,000 on Rota.

During the follow-up interval, 28 new neurologically confirmed cases were reported; 23 patients had parkinsonism-dementia, and 5 had ALS. The only baseline variable associated with an increased risk of parkinsonism-dementia was a preference for traditional Chamorro food.

These findings are consistent with the declining occurrence of ALS in the Marianas, but parkinsonism-dementia continues to occur at a high rate. It is less likely that a long-term deficiency of calcium underlies both ALS and parkinsonism-dementia. Possibly, there are complex interactions between dosage of an environmental toxin, age at exposure, and the protective effects of a Western diet. It may never be possible to define the causes of the epidemic of neurologic disease occurring in the Marianas.

▶ Parkinsonism dementia is still present in these islands, but ALS has tended to disappear. The mystery surrounding this symptom complex continues.

Prevalence and Natural History of Progressive Supranuclear Palsy

Golbe LI, Davis PH, Schoenberg BS, Duvoisin RC (Univ of Medicine and Dentistry of New Jersey–Robert Wood Johnson Med School, New Brunswick; Natl Insts of Neurological and Communicative Disorders and Stroke, Bethesda)
Neurology 38:1031–1034, July 1988　　　　　　　　　　　　　　7–8

Progressive supranuclear palsy (PSP), which is rare and difficult to diagnose, has its onset in late middle age. As in Parkinson's disease, bradykinesia and rigidity are characteristic. Unlike Parkinson's disease, however, PSP usually includes a severely affected gait, supranuclear gaze palsy, and pseudobulbar signs as prominent and early symptoms. Progressive supranuclear palsy is characterized by dementia, emotional incontinence, axial extensor dystonia, poor response to levodopa, and a more rapid course than Parkinson's disease. Because this disorder is often misdiagnosed, its true prevalence is not known. The prevalence of PSP and the sex ratio was determined in 2 counties in central New Jersey.

Neurologists and chronic care facilities were surveyed in and near the 2 counties, which had a combined population of 799,022. Information on patients with PSP was elicited. All of those suspected of having the disorder were examined personally using strict criteria. The prevalence ratio was 1.39/100,000. Data on 50 patients were analyzed.

Median intervals to onset of requiring gait assistance was 3.1 years; visual symptoms became severe within 3.9 years; dysarthria developed within 3.4 years, and dysphagia in 4.4 years; after 8 years a wheelchair was required, and death occurred 9.7 years after onset of symptoms. The prevalence difference between genders was not significant (male to female ratio, 1.2:1). As physicians become better acquainted with PSP, the prevalence ratio may increase.

▶ This is the largest prevalence study of this disorder of which I am aware. Progressive supranuclear palsy is not as rare as we thought several years ago. The length of life from onset, 10 years, is surprisingly long.

Dyssynergia Cerebellaris Myoclonica (Ramsay Hunt Syndrome): A Condition Unrelated to Mitochondrial Encephalomyopathies

Tassinari CA, Michelucci R, Genton P, Pellissier JF, Roger J (Univ of Bologna, Italy; School of Medicine, Marseille, France)
J Neurol Neurosurg Psychiatry 52:262–265, February 1989　　　　　7–9

Dyssynergia cerebellaris myoclonica (DCM), or Ramsay Hunt Syndrome, is a rare disorder of action or intention myoclonus with cerebellar signs and epilepsy. The most frequent pathologic change is olivodentatorubral degeneration. The findings in 13 cases of DCM in 8 males and 5 females aged 13–48 years were reviewed. Five patients had affected siblings, and the parents of 6 patients were consanguineous.

The mean age at onset of illness was 10.5 years. Seizures were the initial feature in 10 patients and action myoclonus in 2. Ultimately, 12 pa-

Clinical and EEG Features of DCM and Myoclonic
Epilepsy With Ragged Red Fibers (MERRF)

	DCM*	MERRF†
No of patients:	13	26
Age at onset (years)		
Range	6–15	2–42
Mean	10·4	14·7
Inheritance:		
Autosomal dominant or maternal	−	+ +
Autosomal recessive	+ +	+
Isolated cases	+ +	+
Myoclonus	+ + +	+ + +
Cerebellar syndrome	+ +	+ + +
Seizures	+ + +	+ +
Pes cavus	+	+
Dementia	−	+ +
Deafness	−	+ +
Muscle weakness	−	+ +
Muscle atrophy	−	+ +
Optic atrophy	−	+
Retinitis pigmentosa	−	+
Short stature	−	+
Pyramidal signs	−	+
Increased blood lactate and pyruvate	−	+ +
Muscle with ragged red fibres	−	+ + +
CT:		
Cerebral and cerebellar atrophy	+	+ +
Calcifications	−	+
Waking EEG		
Slow background activity	+	+ +
Spontaneous generalised fast spike-		
and-wave discharges	+ + +	+
Slow diffuse activity	−	+
Photosensitivity	+ +	+

*Cases from present series.
†Cases from literature review.
Key: + + + = always present; + + = very frequently present; + = present in some cases; − = not present (not observed in cases reported to date).
(Courtesy of Tassinari CA, Michelucci R, Genton P: *J Neurol Neurosurg Psychiatry* 52:262–265, February 1989.)

tients experienced clonic and 11, myoclonic, seizures. Eleven patients had a mild cerebellar syndrome. At the time of study, an average of 17 years after the onset of DCM, 1 patient was bedridden and 5 required help with daily activities. Results of muscle biopsies showed no morphological or histochemical abnormalities, and computed tomography scans generally were negative.

The DCM condition differs in several respects from myoclonic epilepsy with ragged red fibers (table). The spectrum of progressive myoclonic epilepsy includes these and many other metabolic and genetic disorders. Ramsay Hunt syndrome is unrelated to the mitochondrial encephalomyopathies, although some presumed instances of DCM without pathologic confirmation may actually represent mitochondrial myopathy.

▶ The title makes the point that there are patients with action myoclonus, epileptic seizures, and a mild cerebellar syndrome who do not have mitochondrial encephalomyopathy. A recent issue of the journal *Movement Disorders* (vol. 4, no. 1, 1989) carries the same argument to greater lengths. The contest is between Marsden and Obeso representing Queen Square and Pamplona on 1 side and F. Andermann, Berkovic, Carpenter, and E. Andermann representing the Montreal Neurologic Institute on the other with the bout summed up by Anita Harding of Queen Square. Part of the discussion concerns nomenclature: does using the term *Ramsay Hunt syndrome* improve or worsen the situation? But there's more to it. I suppose the question resolves to whether, if Baltic myoclonus, Unverricht's disease, Lafora body disease, and mitochondrial myopathy are all eliminated, there are still patients left who have the classic triad of the Ramsay Hunt syndrome. The present authors say there are. Sacquegna and colleagues agree with them, presenting 2 additional cases (1). Harding suggests that we use the term *myoclonic-ataxic syndrome* as a substitute for *Ramsay Hunt syndrome* but believes it won't catch on. She is probably right.

Reference

1. Sacquegna et al: *Ital J Neurol Sci* 10:73–75, 1989.

Long-Term Coenzyme Q$_{10}$ Therapy for a Mitochondrial Encephalomyopathy With Cytochrome *c* Oxidase Deficiency: A ^{31}P NMR Study
Nishikawa Y, Takahashi M, Yorifuji S, Nakamura Y, Ueno S, Tarui S, Kozuka T, Nishimura T (Osaka Univ; Natl Cardiovascular Ctr, Osaka, Japan)
Neurology 39:399–403, March 1989   7–10

A patient with mitochondrial encephalomyopathy and cytochrome *c* oxidase deficiency was given coenzyme Q$_{10}$ (CoQ) for 2 years. The results were monitored with bicycle exercise testing, ^{31}P nuclear magnetic resonance spectroscopy, and somatosensory-evoked potential measurements.

Man, 43, had had eyelid droop and visual problems since age 15 years and difficulty in swallowing and speaking since age 20 years. Limb muscle weakness developed 9 years later. The clinical findings included bilateral blepharoptosis, complete ophthalmoplegia, and retinal degeneration. There also was facial and oropharyngeal weakness and a sensorineural hearing loss. Moderate muscle atrophy was present, and the tendon reflexes were depressed. Electromyography showed myopathic changes in all limb muscles. Electroencephalography showed scattered slow waves. Mild cortical atrophy was noted on computed tomography. A quadriceps muscle biopsy specimen showed myopathic changes with ragged-red fibers. Enlarged mitochondria with paracrystalline inclusions were seen in the muscle fibers. There was low enzyme activity in the mitochondrial electron transport chain. The CoQ content was 22% of control per mitochondrial protein. Treatment with 150 mg CoQ daily lessened fatigability, but the ophthalmoplegia and lid droop were unchanged. Abnormal metabolic responses to exercise were less evident during treatment. Postexercise recovery of the ratio of muscle phosphocreatine to inorganic phosphate was accelerated. In addition, somatosensory-evoked potential abnormalities resolved during CoQ therapy.

It appears that CoQ is a useful approach to the long-term treatment of mitochondrial encephalomyopathies. The abnormal redox state was normalized in this patient, and somatosensory conduction velocity was increased.

▶ Well, our biochemist is educating me about coenzyme Q_{10}. It does seem to be a necessary coenzyme in mitochondrial function. It can be bought at a reasonable cost in the local health food store. Although one is given a free booklet on its benefits, it is not a popular item. Because Ihara et al. (1) also report successful therapy of this disease with coenzyme Q_{10} and idebenone, the treatment of mitochondrial disease with this substance is crying for a double-blind study. For those of you who wonder what is going on with these disorders of energy metabolism of the nervous system, have a look at the review by Blass, Sheu, and Cedarbaum (2).

References

1. Ihara et al: *J Neurol Sci* 90:263–271, 1989.
2. Blass, Sheu, Cedarbaum: *Rev Neurol (Paris)* 144:543–563, 1988.

Mitochondrial DNA Mutation Associated With Leber's Hereditary Optic Neuropathy
Wallace DC, Singh G, Lott MT, Hodge JA, Schurr TG, Lezza AMS, Elsas LJ II, Nikoskelainen EK (Emory Univ; Turku Univ, Turku, Finland)
Science 242:1427–1430, Dec 9, 1988   7–11

Leber's hereditary optic neuropathy (LHON) is a maternally inherited form of central optic nerve death associated with acute bilateral blindness. Peripapillary microangiopathy and cardiac dysrhythmia also are frequent features. Expression is variable in most pedigrees, but transmission is exclusively maternal. Human mitochondrial DNA is maternally inherited.

A mitochondrial DNA replacement mutation that correlated with LHON in multiple families was identified. The mutation converted a highly conserved arginine to a histidine at codon 340 in the reduced nicotinamide adenine dinucleotide dehydrogenase subunit 4 gene and eliminated an Sfa NI site. Nine of 11 LHON pedigrees lacked the Sfa NI site; all 45 control samples retained this site. There is excellent correlation between LHON and loss of the Sfa NI site between maternal lineages. However, the association of loss of the Sfa NI site with optic atrophy and cardiac dysrhythmia within pedigrees is much less clear.

This mutation may be necessary but not sufficient for overt symptoms of LHON to occur. Additional factors may be involved in expression of the mutant phenotype. If environmental stresses such as smoking are among them, treatments that increase cellular respiratory metabolism might lower the risk of symptoms in family members not yet affected.

▶ It is with wonderment that one looks at the accomplishments of the laboratory in genetic diseases these days. Here is a disease that has been clarified by these scientists. A recent note by Parker, Oley, and Parks (1) finds the biochemical defect in Leber's to be that of mitochondrial electron transport activity (NADH-Q1 oxidoreductase activity). It is inherited through mitochondrial inheritance and thus from the mother (the ovum contains most of the mitochondria) and shows up most often in male offspring. The authors say that what they have found provides "a simple diagnostic test." One suspects that even though this may be simple to them it will not translate into an available test for some time.

Reference

1. Parker, Oley, Parks: *N Engl J Med* 320:1331–1333, 1989.

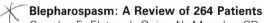

Blepharospasm: A Review of 264 Patients
Grandas F, Elston J, Quinn N, Marsden CD (King's College Hosp; Moorfields Eye Hosp, London)
J Neurol Neurosurg Psychiatry 51:767–772, June 1988   7–12

Blepharospasm—repetitive, involuntary, sustained contractions of orbicularis oculi—is now thought to be a neurologic disease. Possible precipitants and inheritance of the disease, its natural history and chances of remission, and the outcome of various treatments were investigated.

Two hundred sixty-four patients with blepharospasm were studied. Mean age of onset was 55.8 years; a female preponderance of 1.8 : 1 was noted. Dystonia elsewhere was found in 78% of the patients, usually in the cranial-cervical region, and seemed to follow a somatotopic progression. A family history of blepharospasm or dystonia elsewhere was noted in 9.5% of the patients, which suggests a genetic predisposition. Ocular lesions preceded the onset of blepharospasm in 12.1% of the cases.

Response to drug treatment was inconsistent, although initial improvement was observed in one fifth of the patients treated with anticholinergics. Twenty-nine bilateral facial nerve avulsion operations were done with benefit in 27 cases; however, 22 suffered recurrences on average 1 year after surgery. Botulinum toxin injections were used to treat 151 patients. Significant improvement was noted in 118. The mean duration of benefit was 9.2 weeks; the most common side effects were transient ptosis and diplopia.

The cause of bleopharospasm is not known. A minority of patients in this series had a family history of a similar disorder, which suggests a genetic predisposition. Electrophysiologic studies have revealed enlargement and prolongation of the R2 component, with an enhanced recovery cycle of the R2 after paired stimulation. This suggests that the lower brain stem pathways responsible for the blink reflex are intact, but that the interneurons conveying the late R2 component are hyperexcitable or disinhibited.

▶ Blepharospasm is another of neurology's minor but deep mysteries. The authors find it to have sometimes a genetic tendency, an onset after an ocular lesion, and a spread of the movement usually beyond the upper facial nerve area.

This large and careful review will probably stand as a landmark.

A separate analysis (1) gives the neuropathologic findings of 4 patients with cranial dystonias, 3 of whom had blepharospasm. In 1 patient with uncomplicated blepharospasm a small angioma was found in the central tegmental tract of the dorsal pons. In the other 3, however, no abnormality was found in cell populations in the areas of interest (striatum, pallidum, thalamus, and brain stem).

A third contribution (2) from essentially the same group of 22 cases of writer's cramp is also of considerable interest. They examined the patients for anxiety disorder and found no evidence that the disorder was associated with writer's cramp. The patients become anxious because they want to write and can't: the anxiety follows and does not precede the cramp.

References

1. Gibb, Lees, Marsden: *Movement Disorders* 3:211–221, 1988.
2. Harrington et al: *Movement Disorders* 3:195–200, 1988.

Cerebral Cavernous Malformations: Incidence and Familial Occurrence
Rigamonti D, Hadley MN, Drayer BP, Johnson PC, Hoenig-Rigamonti K, Knight JT, Spetzler RF (Barrow Neurological Inst, Phoenix)
N Engl J Med 319:343–347, Aug 11, 1988   7–13

A cavernous malformation, defined as an abnormally enlarged collection of vascular channels without brain parenchyma intervening between sinusoidal vessels, is 1 of 4 commonly occurring types of cerebral vascular malformations. These malformations are rare, and a familial incidence, although uncommon, has been described. Cases of this disorder were studied to characterize its incidence in the general population, to identify familial occurrences, and to determine whether magnetic resonance imaging (MRI) is the radiographic diagnostic technique of choice in detection and follow-up.

Twenty-four patients were investigated. Eleven patients had no evidence of a heritable trait and had a negative family history. Thirteen were members of 6 unrelated Mexican-American families. Sixty-four first-degree and second-degree relatives were assessed. Eighty-three percent of the relatives were asymptomatic; 11% had seizures. Magnetic resonance imaging was done in 16 relatives, 5 of whom were asymptomatic. Fourteen of the studies showed cavernous malformations, and 11 studies identified multiple lesions. Magnetic resonance imaging was found to be far more accurate in detecting cavernous malformations than computed tomography and angiography.

Cavernous malformations are more prevalent than previously reported. A familial form of the disorder is also more common than expected, with a high incidence of multiple lesions and an increased frequency among Mexican-American families. Magnetic resonance imaging is the radiographic technique of choice for detecting and following up these lesions.

▶ The authors have found a higher than expected familial incidence of these abnormalities by studying relatives with MRI scans. This is an interesting finding. Also worth reading is a comment on brain vascular malformations in the same issue.

Reference

1. Stein, Mohr: *N Engl J Med* 319:368–369, Aug 11, 1988.

Diagnosis and Treatment of Presymptomatic Wilson's Disease
Walshe JM (Univ of Cambridge; Addenbrooke's Hosp, Cambridge, England)
Lancet 2:435–437, Aug 20, 1988   7–14

Once Wilson's disease is diagnosed in a family, all close relatives must be screened, and treatment should be offered to those in whom the lesion is detected. Preventive medicine can be practiced in asymptomatic siblings with the disease. Little has been published on the diagnosis or treatment of such patients. Diagnosing presymptomatic Wilson's disease can be very easy or very difficult, as illustrated by an experience with 30 patients seen during a 32-year period.

In 90 families with at least 1 proved case of Wilson's disease, all close relatives were assessed and presymptomatic disease was diagnosed in 30 persons. Eleven had at least 1 abnormal physical sign when examined; 7 of these had Kayser Fleischer rings. In an additional 10 patients, the abnormalities of copper metabolism were so pronounced that there was no doubt about the diagnosis. Six patients were not seen until they had been receiving treatment for 2 or more years; for some, much of the evidence on which the diagnosis was based was unavailable. Three patients had only minor histologic abnormalities in the liver and no increase in urinary copper, but other indices of copper metabolism pointed to a diagnosis of Wilson's disease. Two patients had transient neurologic signs after treatment was initiated. Otherwise, all but 1, who died in an accident, have remained well for up to 26 years.

Considering the fatal outcome of untreated Wilson's disease, there is no case for withholding treatment in those known to have the disease, even if they are asymptomatic. The best policy is to start treatment as soon as the diagnosis is made. A smaller maintenance dose of chelating agent is needed than in symptomatic patients. In this series, all but 2 patients who had transitory symptoms have remained well for 2–27 years.

▶ This is a large series, possibly the largest, of relatives of patients with Wilson's disease found to have presymptomatic Wilson's disease. Half had neurologic signs, but others did not, and only careful testing to differentiate them from heterozygotes showed that they were slated to get the disease. The relatives were treated by Walshe and so far all have remained well for up to 26 years. It is good to be assured that we are doing the right thing in treating these normal-appearing people.

Presymptomatic Neuropsychological Impairment in Huntington's Disease
Jason GW, Pajurkova EM, Suchowersky O, Hewitt J, Hilbert C, Reed J, Hayden MR (Univ of Calgary; Univ of British Columbia)
Arch Neurol 45:769–773, July 1988   7–15

The symptoms of Huntington's disease usually do not appear until midlife, but many studies have suggested that more subtle intellectual changes may occur in some persons at-risk before clinical onset. With recombinant DNA techniques and the identification of closely linked DNA markers, it is now possible in some cases to determine whether at-risk persons have a low (HD−) or high (HD+) risk of having inherited the Huntington's disease gene. A neuropsychologic examination was done to determine whether cognitive changes were present in asymptomatic persons at risk for Huntington's disease.

Ten asymptomatic persons at risk for Huntington's disease were assessed as being at high or low risk with the use of linked DNA probes. Neuropsychologic evaluation, done without knowledge of the results of DNA testing, revealed impairments in 5 of 7 persons in the HD+ group. Abnormalities were related to visuospatial abilities or functions associated with frontal lobes. All 3 subjects in the HD− group displayed no neuropsychologic impairment. Differences between the HD+ and HD− groups were confirmed by statistical analyses. Affected parents of the subjects were at least 12 years older when symptoms began.

Clear neuropsychologic impairment may be present in Huntington's disease even when overt symptoms and signs are not expected for many years. Deficits observed were most notable in 2 areas: visuospatial abilities and functions usually associated with the frontal lobes. General intelligence, verbal memory, and language abilities were not affected.

▶ Most Huntington patients have a relatively long history of minor behavioral abnormalities before the chorea begins. Careful observers in families affected by Huntington's disease can predict with some accuracy who in the family is going to have the disorder. Psychologists are beginning to confirm these hunches by testing persons at risk who can be grouped by linkage analysis into those who will or won't eventually have the disease. Now that we can predict development of the disease, we will await a proper presymptomatic treatment to prevent its manifestations, as Walshe has developed for Wilson's disease (Abstract 7–14).

8 Epilepsy

Anticonvulsant Hypersensitivity Syndrome: In Vitro Assessment of Risk
Shear NH, Spielberg SP, with technical assistance of Cannon M, Miller M
(Hosp for Sick Children, Toronto; Univ of Toronto)
J Clin Invest 82:1826–1832, December 1988   8–1

Hypersensitivity to anticonvulsants is rare but can cause severe morbidity or death. The drugs implicated, including phenytoin, phenobarbital, and carbamazepine, are metabolized to hydroxylated aromatic compounds, suggesting that arene oxides resulting from oxidative metabolism are intermediates in the reaction (Fig 8–1). Arene oxides can bind to cellular macromolecules to disturb cell function and initiate immunologic responses.

Lymphocytes from 53 patients suspected of having hypersensitivity reactions, 49 normal subjects, and 10 patients with seizures without adverse reactions were exposed in vitro to drug metabolites generated by a murine hepatic microsomal system. Seven of 10 patients given all 3 drugs had adverse reactions to each, defined as cytotoxicity 3 SD above the control mean. Forty of 50 patients had positive reactions to all 3 drugs. All the drugs caused an eruption, fever, hepatitis, and hematologic abnor-

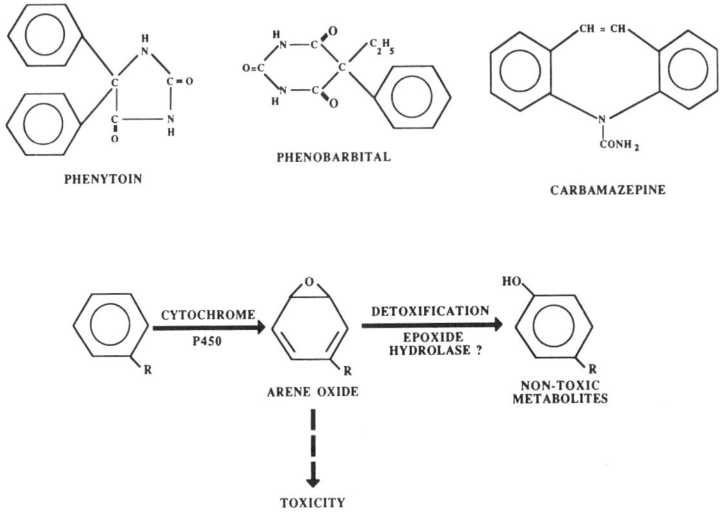

PHENYTOIN   PHENOBARBITAL   CARBAMAZEPINE

Fig 8–1.—Anticonvulsant structures and the proposed metabolic pathway for arene oxide formation. The nontoxic metabolites include parahydroxylated compounds (as shown) as well as other products (e.g., hydroxylated, dihydroxylated, dihydrodiols, and diols). Detoxification is achieved in part spontaneously and in part by epoxide hydrolases. Toxicity is initiated by covalent binding of the reactive metabolites (arene oxides) to cellular macromolecules. The full mechanism of toxicity is unclear. (Courtesy of Shear NH, Spielberg SP: *J Clin Invest* 82:1826–1832, December 1988.)

malities. Cells from the parents of 7 patients had in vitro toxicity intermediate between patient and control values.

The in vitro lymphocyte toxicity assay may aid the diagnosis of adverse anticonvulsant drug reactions. An eventual simpler assay would be a cost-effective means of screening patients who are to receive these drugs.

▶ This is a helpful analysis of patients with clinical sensitivity to these 3 anticonvulsants. The authors point out that the clinical picture is indistinguishable for the 3, all of which have a similar chemical structure. It's likely that, if a patient reacts to 1 of the 3, there may be a reaction to the other 2.

The Lancet (1–2) twice has commented on sodium valproate editorially. The first is a short and inclusive run-through, and concludes that if used as monotherapy in the correct age group its hepatotoxicity is infrequent.

In the second note particular attention is paid to a possible connection of spina bifida to valproate use in pregnant women with epilepsy. The conclusion is that before we accept the connection as valid, more and better studies should be done. But it's enough to make one hesitate when starting a person at risk for pregnancy on the drug.

References

1. *Lancet* 2:1229–1231, Nov 26, 1988.
2. *Lancet* 2:1404–1405, Dec 17, 1988.

Phenytoin-Induced Seizures: A Paradoxical Effect at Toxic Concentrations in Epileptic Patients
Osorio I, Burnstine TH, Remler B, Manon-Espaillat R, Reed RC (Case Western Reserve Univ)
Epilepsia 30:230–234, 1989   8–2

Toxic serum levels of phenytoin have been implicated in worsening of seizures in epileptic patients. This paradoxic effect was examined by reviewing 90 patients seen 96 times in a 6-year period with phenytoin toxicity. They had a serum drug level greater than 20 µg/ml as well as altered consciousness, cerebellar ataxia, dysarthria, or oculomotor abnormality.

Seven patients (7.3%)—all with epilepsy—had seizures when toxic with phenytoin, but in only 2 patients was a causal relationship considered highly probable. In these patients, there was a definite increase in seizure frequency during the period of toxicity. The patients had serum phenytoin concentrations of 93 and 70 µg/ml, respectively. Most epileptic patients with total serum phenytoin levels as high as 85 µg/ml did not have seizures.

Phenytoin in very high concentration will rarely exacerbate seizures or precipitate generalized status in epileptic patients. The true frequency of phenytoin-induced seizures clearly is less than 10%.

▶ Their conclusion is that phenytoin is a very weak convulsant at high concentrations, and we don't really need to worry much about it in normal use.

Alcohol Consumption and Withdrawal in New-Onset Seizures

Ng SKC, Hauser WA, Brust JCM, Susser M (Columbia Univ; Harlem Hosp Center, New York)
N Engl J Med 319:666–673, Sept 15, 1988   8–3

Seizures are thought to result from abrupt withdrawal from alcohol. Little is known about the relation of the duration, magnitude, and type of alcohol use to the risk of incurring seizures. New-onset seizures in a hospitalized population of adults were studied to quantify alcohol as a risk factor and test the withdrawal hypothesis.

Alcohol use before the onset of a first seizure was studied in 308 patients with seizures and 294 controls. The risk of seizures was found to increase with increasing current alcohol use. For seizures occurring without an antecedent event, such as a recent stroke, the adjusted odds ratios increased from threefold at intakes of 51–100 gm of ethanol per day to eightfold at 101–200 gm per day and to almost 20-fold at 201–300 gm per day. For seizures provoked by an antecedent event, the odds ratios were lower and significant only for daily intakes greater than 200 gm. Among ex-drinkers who had abstained for at least 1 year, there was no increased risk. Alcohol withdrawal was not associated with the onset of seizures in this series. Sixteen percent of first seizures among drinkers fell outside the conventionally defined withdrawal period, and the rest showed a seemingly random timing after the last drink.

The relationship of seizures to alcohol use was found to be dose-dependent and apparently causal. Seizures can be interpreted as a disorder induced by the ingestion of alcohol, independently of alcohol withdrawal.

▶ This analysis is credible and threatens one of my time-honored beliefs: that it is the withdrawal from alcohol that causes the seizure and not the steady drinking. Maybe we should reverse our stance of not giving anticonvulsants to alcoholic persons with seizures because they tend to stop taking both the alcohol and the seizure medications at the same time and are therefore in double withdrawal jeopardy. In a discussion in the same issue (1), Simon recommends we differentiate between those in whom seizures occur during withdrawal and those who have seizures while still drinking. So the issue is not settled.

Scheffner and co-workers analyze fatal liver failure in 16 children with valproate therapy in *Epilepsia* (2) and summarize the 100 reported cases worldwide. Ninety percent of the 100 patients were aged less than 20 years, 95% had their first symptoms during the first 6 months of therapy, and 16 were treated with valproic acid alone.

References

1. Simon: *N Engl J Med* 319:715–716, Sept 15, 1988
2. Scheffner et al: *Epilepsia* 29:530–542, 1988.

Electrocerebral Accompaniments of Syncope Associated With Malignant Ventricular Arrhythmias

Aminoff MJ, Scheinman MM, Griffin JC, Herre JM (Univ of California, San Francisco)

Ann Intern Med 108:791–796, June 1988   8–4

Several researchers have made recordings of the electroencephalogram (EEG) and electrocardiogram (ECG) during syncopal episodes. High-voltage delta activity has been reported as one of the most characteristic electrocerebral changes, usually after about 10 seconds from the onset of syncope, and sometimes it is followed by transient electrocerebral silence with subsequent recovery of the EEG. A study was done to examine the electrocerebral and clinical accompaniments of syncope associated with malignant ventricular cardiac arrhythmias.

Fourteen patients with automatic cardioverter defibrillators from previous cardiac arrest or life-threatening cardiac arrhythmia were studied. The intervention involved deliberate induction of cardiac dysrhythmia for routine, postoperative testing of the automatic implantable cardioverter defibrillator. Continuous ECG, EEG, and video recordings were done. Twenty-two episodes of ventricular tachycardia or fibrillation lasting 15–126 seconds were induced, with a definite loss of consciousness in 15 cases and probable loss in 2. In 10 episodes, there were motor accompaniments to the unconsciousness marked by tonic activity or irregular muscle twitching. Patients were usually obtunded or confused up to 30 seconds on regaining consciousness, depending on the duration of induced cardiac dysrhythmia and unconsciousness. Electroencephalographic changes varied. Background slowing was usually followed by a relative loss of electrocerebral activity. In 2 cases, attenuation of background electrocerebral activity followed little or no change in background rhythms. In 5 episodes, EEGs showed no change before loss of consciousness but slowed thereafter in 4 patients.

Conspicuous motor activity may accompany syncope from malignant ventricular arrhythmia and complicate the clinical distinction of syncope from seizures. Postsyncopal confusion was found to last for less than 30 seconds in general. The EEG accompaniments of acute cerebral anoxia resulting in syncope and of the motor accompaniments of syncope are more variable than previously believed, but electrographic seizure activity does not occur.

▶ Aminoff and associates grabbed the chance to study the seizures and EEGs of a group of patients who were purposefully given ventricular arrhythmias to test previously inserted automatic cardioverters. The seizures are different from regular seizures in that the EEG activity is variable, electrographic seizures do not occur, and the postsyncopal confusion lasts for less than 30 seconds.

Functional Hemispherectomy for Treatment of Epilepsy Associated With Hemiplegia: Rationale, Indications, Results, and Comparison With Callosotomy

Tinuper P, Andermann F, Villemure J-G, Rasmussen TB, Quesney LF (McGill Univ, Montreal)
Ann Neurol 24:27–34, July 1988   8–5

Hemispherectomy is effective in arresting seizures that are associated with maximal or almost maximal hemiparesis. However, this procedure has an unacceptable 33% risk of late complications from cerebral hemosiderosis. Anatomically partial but functionally complete hemispherectomy was developed to avoid such complications. The results of the first 14 patients undergoing this procedure with long-term follow-up (4 to 13 years) were reported.

The patients were 5 females and 9 males, aged 3 to 38 years. In the procedure, the frontal or occipital lobes or both were left in place with the blood supply intact, but with connections to commissures and brain stem divided. The parietal and temporal lobes and the central strip were removed. At follow-up examination, 10 patients were free of seizure, 1 had had a single nocturnal seizure, 1 had occasional focal twitching, and 2 had a worthwhile but lesser decrease in the seizure tendency. None of the patients has developed cerebral hemosiderosis to date (Fig 8–2).

In appropriately selected patients, functional hemispherectomy is an effective procedure, preferable to callosotomy or partial hemispherectomy. When there is no independent ictal discharge from the opposite hemi-

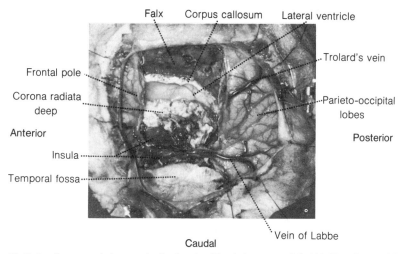

Fig 8–2.—Postremoval photograph after functional hemispherectomy (left side). Note the remaining frontal and parieto-occipital lobes, which have been completely disconnected from the brain stem and corpus callosum, the empty middle fossa (temporal lobectomy), and the resected central region, along with the parasagittal tissue. The corpus callosum is sectioned from the genu to the splenium. The insula is left intact. (Courtesy of Tinuper P, Andermann F, Villemure J-G, et al: *Ann Neurol* 24:27–34, July 1988.)

sphere, arrest of seizures can be expected, resulting in improved cognitive functioning and social behavior and a decrease or discontinuation of anticonvulsant medication. In this series, patients' gait and hand use remained unchanged.

▶ Hemispherectomy has been around for 4 decades but has gone out of fashion, in part because of the long-term cerebral hemosiderosis that results from repeated bleedings from brain movement. Hemosiderosis has a delayed onset with the neurologic deterioration beginning 4–20 years after operation. This group has left the frontal and occipital lobes intact but disconnected from commissures and brain stem and, after following 14 patients for 4–13 years, so far has not seen cerebral hemosiderosis. It looks as though this may be a better way to do the operation.

A supplement to *Epilepsia* (1) carries an update on corpus callosum section by Susan Spencer, a note by Wieser of Zurich on selective amygdalohippocampectomy for temporal lobe epilepsy, and other excellent comments on seizures. It also includes Cesare Lombroso's warm, historical sketch of William G. Lennox.

Reference

1. *Epilepsia* 29(Suppl 2), 1988.

Employers' Attitudes to Epilepsy
John C, McLellan DL (Southampton Univ, Southampton, England)
Br J Ind Med 45:713–715, October 1988   8–6

A person with epilepsy often has trouble getting employment. Studies show that public attitudes toward epilepsy have improved, but finding a job is still hard for 25% to 75% of the 140,000 potential employees with epilepsy in the United Kingdom. A study was done to determine whether there is a relationship between the accuracy of employers' knowledge of epilepsy and the opportunities for employment for people with epilepsy in the Southampton area.

The personnel officer or manager of 52 companies in Southampton were given a questionnaire. Twenty-one of the companies were involved in manufacturing, 2 in heavy engineering, 3 in printing, 7 in retailing, and 6 in transportation. There were 2 dairies, 2 energy boards, 3 educational employers, and 1 bank. The first part of the questionnaire elicited employers' attitudes to a range of illnesses and disabilities, including heart conditions, loss of 1 eye or leg, diabetes, and chronic bronchitis. The second part of the questionnaire elicited knowledge of epilepsy.

Fewer jobs were available for epileptic persons than for people with any of the other disorders. Seventy-two percent of employers said they would not allow an epileptic person to handle machinery, even if he or she had a driver's license. Employers agreed that, compared with other persons with disability, persons with epilepsy would be likely not to take the most time off work. However, 43% of employers erroneously believed that their employers' liability insurance premiums would not cover people with epilepsy, and 17% thought that the Health and Safety at Work Act restricted them from employing persons with epilepsy. Employers tended to underestimate the prevalence of epilepsy and overestimate the frequency of attacks. Unconsciousness was considered an important feature in the condition. Only 50% of employers knew that the accident frequency rate at work for epileptic persons is lower than that for the general population. Fifty-four percent thought epilepsy was associated with lower intelligence, and 6% thought that it was associated with a violent personality. An excessive concern about the medical consequences of epilepsy for the patient was evident.

Employers in the Southampton area are hesitant to hire people with epilepsy. Twenty-five percent stated they had no jobs at all for such people. This was unrelated to the type of employment and related to the size of the company: smaller places were less likely to have jobs for persons with epilepsy. It is easier for people with 1 eye or leg, diabetes, heart disease, or chronic bronchitis to find employment.

▶ Things are improving for epileptic persons seeking work, but there still are attitude problems among employers.

Benign Familial Neonatal Convulsions Linked to Genetic Markers on Chromosome 20

Leppert M, Anderson VE, Quattlebaum T, Stauffer D, O'Connell P, Nakamura Y, Lalouel JM, White R (Univ of Utah; Univ of Minnesota, Minneapolis; Med Univ of South Carolina, Charleston)
Nature 337:647–648, Feb 16, 1989   8–7

A form of epilepsy known as benign familial neonatal convulsions (BFNC) is an incompletely understood disease whose segregation pattern indicates autosomal dominant inheritance with high penetrance. In the expectation that an understanding of molecular basis of BFNC might lead to new therapies, the gene for BFNC was attempted to be localized. A large, 4-generation family, including 19 affected persons, was studied by linkage analysis using the computer program LINKAGE.

Two polymorphic DNA markers on chromosome 20 (CMM6, or D20S19, and RMR6, or D20S20) were tightly linked to the presence of BFNC. Maximum lod scores (log likelihood ratios) were 2.87 and 3.12 for the 2 markers, respectively. Confirmation that these marker loci are on chromosome 20 was achieved by linkage in reference families with another DNA marker, MS1-27 or D20S4, which has been mapped to chromosome 20 using somatic cell hybrids and in situ hybridization.

Mutations at a single locus on chromosome 20 lead to the predisposition, for members of this family, to BFNC. Other families with this clinically heterogeneous disease should be tested for linkage with the same 2 markers to test for genetic heterogeneity. The next step in this research will be the identification of candidate BFNC genes from chromosome 20.

▶ I hope to be alive when the entire genome is finally unraveled. Then the statement that I like to make to students may be confirmed: that there is no disease that does not have some genetic tendency. Of course, there must be many other genes related to the tendency to epilepsy, and when all is said and done, one believes it likely that the majority of the factors leading to epilepsy are genetic.

9 Parkinson's Disease

Parkinson's Disease and Essential Tremor in Families of Patients With Early-Onset Parkinson's Disease
Marttila RJ, Rinne UK (Univ of Turku, Finland)
J Neurol Neurosurg Psychiatry 51:429–431, March 1988   9–1

Whether and to what degree heredity is a factor in Parkinson's disease remains unclear. There incidences of Parkinson's disease and of essential tremor were estimated for the relatives of 52 patients with idiopathic Parkinson's disease beginning before age 45 years. Expected numbers of cases were derived from age- and sex-specific incidence rates in the general population.

The total of person-years observed was 19,093. Three cases of Parkinson's disease occurred among the relatives of index patients: 1 in a parent and 2 in siblings. Essential tremor occurred or had occurred in 10 parents and 3 siblings. Observed rates of Parkinson's disease and essential tremor did not differ significantly from those expected.

These data fail to support either the inheritance of early-onset Parkinson's disease or an association of Parkinson's disease with essential tremor.

► An increased incidence of early onset of Parkinson's disease has been reported in families affected by essential tremor. In this careful study, it appears that essential tremor and early-onset Parkinson's disease have no connection.— R.N. DeJong, M.D.

► Cleeves, Findley, and Koller (1) agree, finding no genetic link between essential tremor and Parkinson's disease in the citizens of London and Chicago. I'm disappointed, believing for decades there was a connection.

Reference

1. Cleeves, Findley, Koller: *Ann Neurol* 24:23–26, 1988.

Parkinsonism Death Rates by Race, Sex, and Geography
Kurtzke JF, Goldberg ID (Georgetown Univ)
Neurology 38:1558–1561, October 1988   9–2

Evidence that Parkinson's disease may be place-related, and thus an environmental disease, has recently emerged in studies comparing Parkinson's disease death rates for whites by U.S. state of residence. A strong north-south gradient, which correlated well with the gradient for multiple sclerosis, has been noted. One researcher raised the question of

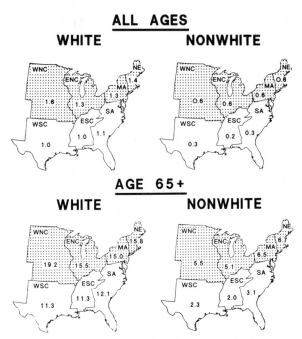

Fig 9–1.—Parkinsonism. Average annual age-adjusted (U.S., 1940) death rates per 100,000 population for all ages, and for age 65+, by color (white and nonwhite), according to residence at death within the eastern 7 of the 9 census regions, U.S., 1959–1961. (Courtesy of Kurtzke JF, Goldberg ID: *Neurology* 38:1558–1561, October 1988.)

whether blacks showed a like geographic gradient. Therefore, Parkinson's disease death rates by sex, race, and geography were explored.

From 1959 to 1961, there were 8,674 deaths in the United States coded to parkinsonism as an underlying cause of death. Of these, 8,439 were of white persons and 235 were of nonwhite persons. Significantly lower Parkinson's disease death rates were found for blacks than for whites. Rates for Oriental Americans were the same as for whites. All racial groups demonstrated a male preponderance. Both whites and blacks had a similar excess of Parkinson's disease death rates among residents of the 4 northern census regions of the United States over their rates for the 3 southern regions (Fig 9–1). In each region, sex and race differences remained the same.

These findings suggest that blacks in the United States appear to be protected against Parkinson's disease, although they share the north-south gradient observed for whites. Thus, race, sex, and geography appear to be independent risk factors for Parkinson's disease, providing further evidence that this may be an acquired, environmental disease.

▶ The search for the cause of parkinsonism becomes ever more interesting. Kurtzke and Goldberg have taken information available to all of us and have found that there are differences in the death rates in the U.S. by race, sex, and geography. A white northern male is more likely to get parkinsonism. The authors believe race, sex, and geography are independent risk factors. In a previous publication (1) Lux and Kurtzke point out the similarity in the north-south gradient of parkinsonism and multiple sclerosis and conclude that it is likely both are environmental illnesses. We could not agree more, but what are the environmental factors?

Teravainen et al. (2) concluded that parkinsonism was apparently coming on at an earlier age in both Helsinki and Vancouver, British Columbia. Rajput et al. (3) studied Parkinson's disease patients with early onset (before the age of 40) and noted that those affected were more likely to have lived in rural rather than urban Saskatchewan. They think that something in the rural environment, possibly well water, is related to the disease (see discussion of ALS in Abstract 10–6 of this issue). Eldridge has suggested that parkinsonism is acquired during intrauterine life. Mattock, Marmot, and Stern (4) have noted that patients with parkinsonism born between 1892 and 1929 have an unusual tendency to occur in clusters, during years close to the influenza pandemics of the same period. This reminds me of the study several years ago from King County, Seattle, that reported the association between the influenza pandemic and the Von Economo encephalitis pandemics of 1918–1925.

Mattock, Marmot, and Stern wonder whether "intrauterine influenza may be cytotoxic to the developing fetal substantia nigra" and consider that "an affected individual may be born without evidence of disability but with limited striatal neurochemical reserves and a reduced nigral cell count."

It is known, of course, that toxins can also injure the cells of the substantia nigra and MPTP is the most prominent current candidate. A review by Langston (5) is thought-provoking. Perry, Jones, Hansen, and Wall (6) point out that the only substances found in the human diet that are MPTP analogues are 2-phenylpyridine (2-PP) and 3-phenylpyridine (3-PP), both of them present in tea. They have done us all a real service by exposing black mice to these 2 substances and finding that neither lowered dopamine or its metabolites in the striatum. So, back to the old teapot. Anyway, if tea were the culprit, England should have 10 times more cases of parkinsonism than Germany.

References

1. Lux, Kurtzke: *Neurology* 37:467–471, 1987.
2. Teravainen et al: *Can J Neurol Sci* 13:317–319, 1986.
3. Rajput et al: *Can J Neurol Sci* 13:312–316, 1986.
4. Mattock, Marmot, Stern: *J Neurol Neurosurg Psychiatr* 51:753–756, 1988.
5. Langston: *Eur Neurol* 26(Suppl 1):2–10, 1987.
6. Perry, Jones, Hansen, et al: *J Neurol Sci* 85:309–317, 1988.

No Parkinsonism After Acute Paraquat Poisoning

Zilker T, Fogt F, von Clarmann M (Technischen Universität München, Munich, West Germany)
Klin Wochenschr 66:1138–1141, November 1988   9–3

The phenylpyridine derivatives N-methyl-4-phenyltetrahydropyridine (MPTP) and its metabolite 1-methyl-4-phenylpyridine (MPP+) are highly

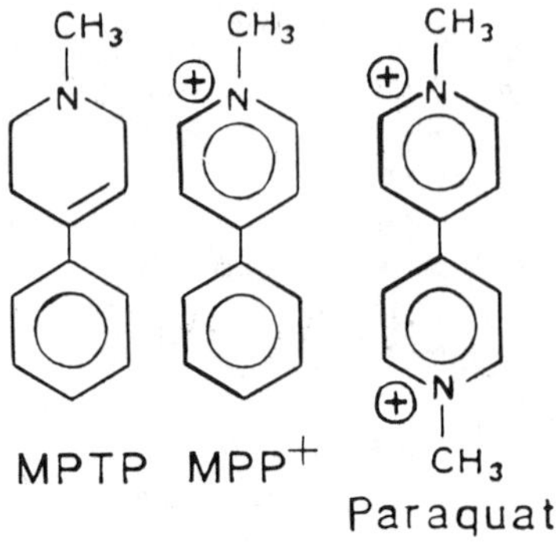

Fig 9–2.—Structural similarity between paraquat and MPTP and MPP+, respectively. (Courtesy of Zilker T, Fogt F, von Clarmann M: *Klin Wochenschr* 66:1138–1141, November 1988.)

neurotoxic chemicals, which cause irreversible parkinsonism in exposed animals and human beings. The herbicide paraquat structurally resembles MPTP and MPP+ (Fig 9–2). Paraquat is extremely toxic. Ingestion of as little as 4 gm of paraquat leads to acute oliguric reversible renal failure, reversible hepatitis, and rapidly progressing irreversible pulmonary failure caused by pulmonary fibrosis, which develops within 1–2 weeks.

Previous investigators suspected a high correlation between the use of herbicides and the occurrence of parkinsonism, which led them to question whether paraquat affects the central nervous system. To address this issue, the records of 32 patients who were treated for paraquat poisoning during a 13-year period were reviewed retrospectively and the survivors were asked to come in for neurologic reevaluation. All 6 patients who had had accidental dermal contact with paraquat survived; 3 came in for reexamination. Only 3 of 19 patients who had deliberately taken paraquat in a suicide attempt survived; all 3 came in for reexamination. Four of 7 patients who had accidentally swallowed paraquat survived, 1 of whom came in for reexamination.

Neurologic reevaluation revealed that none of the 7 patients had any signs of neurologic impairment. Only 1 woman who had survived her suicide attempt and had been treated for 8 years with neuroleptic and antidepressive drugs because of her psychiatric illness had severe tardive dyskinesia, which was attributed to her long-term drug therapy. Survivors of acute paraquat poisoning do not have central nervous system sequelae. Therefore, the observed correlation between exposure to paraquat-containing herbicides and the occurrence of parkinsonism should be considered coincidental.

▶ This pretty much lays to rest the fear that paraquat in our food chain might be responsible for parkinsonism because of its chemical similarity to MPTP and MPP. The authors had followed a large series of patients exposed to paraquat, including 19 who had ingested it in a suicide attempt. Three of them survived and were followed for some years. No parkinsonism appeared in them or in those who had dermal contact in their work.

Case-Control Study of Early Life Dietary Factors in Parkinson's Disease

Golbe LI, Farrell TM, Davis PH (Univ of Medicine and Dentistry of New Jersey, New Brunswick; Louisiana State Univ, Shreveport)
Arch Neurol 45:1350–1353, December 1988   9–4

Some elements of the amyotrophic lateral sclerosis–parkinsonism–dementia complex of Guam are produced in monkeys by giving L-β-methylamino-alanine, derived from the false sago palm. Patients with idiopathic Parkinson's disease (PD) were surveyed to determine preferences for fruits and vegetables eaten raw, because L-β-methylamino-alanine is most abundant in seeds and is heat labile. Same-sex siblings of the patients constituted a control group.

Eighty-one patients with PD participated in the study. No food item was associated with the presence of PD, but preferences for nuts, salad oil or dressing, and plums were associated with the absence of disease (table). These items have a higher vitamin E content than the other 14 items inquired about.

This study fails to support a role for L-β-methylamino-alanine in PD, but it suggests that vitamin E, as an antioxidant, may protect against the disease.

▶ So to prevent the development of parkinsonism we should eat nuts (not peanuts), salad oil made from seeds, and plums; take vitamin E; and smoke. Choosing our ancestors correctly seems to be only minimally beneficial. One

Case-Control Pairs Discordant for Preference (Relative to Spouse) for Various Fruits and Vegetables

	Pt > Sib	Pt < Sib	Odds Ratio	P
Bananas	16	12	1.3	NS
Blueberries	13	21	0.62	NS
Cherries	12	14	0.88	NS
Cucumbers	11	19	0.58	NS
Grapes	7	3	2.3	NS
Melon	5	14	0.36	NS
Mustard	11	20	0.55	NS
Nuts (other than peanuts)	7	18	0.39	<.05
Olives	14	20	0.7	NS
Peaches	7	3	2.3	NS
Pears	7	14	0.5	NS
Pickles	9	19	0.47	NS
Plums	4	17	0.24	<.05
Raisins	12	17	0.24	NS
Salad oil or dressing	8	24	0.33	<.05
Strawberries	5	12	0.42	NS
Tomatoes	19	13	1.46	NS

Abbreviations: Pt > Sib, patient more likely than sibling to eat item; *Pt < Sib,* patient less likely than sibling to eat item; *NS,* not significant. (Courtesy of Golbe LI, Farrell TM, Davis PH: *Arch Neurol* 45:1350–1353, December 1988.)

has the distinct impression that the major factor causing this disease is not genetic, that it must be something in the environment. Its nature is still unknown. It must be discoverable. So to those of you asking questions of patients, a word of encouragement: Keep it up; the answer is still out there somewhere.

Lisuride, a Dopamine Agonist in the Treatment of Early Parkinson's Disease
Rinne UK (Univ of Turku, Finland)
Neurology 39:336–339, March 1989   9–5

Early use of a dopamine agonist in conjunction with levodopa might improve the response in patients with Parkinson's disease. This approach was tested in 90 patients with idiopathic Parkinson's disease, none of whom had received levodopa previously. Patients were randomized to receive levodopa or lisuride alone, or both drugs together, from the outset. If the response to lisuride was inadequate after 3 months, levodopa was added. Lisuride was given in an initial daily dose of 0.05 mg, or 0.025 mg when combined with levodopa, 50 mg.

Lisuride alone was less effective than levodopa during the first 3 months, and only a few patients had definite long-term improvement. Combined treatment was more effective, and adding levodopa to lisuride improved the therapeutic response. Patients given levodopa alone had more fluctuations in disability during 4 years of follow-up. End-of-dose failure was less prevalent when both drugs were used together. Severe nausea sometimes was a problem when lisuride was administered. Four patients were withdrawn from combined treatment because of psychiatric side effects.

Dopamine agonists operate mainly or solely on D-2 dopamine receptors, but stimulation of D-1 receptors as well appears necessary for a good response. Early use of both levodopa and a dopamine agonist allows less levodopa to be used, and this may lower the risk of long-term complications.

▶ The authors conclude that a dopamine agonist such as lisuride with a low dose of levodopa is the proper treatment early in the course of the disease to prevent the later development of end-of-dose failure and dyskinesia.

Practical Application of a Low-Protein Diet for Parkinson's Disease
Riley D, Lang AE (Toronto Western Hosp)
Neurology 38:1026–1031, July 1988   9–6

Levodopa is often given initially with meals to lessen gastrointestinal side effects, but later in the course of treatment, many patients observe deleterious effects on the time to onset of benefit, peak clinical effect, or duration of response when they take this drug close to a meal. Studies have established the utility of protein restriction in stabilizing clinical fluctuations in small numbers of parkinsonian patients on long-term levodopa treatment. The efficacy and practicality of 1 diet in a larger outpatient population with Parkinson's disease (PD) were assessed.

Thirty-eight patients with PD were treated with the protein-restricted diet in addition to their usual drug regimen. The diet involved restriction to no more than 7 gm of protein before the evening meal. This meant that virtually no meat, dairy products, or foods made with flour were permitted. Patients who had previously failed to respond significantly to levodopa did not benefit. Sixty percent of those who experienced fluctuations in response to levodopa improved, obtaining an increase in the ratio of on to off hours. The benefit always occurred within 1 week of initiating the diet. The diet was well tolerated, and there was a low incidence of adverse effects. Side effects that occurred could usually be reversed by reducing levodopa dosages.

This low-protein diet is a simple adjunct to levodopa treatment that can be instituted readily on an outpatient basis. The diet may produce improvement even in patients with fluctuations who have not had optimal benefit from all forms of manipulation of the dosage schedule of levodopa or the addition of newer ancillary agents.

▶ Before the evening meal a limit of 7 gm of protein was allowed. Therefore, breakfast, lunch, and all snacks consisted of soup, fruit, vegetables, sweets, and nondairy liquids. Of their 30 patients, 22 were not resistant to levodopa and 17 of them improved either in an increased on-off time ratio or improved peak motor performance or both.

It would seem worthwhile to try this in those patients with marked on-off difficulty.

Autopsy Findings in a Patient Who Had an Adrenal-to-Brain Transplant for Parkinson's Disease
Peterson DI, Price ML, Small CS (Riverside Gen Hosp, Riverside, Calif; Loma Linda Univ, Loma Linda, Calif)
Neurology 39:235–238, February 1989   9–7

The autopsy findings for a patient given an adrenal-to-brain transplant for Parkinson's disease 4 months before dying were reviewed.

Man, 65, with Parkinson's disease for several years, had responded to carbidopa-levodopa and bromocriptine treatment but was unable to drive, shop, or handle finances. He was disoriented in time but oriented to person and place. Part of the right adrenal gland was transplanted to the right caudate nucleus and putamen. The patient improved for perhaps 2 weeks. Four months postoperatively he was seen in an obtunded state after a seizure, had stuttering speech and Babinski signs, and died in cardiac arrest shortly afterward. Autopsy findings included chronic aspiration that caused mild pneumonia. A piece of orange-yellow

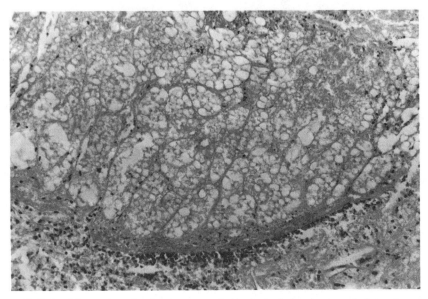

Fig 9–3.—Microscopic section that shows recognizable ghosts of adrenal cortex cells that no longer contain nuclei. There are some inflammatory cells around the transplant and some of these cells have migrated into the transplanted tissue, but no viable adrenal cells are present. The thin layer of glial tissue separates brain tissue and necrotic adrenal tissue. (Hematoxylin-eosin, ×220 before 52% reduction.) (Courtesy of Peterson DI, Price ML, Small CS: *Neurology* 39:235–238, February 1989.)

tissue was seen in the right caudate nucleus, internal capsule, and putamen. Microscopic examination indicated that the entire transplant was necrotic (Fig 9–3), but the graft evidently contained adrenal medullary tissue at the time of transplantation.

Other recipients of adrenal transplants reportedly improved over several weeks to months. However, some trophic factor from injured caudate tissue or altered function of the choroid plexus may have been responsible for the improvement, or surgery may have directly affected the basal ganglia. Much more experience is needed before adrenal transplants can be recommended as an accepted treatment for Parkinson's disease.

▶ This is, to our knowledge, the first report of an autopsy after such a transplant in humans. It appears from this single report that the cautious approach to the results of the transplant surgery for parkinsonism is justified. Allen, Burns, Tulipan, and Parker report their results in 18 transplanted patients. Four of 12 showed improvement 1 year later (1).

Reference

1. Allen, Burns, Tulipan, et al: *Arch Neurol* 46:487–491, May 1989.

Does Cognitive Impairment in Parkinson's Disease Result From Non-Dopaminergic Lesions?

Pillon B, Dubois B, Cusimano G, Bonnet A-M, Lhermitte F, Agid Y (Hôpital de la Salpêtrière, Paris)
J Neurol Neurosurg Psychiatry 52:201–206, February 1989   9–8

It has been proposed that deficient dopaminergic transmission in the central nervous system explains cognitive disorder in Parkinson's disease, but this hypothesis remains controversial. Improvement on levodopa occurs only at early stages of the disease. Parkinsonian motor symptoms in 120 patients were correlated with performance on tests of neuropsychologic function. The patients, all with idiopathic Parkinson's disease, were receiving a mean of 878 mg of levodopa daily and had been treated for about 5 years on the average.

Although memory and intelligence scores were within the means for normal age-matched persons, they were lower than expected from the educational level. All test scores were correlated significantly with the basal motor score. Some of the test scores were correlated with akinesia and rigidity, but none were correlated with tremor. None of the test scores were correlated with the levodopa-responsive motor score, but all were related closely to the residual motor score under levodopa therapy.

Cognitive disturbances in Parkinson's disease appear to be related to nondopaminergic lesions. The lesions responsible for dysarthria and gait impairment may also give rise to cognitive dysfunction. All these features become progressively more difficult to manage as the disease progresses.

▶ This makes good sense. It is believable that the cognitive impairment is not directly related to the dopaminergic dysfunction. It fits with the tendency in therapy for the patient's motor improvement on dopaminergic drugs to occur simultaneously with disimprovement of the mental functioning over time.

10 Neuromuscular Disorders

"Maximal" Thymectomy for Myasthenia Gravis: Results
Jaretzki A III, Penn AS, Younger DS, Wolff M, Olarte MR, Lovelace RE, Rowland LP (Columbia-Presbyterian Med Ctr, New York)
J Thorac Cardiovasc Surg 95:747–757, May 1988   10–1

A combined transcervical-transsternal en bloc thymic resection is based on the wide distribution of thymic tissue in the neck and anterior mediastinum, and on reports of microscopic foci of thymus in pericapsular mediastinal fat. Ninety-five patients having "maximal" thymectomy between 1977 and 1985 were followed up for 6 to 89 months. Seventy-two patients had primary surgery for myastenia gravis without thymoma. Fifteen patients had myasthenia and thymoma, whereas 8 were reoperated on for myasthenia without thymoma.

All but 3 of the 72 patients having primary surgery for myasthenia without thymoma benefited from the operation. No patient was clinically worse, and 46% were in remission without medication at follow-up. The life table remission rate at 89 months was 81%. Two patients with thymoma were in remission, and 9 were free of symptoms on medication. Two of these patients died in crisis 2 and 4 years after operation. All the patients who were reoperated on had residual thymic tissue. None were worse at follow-up, but only 1 patient was in remission. There were no operative or hospital deaths and no phrenic or recurrent nerve injuries, and no patient became hypoparathyroid. Seven major postoperative complications occurred.

Maximal thymectomy is an appropriate operation for patients with generalized myasthenia gravis. The same approach is used at reoperation if severe symptoms persist or recur after primary surgery. Complete removal of coexisting thymic tissue is indicated in the presence of thymoma, with or without myasthenia gravis.

▶ S.H. Subramony, M.D., Associate Professor of Neurology, Department of Neurology, University of Mississippi Medical Center, Jackson, writes the following comment.

▶ This article supports the concept that the more complete the removal of thymic tissue, the better the ultimate result achieved. The reported remission rates for such an aggressive approach to removing thymic tissue are greater than those reported for more classical procedures. However, the surgeons seem divided on the issue of how to achieve such removal, i.e., with "maximal thymectomy" as reported here with an "extended" thymectomy that removes thymic tissue scattered in the mediastinum, or with newer techniques of the transcervical procedure. One has to consider the increased risk of morbidity such as phrenic nerve injury with such an aggressive approach as well.—S.H. Subramony, M.D.

Resistance to Succinylcholine in Myasthenia Gravis: A Dose-Response Study

Eisenkraft JB, Book WJ, Mann SM, Papatestas AE, Hubbard M (Mt Sinai School of Medicine, New York)
Anesthesiology 69:760–763, November 1988   10–2

Some patients with myasthenia gravis appear to be resistant to succinylcholine. Dose-response relations were examined in 5 patients scheduled for thymectomy and in 10 normal persons. Succinylcholine was given in an initial dose of 0.15 mg/kg, followed by incremental boluses of 0.1–0.2 mg/kg and an infusion to replace eliminated drug.

No complications occurred in the patients or normal persons. The dose-response curve for myasthenic patients was to the right of that for normal persons, and the slopes and intercepts of mean dose-response curves differed by group. The ED_{50} and ED_{90} values for succinylcholine also differed significantly. Four of the 5 myasthenic patients had fade in the train-of-4 response, which was never seen in the normal group.

Patients with myasthenia gravis are indeed resistant to succinylcholine. If rapid intubation is necessary, a dose of at least 1.5–2 mg/kg may be required for a rapid onset of good intubating conditions. One possible explanation for this resistance is a decreased number of acetylcholine receptors at the motor end plate.

▶ This is quite a suprise. I had always assumed myasthenic patients were more sensitive to succinylcholine and had tried to forbid its use during thymectomy but had not succeeded. Succinylcholine is apparently safe to use for endotracheal intubation in myasthenia.

The Lambert-Eaton Myasthenic Syndrome: A Review of 50 Cases

O'Neill JH, Murray NMF, Newsom-Davis J (Natl Hosp for Nervous Diseases; Royal Free Hosp, London)
Brain 111:577–596, June 1988   10–3

The Lambert-Eaton myasthenic syndrome (LEMS) is a disorder of neuromuscular transmission, first clinically recognized in association with lung cancer and later in patients in whom no neoplasm could be found. The clinical and electrophysiologic features of 50 patients with LEMS were analyzed.

Among 25 patients with carcinoma, 21 had small cell lung cancer (SCLC), which was evident within 2 years of onset of LEMS symptoms in

20 patients and at 3.8 years in 1 patient (Fig 10–1). Of 25 patients without carcinoma, 14 had histories of LEMS lasting more than 5 years. The dominant neurologic features were similar in both the cancer and non-cancer groups and consisted of proximal lower limb weakness in all patients, depressed tendon reflexes in 92% with posttetanic potentiation in 78%, autonomic features in 74%, and mild to moderate ptosis in 54%. The compound evoked muscle action potential amplitude in the abductor digiti minimi was less than the lower limit of control values in 48 of the patients, and the increment following maximum voluntary contraction was greater than the upper limit of control values in 48. Single fiber electromyographic anomalies were detected in 29 of 29 patients examined. A patient presenting with LEMS has a 62% risk of having an underlying SCLC. This risk drops sharply after 2 years and becomes very low at 4 to 5 years. In SCLC cases antigenic determinants on tumor cells can initiate the autoimmune response, often early in the course of the malignancy, but the association of LEMS with tumors other than SCLC may be fortuitous.

▶ This is a superb analysis of 50 cases of the Lambert-Eaton myasthenic syndrome. The original 100% association with small cell carcinoma of the lung is now down to 62%. Single fiber EMG analysis was positive in 29 of 29 patients in whom it was tried. It is good that progress is being made on this peculiar disorder. I clearly remember seeing a patient with this in 1952 during my internship, before the disease had been described. The patient was an old railroad engineer of whom I had become fond. He had lung cancer, ptosis, gener-

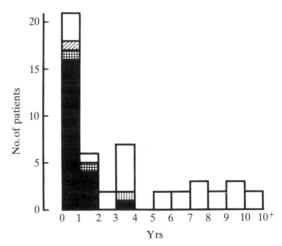

Fig 10–1.—Duration of symptoms of LEMS at time of tumor detection in the patients with detected carcinoma and at final follow-up in patients with no carcinoma detected (NCD). *Solid bars* = small cell lung carcinoma; *vertical hatching* = breast carcinoma; *horizontal and vertical hatching* = thoracic tumor of undetermined histology; *open bars* = NCD patients. Tumor diagnosis preceded symptoms of LEMS by 2 months in the case with adenocarcinoma, but the result has been included in the data for year 1. (Courtesy of O'Neill JH, Murray NMF, Newsom-Davis J: *Brain* 111:577–596, June 1988.)

alized weakness, and dyspnea. One day while struggling to breathe he turned and said, "That was my last breath." He was right.

Characterization of Dystrophin in Muscle-Biopsy Specimens From Patients With Duchenne's or Becker's Muscular Dystrophy
Hoffman EP, Fischbeck KH, Brown RH, Johnson M, Medori R, Loike JD, Harris JB, Waterston R, Brooke M, Specht L, Kupsky W, Chamberlain J, Caskey CT, Shapiro F, Kunkel LM (Harvard Med School; Howard Hughes Med Inst, Boston; Univ of Pennsylvania; Muscular Dystrophy Group Labs, Newcastle-upon-Tyne, England; Washington Univ, St Louis; et al)
N Engl J Med 318:1363–1368, May 26, 1988   10–4

Deficiency of the protein dystrophin is the likely cause of Duchenne's muscular dystrophy. The relationship between clinical phenotype and dystrophin status was studied in muscle biopsies from 103 patients with neuromuscular disorders, including 38 with Duchenne's dystrophy, 7 with intermediate dystrophy, 18 with Becker's dystrophy, and 40 with other disorders.

Thirty-eight of 40 patients with other neuromuscular disorders had normal dystrophin phenotypes. Of 63 patients with a diagnosis of Duchenne's, Becker's, or intermediate dystrophy, 58 had a clearly abnormal dystrophin phenotype. The clinical severity was correlated with the dystrophin assessment. A majority of patients with Duchenne's dystrophy had no detectable dystrophin, whereas most of those with Becker's dystrophy had nearly normal levels of dystrophin of abnormal size.

Assay of dystrophin should prove useful in delineating myopathies that overlap clinically with the Duchenne's and Becker's dystrophies. Detection of qualitative and quantitative changes in the protein should be diagnostically useful.

▶ I had the happy privilege of listening to Dr. Kunkel give part of this spectacular success story at a recent meeting of the American Academy of Neurology.

As I write, the National Telethon is on to raise more money for muscular dystrophy. The effort is still necessary because, although this represents a genuine breakthrough, methods will have to be found to treat the disease, which may take years.

For a short, understandable, and fascinating account, please read Rowland's editorial, "A Triumph of Reverse Genetics and the End of the Beginning," in the same issue (1). It is a superbly written piece by an insider in the world of muscle.

Reference

1. Rowland: *N Engl J Med* 318:1392–1394, May 26, 1988.

Genetic Abnormalities in Duchenne and Becker Dystrophies: Clinical Correlations

Medori R, Brooke MH, Waterston RH (Washington Univ, St Louis)
Neurology 39:461–465, April 1989   10–5

Patients with the allelic Duchenne (DMD) and Becker (BMD) muscular dystrophies show much heterogeneity in their clinical course, making prognosis and evaluation of new therapies difficult. Previous work suggests that this clinical heterogeneity is resulting from molecular heterogeneity at the DMD/BMD locus. To test this hypothesis, 49 patients with muscular dystrophy were analyzed in an attempt to correlate DNA alterations at this locus with the clinical course of the disease. Patients included 32 males with classic DMD, 2 females with DMD, 7 patients with BMD, 4 males with mild DMD, and 2 each normal males and females. Restriction fragments of genomic DNA were probed with 6 different fragments spanning the entire 14-kilobase complementary DNA.

Of the 32 male patients with DMD, 14 had an internal deletion in the center of the gene in exon 7. These 14 had milder clinical manifestations than the other 18 male patients with DMD in whom no deletions were detected. Dystrophin was absent in patients in both of these groups. Of the patients with mild DMD or BMD, 4 showed no deletions. The other 7 had deletions in the 5´ portion of the gene. Three of these 7 patients had dystrophin of a lower than normal molecular weight.

A "hot spot" for deletions occurs in the central portion of the DMD-BMD gene, the only region in which deletions were found among classic male patients with DMD. However, only 14 of 32 of these patients showed deletions. Presumably the others have smaller mutations, which will require more sensitive methods to detect. The presence of 5´-end deletions in patients with BMD and mild DMD implies that dystrophin molecules lacking amino terminal portions may be partially functional. Additional studies with more patients may permit increased predictive value of DNA analysis.

▶ This article, one just following it by Baumbach and co-workers (1), another in the *Lancet* by Norman, Coakley, Thomas, and Harper (2), and the discussion by Fischbeck in *Neurology* (3) leave me nearly totally confused. The only thing that seems still stable is that Becker's dystrophy and Duchenne type dystrophy are separate diseases even though their genetic abnormality is similar, overlapping, and not yet clear. Or are they?

References

1. Baumbach et al: *Neurology* 39:465–474, 1989.
2. Norman, Coakley, Thomas, et al: *Lancet* 1:466–468, March 4, 1989.
3. Fischbeck: *Neurology* 39:584–585, 1989.

Motor Neuron Disease in the Province of Ferrara, Italy, in 1964–1982

Granieri E, Carreras M, Tola R, Paolino E, Tralli G, Eleopra R, Serra G (Univ of Ferrara, Italy)
Neurology 38:1604–1608, October 1988   10–6

Motor neuron disease, an abiotrophic-degenerative disease of adult life and of unknown etiology, involves motor systems of the nervous system. It includes 3 clinical variants: amyotrophic lateral sclerosis, progressive bulbar palsy, and progressive muscular atrophy. A descriptive and analytic study was done to assess the disease's geographic distribution in 1 territory in northern Italy and to explore its association with antecedent events and putative risk factors.

Seventy-two patients were included. The mean incidence per year from 1964 to 1982 was 0.98 cases per 100,000. At the end of 1981, the prevalence rate was 3.95/100,000. In this 19-year study period, the average mortality was 0.83/100,000/year. The disease was more common among men, among persons aged 50 to 70 years, and among residents of rural areas engaged in agricultural work. A retrospective case-control study confirmed the significantly greater frequency of motor neuron disease among farmers and persons living in rural areas and revealed that the disease was more common among lower social classes, to which most unskilled and heavy laborers belong. A significantly increased risk for motor neuron disease was also found among patients with previous histories of trauma, although confounding variables may account for this observed association.

▶ This survey found that ALS is more common among rural agricultural workers, a finding present in our Mississippi analysis of many years ago. This is not true of all studies of ALS, possibly because of the increasing urbanization of the world.

Williams, Floate, and Leicester (1) have analyzed their Australian kindred with motor neuron disease and believe that ALS may be more often familial than previously thought, with its apparent low penetrance a result of late onset. The same could be said for other possibly genetic late-onset diseases such as Alzheimer's. I suspect there is some truth in it.

Martyn, Barker, and Osmond (2) again raise the question of the relationship between poliomyelitis and motor neuron disease. They find a geographic (England) correlation of the notification rates for polio in the 1930s with the occurrence of motor neuron disease during 1968–1978. Polio and later ALS have a correlation coefficient of 0.42, which is higher than any other childhood disease. But a later letter in *The Lancet* (3) by Sood and Nag notes that what may be true in England and Wales is not true in India. India has a high incidence rate of poliomyelitis (70,000 cases every year), but the occurrence of motor neuron disease is the same there as in the rest of the world.

Vaccination for polio has been available for more than 30 years, and while the WHO is considering its total elimination from the western hemisphere, the incidence rate of ALS may be going up.

Of course correlation does not mean causation. One wonders whether the relationship between the 2 is through a common susceptibility rather than one causing the other, a hereditary susceptibility to both.

Reference

1. Williams, Floate, Leicester: *J Neurol Sci* 86:215–230, 1988.
2. Martyn, Barker, Osmond: *Lancet* 1:1319–1321, June 11, 1988.
3. Sood, Nag: *Lancet* 2:393, Aug 13, 1988.

No Association of Amyotrophic Lateral Sclerosis With Cancer

Zisfein J, Caroscio JT (Mt Sinai Med Ctr, New York)
Mt Sinai J Med 55:159–161, March 1988   10–7

Norris and Engel reported cancer in 10% of 130 consecutive patients with amyotrophic lateral sclerosis (ALS). The authors reviewed experience with 347 patients having ALS, followed up for a mean of 2.5 years, in an attempt to confirm this relationship. Twelve patients had cancer or a history of cancer. Five had new cancers diagnosed after the onset of neurologic symptoms. The incidence of new cancers was 0.57%/year compared with a rate of 0.64%/year in subjects aged 55–59 years in the Connecticut Tumor Registry.

The incidence of cancer in patients with ALS does not differ from that in the general population. Cancer screening of newly diagnosed ALS patients, therefore, is unlikely to yield more cases than screening of age-matched persons without ALS.

▶ The authors found no relationship of true ALS to cancer as also did Chio and co-workers (1). This is reassuring because most of us do not go through screening of ALS patients for cancer even though we are aware that the association has been reported.

Reference

1. Chio et al: *J Neurol* 235:374–375, 1988.

Progressive Muscular Atrophy Localized to One Hand: A Monomelic Form of Motorneuron Disease?

Chaine P, Bouche P, Léger JM, Dormont D, Cathala HP (Hôpital de la Salpêtrière, Paris)
Rev Neurol (Paris) 144:759–763, December 1988   10–8

The development of muscular atrophy of 1 hand in the absence of any local cause is generally suspected as being anterior horn cell involvement, because amyotrophic lateral sclerosis (ALS) often starts with unilateral upper extremity muscle symptoms. However, in some patients the condition stabilizes without progressing to more extensive neurologic involvement. This type of isolated ALS usually affects young men. The case reports of 10 young men with unilateral distal ALS limited to an upper extremity are reviewed.

Age at onset ranged from 16 to 27 years. Patients with a prior history of poliomyelitis or other neuromuscular disorders were excluded from the study. None of the patients had a family history of ALS or other neuromuscular disorders. The patients had undergone electromyographic (EMG) and neuroradiologic examinations, including cervical spinal myelography, computed tomography (CT), and magnetic resonance imaging (MRI). Six patients had previously competed in sports. Most had marked muscle atrophy involving the entire hand, similar to that seen in Aran-

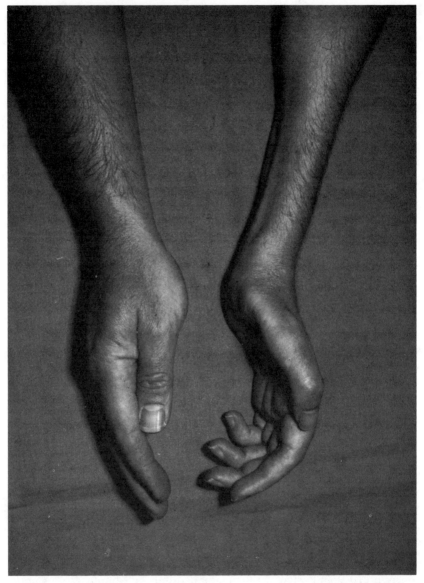

Fig 10−2.—Hands and forearms of patient. (Courtesy of Chaine P, Bouche P, Léger JM, et al: *Rev Neurol (Paris)* 144:759−763, December 1988.)

Duchenne muscular atrophy (Fig 10−2). The muscular deficit involved all the small hand muscles and often the flexors and extensors of the wrist. Eight patients reported increased vasomotor symptoms with exposure to cold.

All patients had normal findings on myelographic and CT examinations. Three of 6 patients who underwent MRI had significant thinning of the cervical spinal cord, which appeared most prominent at C7-C8. However, none had evidence of a central medullary lesion. Seven patients had extensive laboratory work-ups, which generally yielded normal findings except for 4 patients whose muscular enzyme levels were elevated to 1.5 times normal values. Results of viral studies were negative in all cases. Findings of EMG studies were consistent with anterior horn cell involvement. After a follow-up of 1–3 years, the condition has stabilized in 9 of the 10 patients.

The findings for these 10 patients support the data reported by other investigators, which suggest that unilateral isolated ALS of the upper extremity is a distinct monomelic form of motor neuron disease with a benign evolution and prognosis. The differential diagnosis is confirmed in the presence of unilateral, isolated, nonprogressive involvement and definitive stabilization of the condition after 1–3 years of exacerbation.

▶ S.H. Subramony, M.D., Associate Professor of Neurology, Department of Neurology, University of Mississippi Medical Center, Jackson, comments.

▶ This disorder, variously called benign monomelic amyotrophy and juvenile segmental spinal muscular atrophy, is being reported increasingly from different parts of the world. Several cases have been reported from Japan (1), India (2), England (3), and now France. The disease appears characterized by focal wasting of hand and forearm muscles, often sparing the brachioradialis; fasciculations in the involved limbs; cramps; and tremor. The age of onset is typically less than 40 years, and bulbar involvement and definite upper motor neuron involvement are lacking, differentiating it from ALS. Electromyography and MRI scanning of the neck are extremely important diagnostic procedures and are useful in ruling out other lesions such as chronic brachial plexopathies and compressive and cavitary lesions of the spinal cord.

It is not clear from the literature whether the disease remains confined to 1 upper extremity or can be very indolently progressive after an initial period of relatively rapid progression. Thus, in previous reports, the involvement of proximal upper extremity muscles becomes more frequent with longer follow-up. The number of limbs involved has also been correlated with the years of follow-up, and often EMG reveals evidence of disease in asymptomatic contralateral limbs, suggesting that there may be gradual progression.— S.H. Subramony, M.D.

References

1. Sobue et al: *Ann Neurol* 3:429–432, 1978.
2. Singh et al: *Arch Neurol* 37:297–299, 1980.
3. Harding et al: *J Neurol Sci* 59:69–83, 1983.

The Late Sequelae of Poliomyelitis
Howard RS, Wiles CM, Spencer GT (St Thomas' Hosp, London)
Q J Med N Series 251:219–232, March 1988   10–9

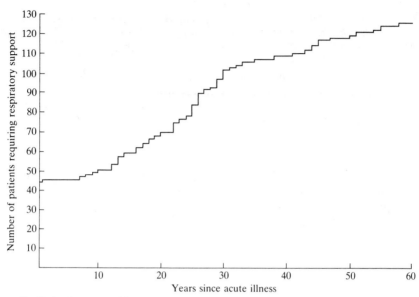

Fig 10–3.—Latent period between the acute illness and the requirement of new respiratory support (43 patients required continuous respiratory support). (Courtesy of Howard RS, Wiles CM, Spencer GT: *Q J Med N Series* 251:219–232, March 1988.)

Patients with histories of poliomyelitis sometimes deteriorate after a prolonged time of stability. Data on 209 patients were reviewed a mean of 34 years after their original illnesses. Many of the patients were referred for respiratory management.

Seventy-eight percent of patients had late functional deterioration, a majority of them because of purely respiratory factors. Twenty patients had new neurologic signs, and 39 deteriorated wholly or partly because of orthopedic problems. A combination of factors was responsible in 31 cases. Respiratory deterioration most often was caused by nocturnal alveolar hypoventilation, sometimes associated with progressive scoliosis. Eighty-six patients required respiratory support a mean of 28.5 years after acute illness (Fig 10–3). No patient had motor neuron disease or postpoliomyelitis muscular atrophy. Fifty patients died, most often of respiratory difficulty.

Late sequelae after poliomyelitis are frequent. Important causes of deterioration may be avoidable or treatable. Patients with chest infection or new respiratory symptoms require careful management because respiratory failure may develop rapidly.

▶ Progressive functional deterioration following poliomyelitis has been reported after a long period of disability. The authors reported that late functional deterioration developed in 78% of the patients they saw. This development was due to purely respiratory factors in 99 cases, new neurologic signs in 20 cases, and orthopedic problems in 17 causes. Thirty-one patients deteriorated because of a combination of factors. This series shows that late sequelae following poliomyelitis are common. The major causes could be avoided, and in particular, those in whom chest infections or new respiratory symptoms develop should be treated with caution as respiratory failure may rapidly supervene.— R.N. DeJong, M.D.

Mortality in Alcoholics With Autonomic Neuropathy

Johnson RH, Robinson BJ (John Radcliffe Hosp, Oxford, England; Wellington School of Medicine, Wellington, New Zealand)
J Neurol Neurosurg Psychiatry 51:476–480, 1988   10–10

Chronic damage to the vagus nerve may be found in alcoholic polyneuropathy. The role of abnormal autonomic function in the prognosis of chronic alcoholism was studied in 79 chronically alcoholic men followed for up to 7 years (mean, 5.5 years). They were aged 52 years, on average, when first evaluated and had abstained from drinking alcohol for a mean of 4 months. Vagal function was assessed by postural change in blood pressure, the Valsalva maneuver, deep breathing, and intravenous atropine injection.

Thirty-two patients had no vagal neuropathy. Twenty-five had 1 abnormal test result, whereas 22 had 2 or more abnormal results of vagal function tests. The groups did not differ in reported alcohol consumption, liver damage, or central or peripheral nerve damage. Survival at 7 years was 91% for patients without vagal neuropathy, 66% for those with 1 abnormal test result, and 79% for those with 2 or more abnormal test results. Deaths from cerebrovascular diseases were more frequent in the total group than expected in a general age-matched population.

Vagal neuropathy in chronically alcoholic men is associated with increased mortality compared with the general population. A majority of deaths in the present series were sudden or unexplained; several were ascribed to stroke. A reduced effective intravascular volume might be a factor in alcoholic men with vagal neuropathy and liver damage. Apnea and hypopnea are more frequent in alcoholics with central nervous system damage and vagal neuropathy.

▶ It's peculiar that vagal neuropathy does not appear to be associated with other central or peripheral neuropathy in alcoholism. It is, however, associated with shorter survival. The authors wonder whether it might in fact be directly related to the earlier death through an effect on the cardiovascular system.— R.N. DeJong, M.D., and R.D. Currier, M.D.

Postmarketing Surveillance for Neurologic Adverse Events Reported After Hepatitis B Vaccination: Experience of the First Three Years

Shaw FE Jr, Graham DJ, Guess HA, Milstien JB, Johnson JM, Schatz GC, Hadler SC, Kuritsky JN, Hiner EE, Bregman DJ, Maynard JE (Ctrs for Disease Control, Atlanta; Food and Drug Administration, Rockville, Md; Merck Sharp and Dohme Research Labs, West Point, Penn)
Am J Epidemiol 127:337–352, February 1988   10–11

The plasma-derived hepatitis B vaccine has been commercially available since June 1982. During the 3 years between its introduction into the market and May 31, 1985, an estimated 850,000 persons were inoculated with the vaccine. Because other viral vaccines have been linked to neurologic illnesses, a study was done to assess the possible relationship between the occurrence of neurologic diseases and hepatitis B vaccination.

During the 3-year study period, 41 patients aged 23 to 66 years reported experiencing neurologic adverse events after hepatitis B vaccination. Five patients had convulsions, 10 had Bell's palsy, 9 had Guillain-Barré syndrome, 5 had radiculopathy, 3 had brachial plexus neuropathy, 5 had optic neuritis, and 4 had transverse myelitis. Twenty-one of the 41 cases occurred after the first vaccine dose, 15 after the second dose, and 5 after the third dose. Seventeen (68%) of 25 patients for whom hospitalization status was listed required hospitalization. None of the patients died. Five patients reported new-onset convulsions after vaccination with hepatitis B vaccine, but 1 patient had a previous history of epilepsy and 1 patient's seizure was associated with alcohol ingestion.

Because all adverse effects were self-reported, validation of the diagnoses proved problematic. Many factors important in judging the results of the study could not be measured. Although Guillain-Barré syndrome was reported significantly more often than expected, no conclusive epidemiologic association could be made between any of the reported neurologic adverse events and the hepatitis B vaccine. However, even if such an association were to be confirmed, the benefits of vaccination in persons at high risk for infection with hepatitis B virus would well outweigh the risk of any neurologic adverse event.

▶ I once talked with a physician, a fellow radio amateur, on the air about his Guillain-Barré syndrome, which he was quite certain was caused by hepatitis B vaccination. Although the association of Guillain-Barré is significant, the authors conclude "no conclusive association can be made between any neurologic adverse event and the vaccine." They further say (and who would disagree?) that even if such an association did exist the preventive benefits of the vaccine in persons at high risk for hepatitis B would unequivocally outweigh the risk of any neurologic adverse event. There were 9 patients with Guillain-Barré syndrome out of 850,000 persons receiving vaccinations.

Prognosis of Acute Polyneuritis Requiring Artificial Ventilation
Krull F, Schuchardt V, Haupt WF, Mewes J (Univ of Cologne; Rheinische Landesklinik, Bonn, West Germany)
Intensive Care Med 14:388–392, 1988   10–12

An estimated 10% to 23% of patients with acute Guillain-Barré syndrome (GBS) require mechanical ventilation for respiratory failure. A decade ago, these patients had a mortality of about 20% to 26%. Fifty-six cases of GBS patients seen during 1970–1983 who required artificial

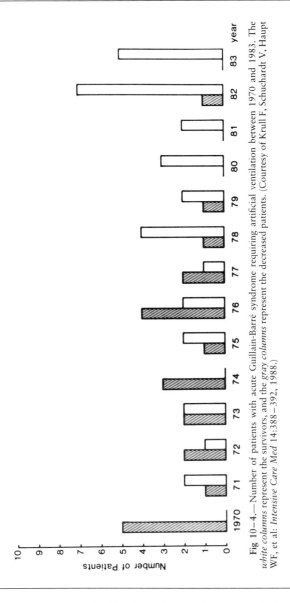

Fig 10–4.—Number of patients with acute Guillain-Barré syndrome requiring artificial ventilation between 1970 and 1983. The *white columns* represent the survivors, and the *gray columns* represent the decreased patients. (Courtesy of Krull F, Schuchardt V, Haupt WF, et al: *Intensive Care Med* 14:388–392, 1988.)

ventilation were reviewed. Indications for intubation included a vital capacity of less than 15 ml/kg and arterial hypoxemia. Early intubation is favored where respiratory function is deteriorating rapidly. Intermittent positive-pressure ventilation is used.

Plasmapheresis and other immunosuppressive measures were not used in these patients. Mortality declined from about 60% in 1970–1978 to less than 10% in 1979–1983. Fewer severe complications occurred in the latter period. The difference in mortality between the 2 periods was significant (Fig 10–4).

Improved supportive care can lower mortality among patients with GBS who require mechanical ventilation. Mortality in such patients has declined substantially during recent years.

▶ I understand A.B. Baker, M.D., was once heard to say that no one with Guillain-Barré syndrome should die, but even in the best of hands the mortality rate is around 5%. Improved ventilatory care as noted in the report is responsible for most of the improvement over the years.

11 Multiple Sclerosis

Multiple Sclerosis in the Faroe Islands: IV. The Lack of a Relationship Between Canine Distemper and the Epidemics of MS
Kurtzke JF, Hyllested K, Arbuckle JD, Bærentsen DJ, Jersild C, Madden DL, Olsen Á, Sever JL (VA Med Ctr, Washington, DC; Georgetown Univ; Roskilde Hosp, Whitinsville MA, Veterinary Office, Tórshavn, Faroe Islands; Aalborg Hosp, Aalborg, Denmark; et al)
Acta Neurol Scand 78:484–500, 1988   11–1

Multiple sclerosis (MS) developed in 32 native residents of the Faroe Islands between 1943 and 1973 in 3 distinct epidemics. The number of patients declined from 20 in the first epidemic to 9 in the second and 3 in the third. Sera were obtained from 12 MS patients and 112 controls to explore the possible relationship between MS and canine distemper (CD). No increase in CD antibody titers was found in the MS group. Only 1 patient reported owning a dog with CD, and the occurrence of CD in different villages did not correlate with the occurrence of MS.

The epidemics of MS in the Faroe Islands was not demonstrably related to the presence of CD or sick dogs.

▶ Kurtzke, Hyllested, and co-workers have very carefully analyzed the question of canine distemper as a cause of multiple sclerosis during the now famous outbreak in the Faroe Islands during the following World War II.

As a matter of interest an entire issue of the journal of *Neuroepidemiology* (vol. 7, no. 4, 1988) is devoted to the question of whether there really was an epidemic of multiple sclerosis in the Faroe Islands. Poser and associates say there was not, and Kurtzke says there was. Geoffrey Dean recommends that the verdict of "unproven" be reached. One thing is certain: never have so many articles owed their genesis to so few cases of any disease.

The Contribution of Mortality Statistics to the Study of Multiple Sclerosis in Australia
Hammond SR, English DR, de Wytt C, Hallpike JF, Millingen KS, Stewart-Wynne EG, McLeod JG, McCall MG (Univ of Sydney; Univ of Tasmania; Greenslopes Repatriation Hosp, Brisbane; Royal Adelaide Hosp, Adelaide; Royal Perth Hosp, Perth, Australia; et al)
J Neurol Neurosurg Psychiatry 52:1–7, 1989   11–2

A strong association between disease frequency and geographic latitude has been shown in prevalence surveys of multiple sclerosis (MS). This association was first demonstrated with the use of mortality statistics. An epidemiologic survey of MS was conducted in 5 areas of different geographic latitude in Australia.

Analysis of MS mortality data for 1971 to 1980 taken from the 5 surveyed areas confirmed the relationship between increasing disease frequency and increasing south latitude. The striking gradient of disease frequency with latitude seems unlikely to be artifactual. A similar association between disease prevalence and mortality data as to frequency variations with latitude has been shown for the United States and New Zealand.

Comparison with mortality data from 1950 to 1959 showed that there had been a substantial fall in MS mortality in 4 of the 5 surveyed areas. The exception was Western Australia, where MS mortality had remained essentially stable.

The data also confirmed an earlier finding that MS mortality among United Kingdom-born migrants dying in Australia was slightly lower than that among the Australian-born population and very much lower than that of the native United Kingdom population. Thus, migration from the United Kingdom to all but the most southern parts of Australia may lower the risk of MS.

Mortality statistics provide a valuable source of support for data obtained from prevalence surveys of MS.

▶ This study tends to show that persons who migrate from a high-risk area to a low-risk area acquire the risk of the low-risk warmer climate area. Viewing Dean's original studies of migration from the United Kingdom to South Africa in the light of present knowledge of multiple sclerosis and its ability to exist quiescently, one would feel that the older migrants may have, in point of fact, had multiple sclerosis at the time of migration even though they were asymptomatic. Those who were younger at migration tended to acquire the risk of the warmer, lower MS prevalence area.

The present study tends to confirm Dean's findings, but the question remains: what is it about the warmer climate that reduces the risk of multiple sclerosis? Are incidental diseases different, is the diet different, are stresses different?

The Prevalence of Multiple Sclerosis in South East Wales
Swingler RJ, Compston DAS (Univ of Wales, Cardiff)
J Neurol Neurosurg Psychiatry 51:1520–1524, December 1988   11–3

A population-based survey of multiple sclerosis (MS) in the county of South Glamorgan, located in southeast Wales, was performed, and findings were compared with those from other epidemiologic surveys in the United Kingdom.

Five sources were used to arrive at a provisional register of identified MS patients. Of 894 patients on the provisional list, 551 (62%) were alive, 251 (28%) had died, and 92 (10%) could not be traced. Of the 551 living patients, 489 resided in South Glamorgan. Of these 489 residents,

441 had definite, probable, or suspected MS. The diagnosis of MS was rejected in the other 48 (9.9%) patients.

The most recent census estimate of the resident population of South Glamorgan county was 376,718. Therefore, the prevalence of MS on January 1, 1985, was estimated at 441 per 376,718, or 117 per 100,000. Of the 441 MS patients, whose ages ranged from 10 to 85 years, 146 were men and 295 were women (Table 1). The mean age at onset of MS was 32.2 years, and MS was diagnosed on average at the age of 36.4

TABLE 1.—Prevalence of Multiple Sclerosis Per 100,000 by Age and Sex in South Glamorgan

Age group (years)	Male No	Rate	Female No	Rate	Total No	Rate
0–14	0	0·0	1	2·6	1	1·3
15–24	3	9·4	18	58·5	21	33·5
25–34	16	59·8	54	204·4	70	131·6
35–44	30	141·9	57	266·0	87	204·4
45–54	40	191·1	60	280·0	100	236·2
55–64	37	179·0	60	264·0	97	223·5
65–74	19	133·0	31	162·0	50	149·9
75 >	0	0·0	12	81·0	12	55·8
Not known	1	—	2	—	3	—
Total	146	79·6	295	150·6	441	117·0

(Courtesy of Swingler RJ, Compston DAS: *J Neurol Neurosurg Psychiatry* 51:1520–1524, December 1988.)

TABLE 2.—Estimated Incidence of Multiple Sclerosis
in South Glamorgan from 1947 to 1984

Year	Number	Population	Incidence ($/10^5/year$)
1947–49	23	351 294	3·3
1950–52	66	351 294	6·3
1953–55	51	351 294	4·8
1956–58	66	380 267	5·8
1959–61	85	380 267	7·5
1962–64	57	380 267	5·0
1965–67	62	390 269	5·3
1968–70	53	390 269	4·5
1971–73	46	390 269	3·9
1974–76	65	390 269	5·6
1977–79	62	384 042	5·4
1980–82	78	384 042	6·8
1983–84	68	384 042	8·9
1947–84	782	390 269	5·4

(Courtesy of Swingler RJ, Compston DAS: *J Neurol Neurosurg Psychiatry* 51:1520–1524, December 1988.)

years. The mean duration of the disease from onset to the prevalence date was 16.5 years. This number may be doubled to estimate the mean duration from onset to death, which would be 33 years.

The average incidence of MS in South Glamorgan county was estimated at 5.41 per 100,000 per year for the period between 1947 and 1984 (Table 2). The estimated average incidence rate has significantly increased over the past 4 decades, but this increase may well result from better methods of ascertainment. The current prevalence is similar to that found in a recent survey from the southeast of England, but significantly lower than the recently revised data on MS prevalence from Aberdeen, Scotland.

▶ This is a reasonable study of a definite population showing that the prevalence rate of multiple sclerosis has risen over the last 40 years. Well, if the prevalence rate is rising and the death rate is decreasing how can that be? Simple: the patients must be living longer, which other studies confirm. Eventually, of course, the incidence rate and the death rate will be equal.

Amplification and Molecular Cloning of HTLV-I Sequences From DNA of Multiple Sclerosis Patients
Reddy EP, Sandberg-Wollheim M, Mettus RV, Ray PE, DeFreitas E, Koprowski H (The Wistar Inst, Philadelphia; Univ of Lund, Sweden)
Science 243:529–533, Jan 27, 1989   11–4

Although no direct correlation has been established between retroviruses and human neurologic disorders, some recent evidence suggests human T-lymphotropic virus type 1 (HTLV-1) involvement. To investigate an association between HTLV-1 and multiple sclerosis (MS), the polymerase chain reaction was used to amplify viral sequences in peripheral blood mononuclear cells from 6 MS patients and 20 healthy controls. The amplified sequences were then cloned and sequenced for identification.

Viral sequences were amplified in all 6 MS patients, and HTLV-1 positive clones were obtained from this material. Sequence determination confirmed the identification. One of the 20 healthy controls also had detectable HTLV-1 material in his sample. Peripheral blood mononuclear cells were cultured from the patients, and both the adherent and the nonadherent cells were separately analyzed for HTLV-1 sequences. Viral material was found primarily in the adherent cells.

These results indicate a possible association between HTLV-1 positive sequences in cells from MS patients and the development of their disease. As the viral sequences were primarily detected in adherent cells, this virus may be an HTLV-1 variant that primarily infects monocytes and macrophages.

▶ This may be an important contribution to the etiology of multiple sclerosis, but questions arise. How were these Swedish patients selected? It is noted that 2 of the 6 had a positive HTLV-1 antibody and 1 had a questionably positive antibody. The chance of this happening in 6 randomly selected MS patients is quite small. All of the patients had moderate mononuclear pleocytosis in the cerebrospinal fluid, which also is unusual. One had an MRI scan that was said to be compatible with MS, but what about the other 5? It would be of interest now to study 6 randomly selected patients with definite MS from the Philadelphia area with negative HTLV-1 titers, normal cerebrospinal fluid cell counts, and classic MRI scans.

Four Formulas for Calculating Cerebrospinal Fluid Immunoglobulin G Abnormalities in Multiple Sclerosis: A Comparison
Goren H, Valenzuela R, Williams GW, Bocci L, Slaughter S (Cleveland Clinic Found)
Cleve Clin J Med 55:433–438, October 1988   11–5

Various formulas have been developed to improve evaluation of cerebrospinal fluid for diagnosis of multiple sclerosis (MS). These include the Tourtellotte formula for measuring central nervous system immunoglobulin G (IgG) synthesis, the Schuller formula for measuring local IgG synthesis, the IgG index, and the IgG-albumin ratio. The predictive values of these measurements in MS were compared. Serum and cerebrospinal fluid IgG was measured by laser immunonephelometry in patients known to have MS, those with probable MS, those with possible MS, patients with other nonneurologic disease, and those with other nonimmunologic neurologic disease.

Results of all 4 formulas showed significantly higher values in the definite multiple sclerosis group than in the other patients, as shown by the Wilcoxon rank-sum test. Tourtellotte's formula was the most sensitive of the formulas, whereas Schuller's formula was only slightly more specific, according to McNemar's test of symmetry. When clinical performance was compared by receiver operating characteristic curves, little difference was noted among the formulas.

It is not yet possible to say which of the formulas is best. The data from this and an earlier study indicate that Schuller's formula, the IgG index, and IgG-albumin ratio are less sensitive than Tourtellotte's formula, but there is little difference among them in regard to specificity.

▶ The authors find that Tourtellotte's formula is possibly the most sensitive and Schuller's the most specific, but there is little difference among the 4. They are all more or less equal. We can apparently rely on whatever formula our laboratory uses.

Benign Versus Chronic Progressive Multiple Sclerosis: Magnetic Resonance Imaging Features
Koopmans RA, Li DKB, Grochowski E, Cutler PJ, Paty DW (Univ of British Columbia, Vancouver)
Ann Neurol 25:74–81, January 1989   11–6

The results of magnetic resonance imaging (MRI) in 32 patients with benign multiple sclerosis (MS) were compared with those in 32 others with the chronic progressive form of MS. The groups were matched for age, sex, and duration of illness. In the latter patients neurologic function had progressively declined over more than 6 months. Patients with benign disease had low disability scores and had been ill for 10 years or longer.

Computer-assisted quantification of MR images indicated a higher mean lesion load in chronic progressive MS than in benign MS patients. About one fifth of patients with benign MS, however, had a lesion load higher than the chronic progressive patients. More infratentorial lesions were found in chronic progressive patients. In addition, such patients tended to have more confluent lesions. Patients with benign MS had a larger number of asymptomatic infratentorial lesions.

Distinct characteristic differences in MR findings were noted between patients with benign MS and those with chronic progressive disease. However, whether MR imaging will prove helpful in characterizing patients shortly after the onset of disease is uncertain.

▶ The chronic multiple sclerosis patients were more likely to have more lesions, more confluency of lesions, and more lesions below the tentorium, all of which makes sense.

Pain Syndromes in Multiple Sclerosis
Moulin DE, Foley KM, Ebers GC (Univ of Western Ontario, London, Ont; Mem

Sloan-Kettering Cancer Ctr, New York)
Neurology 38:1830–1834, December 1988   11–7

Charcot knew that pain is a part of multiple sclerosis, but reported rates of this complication vary widely. To detail the clinical characteristics of patients experiencing pain, 159 patients were observed in a multiple sclerosis clinic.

Fifteen (9%) patients had acute pain at some time during their illness. Chronic pain syndromes occurred in 48% of patients, and 55% of the total population had pain of some type. Patients with pain did not differ from those without pain with respect to age, duration of disease, or degree of disability, but female patients were overrepresented in the group with pain. Seven patients with acute pain had trigeminal neuralgia. The major chronic pain syndromes were dysesthetic limb pain, back pain, and painful leg spasms. Three patients had visceral pain. Only 4 patients had a history of migraine, but 16% of the population had frequent tension-type headaches.

Chronic pain is common among patients with established multiple sclerosis. Treatment must be individualized. Paroxysmal pain is best managed with anticonvulsant drugs. Chronic dysesthetic pain does not often respond to tricyclic antidepressants. Back pain is initially treated with nonsteroidal anti-inflammatory drugs and aggressive physical measures. Painful leg spasms may respond to muscle relaxants or a brief course of steroids.

▶ Probably like most neurologists, I have tried to deny that multiple sclerosis is a painful disease. But you can't fool the patients, and they have told me differently over the years. These authors have analyzed the type and distribution of the pain and have suggested appropriate therapy for the various types.

One of the toughest questions we are asked by patients when they are first diagnosed is, How will I do in the future? Many attempts have been made to answer the question. A study from Norway (1) now tries again. Vertigo near or at onset, a progressive course, and older age at onset are associated with a shorter life. The latter factor was not corrected for the expected shorter survival of older persons, so it may not be meaningful. Why vertigo at onset should shorten life is unclear. The progressive course I would agree with, but I wonder how many of the patients with steady progression at onset have had a silent onset many years before. Larger MRI experience will answer that question some day.

Reference

1. Rise et al: *J Clin Epidemiol* 41:1031–1036, 1988.

Double-Masked Trial of Azathioprine in Multiple Sclerosis
British and Dutch Multiple Sclerosis Azathioprine Trial Group (Guy's Hosp, London)
Lancet 1:179–183, July 23, 1988   11–8

The resemblance of multiple sclerosis (MS) to the experimental autoimmune condition chronic relapsing experimental allergic encephalomyelitis has led to trials of immunosuppressive treatment in the human disease. The most widely used agent was azathioprine. In 1982, a multicenter trial lasting 3 years was begun to test the efficacy of azathioprine in treating MS.

By random assignment, 354 patients with MS received either azathioprine, 2.5 mg/kg daily, or placebo. During the 3-year follow-up, only small differences between the groups emerged. The mean deterioration in Kurtzke disability score was 0.62 in the azathioprine group and 0.80 in the placebo group at 3 years. In the ambulation index, the mean deterioration was 0.84 and 1.25, respectively. After 3 years, there were slightly fewer relapses in the azathioprine group than in the placebo group, but the difference of 0.3 was not statistically significant.

These results show a small beneficial effect from azathioprine. This benefit was so small that the use of azathioprine cannot be generally recommended for most patients with MS. Analysis of subgroups (by age, sex, severity, rate of progression, HLA status, and relapsing or progressive course) did not reveal any that have shown clear clinical benefit.

▶ This was a long and large trial and probably will not be bettered. It tends to be believable and fits in with one's own clinical experience: azathioprine probably does some good but may not be worth the worry over the blood count, etc.

A recent note by Milanese and associates from Milan (1) does not confirm recent reports that intrathecal interferon-β reduces the exacerbation rate in multiple sclerosis. They found that the rate in the treated group was slightly higher than the placebo group. Rosenberg and Appenzeller (2) in a small trial find that amantadine does appear to be effective against the fatigue so common in MS.

Nelson, Franklin, and Jones in *JAMA* (3) note that whether the MS mother breast-feeds or not makes very little difference in the exacerbation rate.

References

1. Milanese et al: *Lancet* 2:563–564, Sept 3, 1988.
2. Rosenberg, Appenzeller: *Arch Neurol* 45:1104–1106, 1988.
3. Nelson, Franklin, Jones: *JAMA* 259:3441–3443, June 17, 1988.

Double-Blind Randomized Trial of ACTH Versus Dexamethasone Versus Methylprednisolone in Multiple Sclerosis Bouts: Clinical, Cerebrospinal Fluid, and Neurophysiological Results

Milanese C, La Mantia L, Salmaggi A, Campi A, Eoli M, Scaioli V, Nespolo A, Corridori F (Istituto Neurologico "C Besta," Milan, Italy)
Eur Neurol 29:10–14, 1989   11–9

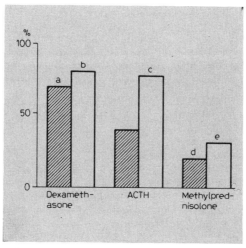

Fig 11–1.—*Diagonally striped column* = improved patients at day 7 of treatment; *white column* = improved patients at day 30 from treatment onset. A significantly greater percentage of improvement at day 7 is seen in dexamethasone- than methylprednisolone-treated patients (*a* vs. *d: P* = .024), and at day 30 in both dexamethasone- and ACTH- than methylprednisolone-treated patients (*b, c* vs. *e: P* = .024). (Courtesy of Milanese C, La Mantia L, Salmaggi A, et al: *Eur Neurol* 29:10–14, 1989.)

Twenty-four patients with clinically definite multiple sclerosis (MS) and 4 with early probable MS participated in a double-blind trial of steroids and adrenocorticotropic hormone (ACTH). Two patients with optic neuritis also were included. All patients had new signs or symptoms or definite worsening of existing features after being stable for at least 1 month. Initial doses were 50 units of ACTH, 8 mg of dexamethasone, and 40 mg of methylprednisolone daily. All medications were tapered over the 2-week treatment period.

Clear differences related to treatment were observed, with the most impressive findings in the dexamethasone group (Fig 11–1). The effects were unrelated to the interval from the onset of the episode to treatment or to the functional system affected. Neurophysiologic parameters and the cerebrospinal fluid were not significantly altered by treatment. The appearance of new lesions on radiography was not related to clinical deterioration.

Low doses of steroids, especially dexamethasone, can promote recovery from episodes of MS in patients with nonprogressive illness. It would seem best to reserve high-dose intravenous methylprednisolone for patients who fail to respond to ACTH or low doses of steroids.

▶ This study is of interest and was necessary. The whole question is, I suppose, whether the dosages of the drugs used were truly equivalent. Why is it that a person who has failed dexamethasone or prednisone or methylprednisolone treatment can then be given ACTH intravenously and will improve? Is it just a matter of the larger dosage? It would not seem reasonable to throw ACTH out yet.

Quantitative Magnetic Resonance Imaging in Multiple Sclerosis: The Effect of High Dose Intravenous Methylprednisolone
Kesselring J, Miller DH, MacManus DG, Johnson G, Milligan NM, Scolding N, Compston DAS, McDonald WI (Natl Hosp for Nervous Diseases, London; Univ of Wales, Cardiff)
J Neurol Neurosurg Psychiatry 52:14–17, 1989   11–10

Corticosteroid therapy in patients with multiple sclerosis (MS) effectively reduces the duration of an episode of acute exacerbation but does not alter the long-term clinical outcome. It has been suggested that the resolution of the characteristic edema of the early MS lesion is responsible for the early symptomatic improvement. This study was done to evaluate the effects of methylprednisolone therapy on the magnetic resonance imaging (MRI) appearances of MS brain lesions and to correlate these effects with observed short-term clinical changes.

Fifty clinically stable, ambulatory patients, aged 22 to 58 years, with definite or probable MS underwent MRI of the brain immediately before and 3 to 7 days after the completion of 5 days of intravenous methylprednisolone therapy at doses of 0.5 gm daily. In addition, relaxation times were measured in 12 randomly selected patients and 18 healthy controls.

Forty-nine of the 50 patients had abnormal results of magnetic resonance scans. New lesions in 9 patients were apparent on second magnetic resonance scans, but the new lesions were clinically silent. Although in 7 patients a single preexisting lesion appeared to have become smaller, none of the patients showed resolution of a lesion. Two patients showed a reduction in the size of an abnormal area, but at the same time, a single new lesion developed, confirming that corticosteroids do not rapidly alter the underlying plaque formation process. After treatment, 20 patients were clinically improved, 25 patients were unchanged, and 5 had deteriorated. Before treatment, all patients showed elevated values in normal-appearing white matter but not in cortex when compared with normal controls. After treatment, patients showed a significant reduction in T_1 and T_2 in cortex and in T_1 alone in normal-appearing white matter.

Because the increased brain water content in normal-appearing white matter of MS patients was significantly reduced by high-dose methylprednisolone therapy, the rapid symptomatic improvement observed after corticosteroid treatment in 20 of the 50 patients may have resulted from the resolution of brain edema.

▶ This is another confirmation that steroids, although they may cause improvement in a major portion of the patient's acute symptoms, may allow new lesions to develop at the same time, much to everyone's disappointment.

Multiple Sclerosis: The Lipid Relationship
Swank RL, Grimsgaard A (Oregon Health Sciences Univ, Portland)
Am J Clin Nutr 48:1387–1393, December 1988   11–11

There is some evidence for a relationship between multiple sclerosis and the consumption of saturated fatty acids of animal origin. The authors related differing levels of fat and oil consumption to disability and mortality in 150 patients with an exacerbating-remitting course. The low-fat diet was modified over the years, and not all patients followed the recommended diet.

Mortality in patients whose daily fat consumption was less than 20 gm and averaged 17 gm was 31%, and clinical deterioration was slight. With higher daily intakes of fat, averaging either 25 or 41 gm, serious disability occurred and mortality was about 80% during the 35-year observation period (Fig 11–2). Treatment before severe disability developed improved the outlook. Female patients tended to do better than male patients. Oil intake tended to be related inversely to both fat intake and the rate of clinical deterioration.

High sensitivity to animal fat suggests its involvement in the development of multiple sclerosis. These fats aggregate blood cells, thereby slowing the circulation and reducing oxygen availability to the brain. Sur-

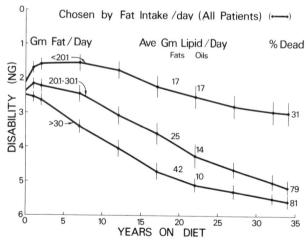

Fig 11–2.—Patients grouped by fat intake per day: average rate of deterioration of MS with 95% confidence limits *(vertical lines)* and percentage of deaths at the end of the study for 3 groups of patients *(solid lines)*. The average daily fat and oil intakes are indicated above each solid line, and percentage of deaths at the end of each solid line. (Courtesy of Swank RL, Grimsgaard A: *Am J Clin Nutr* 48:1387–1393, December 1988.)

rounding regions might be acidified and lysing enzymes might be activated, increasing the permeability of the blood-brain barrier.

▶ This is your payoff for hiring drudges like me and others in the Chicago office to go through stacks of publications. This 40-year follow-up of Swank's MS patients is in the *American Journal of Clinical Nutrition,* of all places. We thank Dr. Swank for giving us this long-term follow-up on a group of patients who have faithfully reported to him over the 40-year period.

There could be several reasons why the relationship between low-fat diet and slower course of MS is true, aside from the one that Swank (and I) tend to believe: that the diet actually does some good for multiple sclerosis. For instance, the diet may simply cut down on deaths from vascular disease.

For the past several years I have been taking a diet history on MS patients who have done either particularly well or particularly poorly. Those who seem to do well are near vegetarians, and those who don't are cheeseburger eaters. So I have been recommending the Heart Association's low saturated fat diet to all. And stopping smoking.

Bates and co-workers (1) report a large double-blind 2-year trial of long-chain n-3 polyunsaturated fatty acids (10 gm/day of max EPA oil, a fish oil) vs. the same amount of olive oil. Both groups were advised to avoid saturated fats in their diet. The fish oil group did better, but not significantly so. Of course, both groups may have done better than usual; there was no untreated control group. Nevertheless, what harm can come to someone by going on a low-fat diet?

Reference

1. Bates et al: *J Neurol Neurosurg Psychiatry* 52:18–22, 1989.

The Natural History of Multiple Sclerosis: A Geographically Based Study—I. Clinical Course and Disability
Weinshenker BG, Bass B, Rice GPA, Noseworthy J, Carriere W, Baskerville J, Ebers GC (Univ of Western Ontario, London, Ont)
Brain 112:133–146, 1989   11–12

A follow-up study of 1,099 consecutive multiple sclerosis (MS) patients was carried out during 1972–1984. A geographically based group of 196 patients, 90% of all those from Middlesex County, was analyzed separately, as was a group of 197 patients seen from the outset of MS. The overall average duration of disease was 12 years. The patients followed from the outset were seen for a mean of 4.2 years.

One third of the total population and 28% of patients from Middlesex County had progressive disease from the outset. Among patients with MS for 6–10 years, progressive MS developed in 30% to 40% of patients with initially remitting illness. A bimodal distribution of disability was apparent on cross-sectional analysis, with peaks occurring at no disability level and at the level that aid was needed for walking. The median time to reach the latter point was 15 years overall and 9½ years for patients followed from disease outset. Eighty-seven percent of patients followed for up to 40 years were still alive, although ascertainment of patients with this length of MS duration was incomplete. Only 1 patient followed from disease onset died of causes related to MS. Sixteen patients in all (1.5%) died of MS-related causes.

These data should prove helpful in planning clinical trials and estimating the size of a study group needed to demonstrate a given degree of patient benefit.

▶ We commented above on Swank's low-fat diet group that had done so well (Abstract 11–11), with more than 80% alive after 40 years, and now we hear that may be normal. Is one forced to the conclusion that members of Swank's high-fat diet group were killing themselves off prematurely; in other words, the control group did poorly and the treatment group did as expected?

A recent study of MS survival from Germany finds a shorter average survival of 35–40 years after onset of symptoms and further notes that the shorter survival in males and those older at onset are nonspecific and simply reflect the fact that males in general and older persons in general don't live as long (1).

Reference

1. Poser S, Kurtzke JF, Poser W, et al: *J Clin Epidemiol* 42:159–168, 1989.

Severely Threatening Events and Marked Life Difficulties Preceding Onset or Exacerbation of Multiple Sclerosis
Grant I, Brown GW, Harris T, McDonald WI, Patterson T, Trimble MR (Univ of California, San Diego, La Jolla; Univ of London; Natl Hosps, Queen Square and Maida Vale, London)
J Neurol Neurosurg Psychiatry 52:8–13, January 1989   11–13

Do stressful life circumstances in fact influence the onset and course of multiple sclerosis (MS)? Using the Life Events and Difficulties Schedule, data on life circumstances were obtained in 39 patients with early MS and 40 controls matched for age, sex, marital status, and socioeconomic status. The patient group included 29 women and 10 men aged 36 years, on average.

In 75% of the patients marked life adversity was experienced in the 6 months before onset of disease compared with one third of the controls. Severely threatening events occurred much more frequently in the patient group. The excess of marked life stress in a patient was most evident in the 6 months before disease onset (Fig 11–3). Marked adversity was associated with both first-episode and relapsing MS patients. Reports of marked adversity did not correlate with disability ratings at the time of the interview.

A temporal relationship between marked life adversity and the onset of MS is evident, but whether that relationship is a causal one was not es-

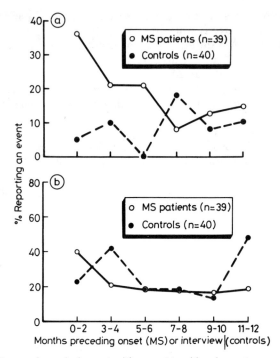

Fig 11–3.—Report of severely threatening life events (a) and less threatening events (b) by multiple sclerosis *(MS)* patients and controls. (Courtesy of Grant I, Brown GW, Harris T, et al: *J Neurol Neurosurg Psychiatry* 52:8–13, January 1989.)

tablished. There is, however, neuroimmunologic evidence that stress can lead to altered immune status, and good evidence also exists for immunologic abnormalities in MS.

▶ This article will be interesting not only to us but to the legal fraternity when approached by patients for help in litigation related to such events and worsening of their multiple sclerosis.

I suspect it is true. It simply happens too often in practice to be ignored, but proof is difficult.

12 Infections of the Nervous System

Dexamethasone Therapy for Bacterial Meningitis: Results of Two Double-Blind, Placebo-Controlled Trials
Lebel MH, Freij BJ, Syrogiannopoulos GA, Chrane DF, Hoyt MJ, Stewart SM, Kennard BD, Olsen KD, McCracken GH Jr (Univ of Texas, Dallas)
N Engl J Med 319:964–971, Oct 13, 1988   12–1

The case fatality rates for infants and children suffering from bacterial meningitis range from 5% to 10%, and as many as 50% of those who survive have long-term complications. Two prospective double-blind, placebo-controlled trials were done to assess the efficacy of dexamethasone therapy in addition to either cefuroxime or ceftriaxone.

Two hundred infants and children were enrolled in the studies. Ninety-eight patients received placebo, and 102 received dexamethasone, 0.15 mg/kg, every 6 hours for 4 days. The mean increase in the cerebrospinal fluid concentration of glucose and the reductions in lactate and protein levels after 24 hours of treatment were significantly greater in those who received dexamethasone than in those who received placebo. In the first study, 1 patient in the placebo group died. Compared with the placebo group, patients who received dexamethasone became afebrile earlier and were less likely to acquire moderate or more severe bilateral sensorineural hearing loss. Twelve children in the 2 placebo groups (14%) suffered severe or profound bilateral hearing loss that required the use of a hearing aid, compared with 1 (1%) in the 2 dexamethasone groups.

▶ This trial has been a long time coming and is welcome now that it's here. It indicates that a short course of dexamethasone is beneficial in infancy and childhood meningitis, reducing not only the duration of the febrile period but also the postmeningitic deafness. A thoughtful analysis by Arnold Smith in the same issue (1) is worth reading, as is a comment by Tuomanen (2) sent by Paul Hyman. Tuomanen clarifies the situation by explaining that it is the breakdown products of the killed bacteria that cause the inflammatory response and thus the secondary effects that may last a lifetime.

References

1. Smith A: *N Engl J Med* 319:1012–1013, Oct 13, 1988.
2. Tuomanen E: *Ann Intern Med* 109:690–692, Nov 1, 1988.

Fulminant Bacterial Meningitis Without Meningeal Signs
Callaham M (Univ of California, San Francisco)
Ann Emerg Med 18:90–93, January 1989   12–2

Meningitis must often be considered in patients who present with fever, myalgia, and headache. As these symptoms are common, the absence of stiff neck is often considered to be an indication to rule out meningitis. Meningeal signs, especially in alert patients, are not discussed much in the literature, which implies that neck stiffness is usual except in immunosuppressed patients, the elderly, or infants. Two adults and a child presented with bacterial meningitis with no meningeal signs.

Alterations of mental status or a stiff neck were not evident on presentation in the first patient, a woman aged 41 years. The neck was still supple on her second visit, although her mental status had deteriorated. The second patient, a man aged 41 years, showed subtle alterations of mental status attributed to earlier pain medication and to fatigue. The patient's neck did not become stiff for 16 hours after hospitalization. The third patient, a boy aged 4 years, showed alterations of mental status attributed to head trauma, but no neck stiffness. Infection was noted, but the focus was not located for 19 hours. All 3 patients had vomiting, and 2 had fever. Lumbar puncture showed elevated protein levels, very low glucose values; Gram's staining demonstrated *Streptococcus pneumoniae* in 2 patients. All 3 patients died.

Fatal bacterial meningitis in nonimmunosuppressed adults may have a subtle presentation. Lumbar puncture should be performed in patients with headache and subtle alterations of mental status when the cause is in serious doubt.

▶ It is hard to believe that meningitis can be present without meningeal signs until one has seen it. These patients did not appear seriously ill when first seen but soon became ill, and treatment in all 3 cases was too late to save the patients' lives. A possible clue is that all 3 patients had high white counts. What other clues are there?

Late Progression of Post-Encephalitic Parkinson's Syndrome
Calne DB, Lees AJ (Univ of British Columbia; Natl Hosp for Nervous Diseases, London)
Can J Neurol Sci 15:135–138, May 1988   12–3

The very late course after encephalitis lethargica, contracted in the pandemic of 1919, remains uncertain. Eleven patients with neurologic deficits who had been hospitalized for longer than 40 years were studied. The patients had a mean age at admission of 22 years and a mean age of 74 when most recently observed.

All the patients had considerable motor disability, but none were severely demented. Three patients had upper motor neuron signs without a definite history of stroke. Several patients had dystonia, and some had contractures. Bradykinesia, rigidity, tremor, and speech problems were present in a majority of patients. Review of past records, photographs, and disability ratings suggested that neurologic disability from basal ganglia damage often increased late in life. Motor function deteriorated most markedly, compared with intellectual and special sensory functions.

Neuronal damage in senescence may result from excessive production or inadequate removal of free radicals. This may also be the final common path of neuron destruction in such degenerative disorders as Parkinson's disease, Alzheimer's disease, and motoneuron disease.

▶ Von Economo's lethargic encephalitis appeared spontaneously in 1919 and seemed to disappear decades later. It was sometimes followed by severe neurologic sequelae. This is an interesting and well-summarized report on the present status of a few survivors.—R.N. DeJong, M.D.

Herpes Zoster Associated Encephalitis: Clinical Findings and Acyclovir Treatment
Peterslund NA (Marselisborg Hosp, Aarhus, Denmark)
Scand J Infect Dis 20:583–592, 1988   12–4

The clinical course of herpes zoster-associated encephalitis (HZAE) in 14 patients was reviewed with regard to treatment with acyclovir. Acyclovir was given to 9 of the patients, all of whom were immunocompetent. Data on 8 previously reported patients given acyclovir were also reviewed, in addition to data on 44 patients not given acyclovir.

The risk of HZAE increased with both dissemination and immunosuppression in this combined series. In contrast, cranial zoster did not much increase the risk. The chief clinical features were disordered mental function and ataxia. About one third of the patients had neck stiffness. Cranial computed tomography was usually normal, but electroencephalography was consistently abnormal. Acyclovir therapy appeared to be beneficial. Signs of HZAE developed in 2 patients who were receiving desciclovir but who recovered during continued treatment.

The pathogenesis of HZAE remains to be clarified, but current evidence favors direct viral invasion. The effects of acyclovir therapy must be continuously and critically assessed; however, a controlled study would entail ethical problems. Current data warrant using acyclovir to treat HZAE.

▶ It's of interest that the CAT scans were generally normal and the EEGs always were abnormal. The duration from the skin lesion to the encephalitis was 15 days in immunosuppressed patients and 5 days in nonimmunosuppressed patients. The spinal fluid is often abnormal. The authors feel that treatment with acyclovir is appropriate and wonder whether a blinded study of its effectiveness is ethical.

Clinical Picture of HTLV-I Associated Myelopathy
Shibasaki H, Endo C, Kuroda Y, Kakigi R, Oda K-I, Komine S-I (Saga Med School, Nabeshima, Japan)
J Neurol Sci 87:15–24, October 1988   12–5

High titers of antibody against HTLV-1 are reported in patients with tropical spastic paraparesis, and a pathogenic relationship is suspected in southern Kyushu, Japan. The authors reviewed 16 consecutive Japanese patients seen during a 6-year period who had progressive spastic paraparesis and increased HTLV-1 titers.

The mean age of the patients was 50 years, and symptoms had been present for a mean of 15 years. A gait disturbance was the usual initial sign; leg stiffness was frequent. The legs were markedly spastic in 5 patients and moderately spastic in 7. Sensory impairment was not marked except for vibratory sensation in 2 patients. Median nerve conduction velocities generally were normal. Difficulty in voiding, with residual urine, was a frequent finding, as was marked urinary frequency. Urodynamic studies demonstrated an overactive detrusor muscle and detrusor-urethral sphincter dyssynergia. Five patients were able to walk without aid. Two patients had adult T cell leukemia-like cells in their spinal fluid. Steroid treatment seemed to improve walking speed to some degree in 9 patients.

The features of HTLV-1–associated myelopathy suggest diffuse lesions in white matter, chiefly involving the thoracic spinal cord. The disorder probably is a chronic diffuse leukomyelitis involving the lateral and to some extent the posterior columns of the cord in a symmetric manner. A distinction from multiple sclerosis may be difficult in areas where the progressive spinal form of disease is common.

▶ I'm not aware of having seen a patient with this disease, but I'm always afraid I'll miss the diagnosis. So far we have not succeeded in getting a report back from the lab. Someone, without fail, helpfully changes the lab order slip from HTLV-1 to HIV-1. So we know the patient does not have AIDS but not whether he or she has antibodies to the tropical spastic paraplegia virus. It's good to have a better understanding of the clinical picture, which these authors have provided.

Neurocysticercosis: Two Hundred Thirty-Eight Cases From a California Hospital
Scharf D (Univ of Southern California)
Arch Neurol 45:777–780, July 1988   12–6

The incidence of diagnosed cases of cysticercosis has almost doubled at the Los Angeles County–University of Southern California Medical Center during the past 5 years. The spread of *Taenia solium* is hematogenous, with the embryo having a predilection for muscle, brain, and eye tissue. The life cycle of *T. solium* is completed when people eat undercooked pork; the encysted embryo is released in the human small bowel and can develop into an adult worm. Cysticercosis results when humans become the intermediate hosts for the larval stage. Patients with cysticercosis seen from 1981 to 1986 were studied.

Two hundred thirty-eight cases were reviewed. Most were young when first seen, but ages ranged from 2 to 82 years. All but 1 patient were Hispanic Americans. Presentation and clinical manifestation varied. Most had seizures at some time. A convulsion was the presenting symptom in 134 cases, and epilepsy was manifest at some point in 147. Fifty-one patients initially had increased intracranial pressures. Seventy-one patients ultimately required ventricular shunting procedures or surgery. Of 56 EEGs obtained, 41 were abnormal.

Mortality and morbidity of neurocysticercosis can be decreased by maintaining a high degree of suspicion in populations at increased risk. Clinical signs and symptoms are protean. In almost every case, the disease follows an individual course depending on the location of the lesion, the load of the parasite, the long-term duration of infection, and individual immunologic response in the host.

▶ Seizures and acute increased intracranial pressure seem to be the most common presenting pictures of neurocysticercosis. Even in a site as remote as ours (Mississippi), we see an occasional patient with this disorder. This is helpful commentary from a center where many patients are seen.

Detection of Human T-Cell Lymphoma/Leukemia Virus Type I DNA and Antigen in Spinal Fluid and Blood of Patients With Chronic Progressive Myelopathy

Bhagavati S, Ehrlich G, Kula RW, Kwok S, Sninsky J, Udani V, Poiesz BJ (State Univ of New York, Brooklyn and Syracuse; VA Med Ctr, Syracuse, NY; Cetus Corp, Emeryville, Calif)
N Engl J Med 318:1141–1147, May 5, 1988   12–7

The cause of chronic progressive myelopathy is unclear in many instances. Recently patients in some countries have been reported to have antibody to HTLV-1. The authors found HTLV-1 DNA or antigen, or both, in the cerebrospinal fluid of 7 patients with chronic progressive myelopathy and in the blood of 11 patients. Twenty-one patients in all had the gradual onset of progressive spastic paraparesis without myelographic evidence of cord compression and without any hereditary degenerative neurologic disorder.

Ten of 13 patients from tropical countries had serum antibody to HTLV-1. A sensitive in vitro enzymatic gene amplification method demonstrated HTLV-1 sequences in fresh peripheral blood mononuclear cells from all antibody-positive patients and in cell cultures of spinal fluid from 3 of these patients. Southern blot hybridization demonstrated virus in cultures of peripheral blood lymphocytes in 3 of 7 patients. Four patients had abnormal magnetic resonance studies, showing in 3 patients multiple foci of increased signal intensity in the periventricular white matter. Seronegative patients had clinical findings similar to those in seropositive patients.

It appears that HTLV-1 is causally associated with many cases of chronic progressive myelopathy in patients from tropical countries. The myelopathy may reflect a direct slow-virus infection of the nervous system, a cytotoxic immune reaction to HTLV-1-carrying cells in the central nervous system (CNS) or a humoral autoimmune disorder in which HTLV-1-infected lymphocytes and CNS cells share common antigenic determinants.

▶ This finding does seem to back up the notion that the myelopathy of HTLV-1 is a chronic viral situation rather than an immune response. There could be some elements of both, or the virus might hang around during the immune response phase. A recent letter (1) by Rosling and associates points out that the epidemic spastic paraparesis (ESP) of rural Africa is not the same as the tropical spastic paraparesis caused by HTLV-1, which also may be found in Africa, among other places. The authors have tested for HTLV-1 antibodies in patients with ESP and found them to be negative. Epidemic spastic paraparesis is from the cyanide in improperly prepared cassava roots, eaten during food shortages in the dry season.

Reference

1. Rosling et al: *Lancet* 1:1222, May 28, 1988.

Neurological Syndromes of Brucellosis
Bahemuka M, Shemena AR, Panayiotopoulos CP, Al-Aska AK, Obeid T, Daif AK
(College of Medicine, Riyadh, Saudi Arabia)
J Neurol Neurosurg Psychiatry 51:1017–1021, August 1988   12–8

Brucellosis is endemic in Saudi Arabia. Because brucellosis may affect the nervous system with resulting diverse and complex symptomatology, the diagnosis in patients presenting with neurologic symptoms may be missed or delayed. Experience in 11 patients diagnosed with brucellosis who presented with symptoms mimicking several neurologic syndromes and diseases was evaluated.

All 11 patients were suspected of brucellosis on the basis of clinical symptoms. Neurologic symptoms and initial diagnoses included transient ischemic attacks, vertigo, cerebrovascular accident, acute confusional state, polyradiculoneuropathy, motor neuron disease, Guillain Barré-like syndrome, cauda equina syndrome, and lateral lumbar disk prolapse. Blood samples were taken for brucella culture and standard agglutination tests for the measurement of *Brucella abortus* and *B. melitensis* titers. Diagnostic investigation included computed tomography, myelography, nerve conduction studies, electroencephalography, and electromyography as indicated. Nine patients also had a spinal puncture for examination of cerebrospinal fluid (table).

Presentation and Neurologic Investigations of 11 Cases of Brucellosis

Case	Type of presentation	Investigation	Result of test
1	Transient ischaemic attacks in the anterior circulation and alternating hemiparesis	CT brain scan	Normal
2	Vertigo, trunkal ataxia and postural hypotension	Audiometry, brainstem evoked potentials, CT brain scan	Normal
3	Cerebrovascular accident (middle cerebral artery territory)	CT brain scan	Normal
4	Acute confusional state	EEG	Slow waves in right parietal area
5	Polyradiculoneuropathy, trunkal ataxia, extensor plantar responses and neurogenic deafness	CT brain scan	Normal
		Nerve conduction studies	Sensorimotor peripheral neuropathy
		Visual evoked potentials	Delayed latencies bilaterally
		Auditory brainstem evoked potentials	None obtained
6	Motor neuron disease (Amyotrophic lateral sclerosis)	Nerve conduction studies	Normal
		EMG of upper and lower limb muscles	Fasciculation potentials with long duration
7	Unilateral brachial radiculopathy	Motor nerve conduction velocities	Normal
		EMG of the right deltoid, biceps and brachioradialis	No resting activity, polyphasic potentials
8	Guillain Barré-like syndrome (Symmetrical polyradiculopathy with no sensory loss)	Nerve conduction studies	Normal
		EMG	Denervation
9	Acute urinary retention, sciatica and perianal hypoalgesia	Lumbosacral radiography	Normal
		Myelogram	Normal
10	Cauda equina syndrome	EMG of tibialis anterior, gastrocnemius and hamstrings	Denervation
		Nerve conduction studies	Normal
11	Lateral lumbar disc prolapse with sphincter dysfunction and myelopathy	Myelography	Complete block at L4/5
		Myelography	Obliteration of the L4 nerve root

(Courtesy of Bahemuka M, Shemena AR, Panayiotopoulos CP, et al: *J Neurol Neurosurg Psychiatry* 51:1017–1021, August 1988.)

Patients with acute disease improved quickly after initiation of adequate antibiotic therapy. However, patients with chronic brucellosis responded poorly to treatment. Five of the blood cultures were positive, 4 of which showed resistance to cotrimoxazole. One patient had a negative blood culture but a positive cerebrospinal fluid culture that was also resistant to cotrimoxazole. Trimethoprim-sulfamethoxazole was given with tetracycline and streptomycin. Rifampicin was not given, as it should be reserved for resistant patients only because tuberculosis is still common in Saudi Arabia.

In countries where brucellosis is endemic, patients who have obscure or unexplained neurologic deficits, even without a definite history of exposure, should alert the clinician to the possibility of brucellosis.

▶ None of the neurologic features of brucellosis would cause me to think of that disorder. This is why infectious disease consultants can make a living: they think of odd things that might cause the patient's symptomatology which ordinarily do not enter our minds.

Creutzfeldt-Jakob Disease in England and Wales, 1980–1984: A Case-Control Study of Potential Risk Factors
Harries-Jones R, Knight R, Will RG, Cousens S, Smith PG, Matthews WB (Radcliffe Infirmary, Oxford, England; London School of Hygiene and Tropical Medicine)
J Neurol Neurosurg Psychiatry 51:1113–1119, September 1988   12–9

Epidemiologic data were obtained from a 5-year survey of Creutzfeldt-Jakob disease (CJD) in England and Wales. Two controls were matched with each patient for age, gender, and hospital. Ninety-three definite cases of CJD were collected in this period, and there were 29 probable cases. Little annual variation in deaths was observed. The mean age at death was 63 years. There was only 1 instance of verified CJD in a relative.

Social class distribution was similar for patients and medical controls, whereas neurologic controls tended to be of higher social status. Patients were more likely than controls to have had herpes zoster during adult life, as well as psychiatric illness requiring treatment. Controls were more likely than patients to have had surgery other than ophthalmic surgery (table). The risk of CJD could not be related to smoking habits or animal

Estimated Odds Ratios and Their 95% Confidence Intervals For the Most Statistically Significant Associations

				Number of		
				Cases	Controls	
Risk factor	Odds ratio	Approximate 95% confidence limits	p value		Neuro	Medical
Surgery at any time	0·6	0·3– 1·00	<0·10	57	68	68
Zoster in adult life	2·6	2·4–	<0·005	6	0	0
Current alcohol	0·5	0·3– 0·8	<0·005	50	71	61
Keeping cats	2·0	1·2– 3·6	<0·01	34	15	27
Pets other than cats/dogs	4·4	1·5–12·7	<0·01	11	3	2
Ferret contact	2·1	1·0– 4·2	=0·05	19	14	8
Mink contact	8·6	0·9–77·9	=0·08*	4	1	0
Dementia in family	3·6	1·8– 7·1	<0·0005	27	11	8

*Unmatched estimates.
(Courtesy of Harries-Jones R, Knight R, Will RG, et al: *J Neurol Neurosurg Psychiatry* 51:1113–1119, September 1988.)

contact. Dementia in close relatives was more frequent among patients than among controls.

It is not more likely that the few positive findings in this study are related to the cause of CJD.

▶ Although the authors downplay it, there was more frequent keeping of cats and other pets and contact with ferrets and mink by the patients than by the controls. Patients were also slightly more likely to have had contact with sheep, fur, and carcasses.

We must get the disease, in the nonfamilial situations, from some animal, human or subhuman. The authors say that "It is unlikely that our few positive findings are related in any way to the etiology of Creutzfeldt-Jakob." It is difficult to agree with them. I think the clues may be valid, and one hopes they will be pursued.

13 Toxins

Characteristics of Freebase Cocaine Psychosis

Manschreck TC, Laughery JA, Weisstein CC, Allen D, Humblestone B, Neville M, Podlewski H, Mitra N (Harvard Med School; Sandilands Rehabilitation Ctr, Nassau, Bahamas; Yale Univ)

Yale J Biol Med 61:115–122, March–April 1988

13–1

Of 106 cocaine-disordered patients hospitalized in 1985 during an epidemic of free-base cocaine abuse in the Bahamas, 29% had psychosis. The onset was acute in 55% of these 31 patients. The mean duration of psychosis was 16 days. Twelve other patients had evidence of past transient psychotic symptoms associated with cocaine intoxication.

Delusions were the most frequent manifestation of psychosis (table). Confused patients had used cocaine more often than the others, were more often violent, and reported more visual and auditory hallucinations. However, psychosis lasted a shorter time in the confused patients. Of 8 patients with a past history of major mental disorder, 5 had psychotic patterns consistent with their preexisting disorder. Psychotic patients had used nearly twice as much cocaine as nonpsychotics had used. Cocaine-related violent behavior was reported in 55% of the psychotic group and 36% of the others.

Psychosis is not uncommon in free-base cocaine abusers. All the classic forms of psychosis are seen. Previous major mental disorder is a risk factor for new and recurrent cocaine-induced psychosis, as is use of a large amount of cocaine. Violent behavior related to cocaine toxicity is seen most often in patients with psychosis.

▶ Cocaine psychosis has been unusual, although case reports have documented its sporadic occurrence. Cocaine hydrochloride, the form of cocaine that is used intravenously, has been implicated in most of these psychotic reactions. In the mid-1970s, the use of cocaine sulfate increased psychiatric presentations. A recent nationwide epidemic of free-base cocaine abuse in the Ba-

Dimensions of Cocaine Psychosis	
Feature	% (*n*)
Delusions*	93 (29)
Perceptual disturbance (Hallucination)*	83 (26)
Disturbed form of thinking	48 (15)
Confusion	42 (13)
Unusual behavior	42 (13)

*Categories include all forms detected in sample, rather than specific types.

(Courtesy of Manschreck TC, Laughery JA, Weisstein CC, et al: *Yale J Biol Med* 61:115–122, March–April 1988.)

hamas has dramatically changed the perception of cocaine psychosis. Major mental disorders and the increased persistence of cocaine use are more common among psychotic patients than nonpsychotic patients. Violent behavior was common among cocaine patients, especially in those with psychosis.

Free-base cocaine psychosis is neither rare nor benign. The use of cocaine during pregnancy may cause spontaneous abortion, premature delivery, fetal growth retardation, and possible congenital anomalies. Newborn infants exposed to cocaine during pregnancy may show signs of central nervous system dysfunction, which can persist for months or perhaps longer.— R.N. DeJong, M.D.

Cocaine Abuse: Neurovascular Complications
Jacobs IG, Roszler MH, Kelly JK, Klein MA, Kling GA (Detroit Receiving Hosp; Wayne State Univ; Harper Hosp, Detroit)
Radiology 170:223–227, January 1989   13–2

Cocaine abuse is associated with many medical complications. Reports of neurovascular complications have increased in recent years. Such com-

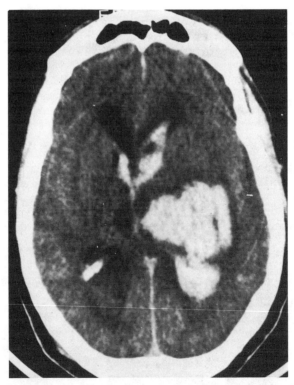

Fig 13–1.— Computed tomographic scan shows spontaneous thalamic hemorrhage with intraventricular extension in a 45-year-old man. (Courtesy of Jacobs IG, Roszler MH, Kelly JK, et al: *Radiology* 170:223–227, January 1989.)

plications consist mostly of subarachnoid hemorrhage, intracerebral hemorrhage, and cerebral ischemia. The increasing popularity of crack and cocaine may make the occurrence of strokes in young adults a common event. The neurovascular complications of cocaine abuse were studied.

The records of 3,712 drug abusers were examined. Thirteen patients had neurologic deficits attributable to cocaine use. The most frequent manifestations were ischemic, occurring in 54% of the patients, who had a mean age of 34.2 years. Twenty-three percent of the patients had subarachnoid hemorrhage, and 23% had intracerebral hemorrhage. Three patients from other centers were added to this group for analysis. Five of 6 patients with head computed tomographic findings of cerebral infarction had subcortical infarcts. Two of 4 patients with a subarachnoid hemorrhage had a congenital intracranial aneurysm. One of 4 patients with an intracerebral hemorrhage had an underlying arteriovenous malformation (Fig 13–1).

Neurovascular complications associated with cocaine abuse were discussed. The mechanism through which such complications occur is not fully understood. The acute hypertensive response that occurs with cocaine use and disordered neurovascular control may play a role.

▶ These 16 patients with strokes induced by cocaine abuse were evenly divided between 8 with cerebral ischemia and 8 with hemorrhage, 4 subarachnoid and 4 intracerebral. Mody and co-workers (1) found about the same proportion in 9 of 14 cocaine abusers with neurologic complications. An article by Nalls and associates (2) showed the CT picture of cocaine intracerebral hemorrhage, which looks much like any other. The angiograms show either microaneurysms or severe narrowing of an artery possibly secondary to vasculitis.

References

1. Mody et al: *Neurology* 38:1189–1193, 1988.
2. Nalls et al: *J Comput Assist Tomogr* 13:1–5, 1989.

Brain Abscess: A Complication of Cocaine Inhalation
Rao AN (New York Infirmary–Beekman Downtown Hosp, New York)
NY State J Med 88:548–550, October 1988   13–3

Recreational cocaine abuse can result in a host of adverse health consequences. Frontal sinusitis from nasal inhalation is well recognized, as is the relationship of frontal sinusitis and brain abscess. A patient was described whose cocaine snorting was associated with the sequential development of frontal sinusitis and a lethal brain abscess.

Man, 31, was found by paramedics in a stuporous condition on a subway platform. Family members reported that he had complained of a "bandlike" headache during the preceding 2 weeks. Neurologic examination revealed a right facial palsy. On his first day of hospitalization, he complained of frontal headaches, and his temperature continued to be 101F. An initial computed tomographic (CT) head scan was negative. On the third day of hospitalization, he complained that his headache was worse, he continued to be febrile, and he subsequently had a grand mal seizure. Sinus radiographs taken on the fifth day revealed opacification of both frontal sinuses and the left maxillary sinus. He remained febrile, and by the eighth hospital day he became more lethargic, stopped eating, and refused a repeat lumbar puncture. On the ninth day, the patient was found unconscious in bed. His pupils were fixed and dilated, and endotracheal intubation and ventilatory support were needed. A repeat CT brain scan revealed a lucency in the left frontal lobe of the brain, with a shift of the right falx cerebri. The patient died on the thirteenth day. At autopsy, acute left frontal sinusitis was found together with an acute abscess of the left frontal lobe and diffuse cerebral edema.

Inhalation of cocaine can result in mucoperichondrial ischemia that can lead to necrosis and infection with adjacent osteitis. Nasal and paranasal sinus symptoms, when otherwise unexplained, should alert clinicians to the possibility of cocaine inhalation. The patient described had sequential development of frontal sinusitis and a lethal brain abscess.

▶ I didn't get the connection between brain abscess and cocaine until the author pointed out that users frequently snort the stuff, which causes necrosis of the nasal tissues. This sometimes leads to a deep sinusitis that can become a brain abscess. Other complications of cocaine have recently been reported. Roth and co-workers (1) show that renal failure and liver dysfunction can result from acute rhabdomyolysis after cocaine use. Lathers and associates show that cocaine can induce seizures, arrhythmias, and sudden death (2). A recent comment by George Silver in *The Lancet* recommending legalization of cocaine since the drug war has been lost was answered by Mayor Koch of New York City (3), who states that a truly effective war on drugs has yet to be launched on the national stage: "It is time to raise the battle flag, not wave the white one."

References

1. Roth et al: *N Engl J Med* 319:673–677, 1988.
2. Lathers et al: *J Clin Pharmacol* 28:584–593, 1988.
3. Koch E: *Science* 242:495, Oct 28, 1988.

Handgun Regulations, Crime, Assaults, and Homicide: A Table of Two Cities
Sloan JH, Kellermann AL, Reay DT, Ferris JA, Koepsell T, Rivara FP, Rice C, Gray L, LeGerfo J (Univ of Washington; Univ of British Columbia; Univ of Tennessee)
N Engl J Med 319:1256–1262, Nov 10, 1988   13–4

About 20,000 persons are murdered in the United States each year, and about 60% of homicides involve firearms. Handguns account for three fourths of all gun-related homicides. To date, no study has separated the effects of handgun control from differences among populations in socioeconomic status, aggressive behavior, violent crime, and other factors. A study was done to investigate the associations among handgun regulations, assault and other crimes, and homicide.

Robberies, burglaries, assaults, and homicides were studied in Seattle and Vancouver from 1980 to 1986. Seattle and Vancouver are similar in many ways (geography, climate, history), but Vancouver has adopted more restrictive regulations of handguns. During the study period, both cities had comparable rates of burglary and robbery. The annual rate of assault was slightly higher in Seattle than Vancouver. However, the rate of assaults involving firearms was found to be 7 times higher in Seattle than in Vancouver. Despite similar overall rates of criminal activity and assault, the relative risk of death from homicide, adjusted for age and sex, was significantly higher in Seattle than in Vancouver. Virtually all of the excess risk could be explained by a 4.8-fold higher risk of being murdered with a handgun in Seattle. Rates of homicide by means other than guns were comparable in the 2 cities.

▶ Last weekend 3 citizens of my city (Jackson: population, 200,000) were killed and 1 was critically injured. Three of these assaults were with handguns, and 1 was with a knife. Americans generally regard Ireland as a violent country because of publicity given the troubles in Northern Ireland over the last 20 years. Seventeen years ago we spent 6 months in Ireland. It is a gentle country, and it is unlikely that 3 persons were injured or killed with handguns in any recent entire year in the Republic of Ireland (population, 3.5 million), where such weapons are prohibited. Holes can be picked in this comparison of Vancouver and Seattle, but an analysis by Mercy and Houk in the same issue of *The New England Journal of Medicine* (1) concludes that "injury from firearms is a public health problem whose toll is unacceptable. The time has come for us to address this problem in the manner in which we have addressed and dealt successfully with other threats to the public health." We are without doubt the most homicidal nation in the history of the planet.

There is a connection between drug use (Abstract 1–10) and homicide in the United States in case you are wondering what this comment is doing in a neurology and neurosurgery publication. At least, that's my excuse.

Reference

    1. Mercy, Houk: *N Engl J Med* 319:1283–1284, Nov 10, 1988.

Neurological Abnormalities Associated With Remote Occupational Elemental Mercury Exposure
Albers JW, Kallenbach LR, Fine LJ, Langolf GD, Wolfe RA, Donofrio PD, Alessi AG, Stolp-Smith KA, Bromberg MB, Mercury Workers Study Group (Univ of Michigan)
Ann Neurol 24:651–659, November 1988   13–5

Mercury-related neurologic abnormalities were assessed in a population of 502 persons, 247 of them exposed occupationally to elemental mercury 20 to 35 years previously. Mercury was used in the plant in producing lithium 6, a weapons component.

Although there were few significant differences between the exposed and nonexposed persons, regression analysis showed significant correlations between increasing exposure, as determined by urinary mercury estimates, and deteriorating neurologic function. Subjects with peak urine mercury levels greater than 0.6 mg/L during exposure had reduced strength and coordination, impaired sensation, increased tremor, and more frequent Babinski and snout reflexes. Exposed persons with polyneuropathy had higher mercury levels than did exposed persons with normal neurologic findings. More than one fourth of those with peak levels greater than 0.85 mg/L had polyneuropathy.

Natural attrition of neurons with advancing age may unmask previously subclinical abnormalities related to exposure to elemental mercury. The present findings support a delayed, remote effect of elemental mercury on the nervous system.

▶ Information about the long-term effect of mercury has been sparse. This is quite a tour de force and represents an enormous amount of work. The authors suggest that the toxic effect of mercury may be delayed for a long period and show up years later as aging of the nervous system takes place. Some of the abnormalities were central (Babinski and snout reflexes), which the authors agree is unexplained. Tremor and polyneuropathy were the main findings.

The long-term effect of organic solvents on the nervous system are recorded by Gregersen (1). Chronic encephalopathy affecting concentration and memory were present in workers exposed 5 and 10 years previously. (See also Mikkelsen et al. [2].)

References

1. Gregersen: *Am J Ind Med* 14:681–701, 1988.
2. Mikkelsen et al: *Acta Neurol Scand (Suppl)* 78:9–143, 1988.

Port Pirie Cohort Study: Childhood Blood Lead and Neuropsychological Development at Age Two Years
Wigg NR, Vimpani GV, McMichael AJ, Baghurst PA, Robertson EF, Roberts RJ (Child Adolescent and Family Health Service, South Australia; Flinders Med Ctr; Univ of Adelaide; Commonwealth Scientific and Industrial Research Organisation [Australia]; Adelaide Children's Hosp, Adelaide, Australia)
J Epidemiol Community Health 42:213–219, September 1988   13–6

The neuropsychologic complications of acute lead encephalopathy have been well documented, but there is still uncertainty about the nature of adverse effects of lesser levels of lead exposure on the neuropsychologic development of young children. Data from the Port Pirie Cohort Study, an ongoing prospective study of the effects of environmental lead in a lead smelter community, were used to examine the relationship between blood lead concentration and child development at age 2 years.

More than 600 children underwent serial blood lead estimations until age 2 years. Interviews were done to elicit information on a range of variables, and formal developmental evaluation was done at age 24 months. Blood lead concentrations determined antenatally, at delivery, and postnatally at 6, 15, and 24 months were negatively correlated with mental development at age 24 months. At 6, 15, and 24 months of age, geometric mean blood lead concentrations were 14.3, 20.8, and 21.2 μg/dl, respectively. When covariates, including maternal IQ, were controlled for, a significant inverse relationship was noted between blood lead concentration measured at age 6 months and mental development at 2 years. There was no such association for psychomotor development. When the quality of home environment was controlled for, the inverse association between blood lead concentration at 6 months and mental development at 2 years persisted, although less strongly.

A child with a blood lead concentration of 30 μg/dl at age 6 months was estimated to have a deficit of 3.3 points (about 3%) on the Bayley Mental Development Scale compared with a child with a blood lead concentration of 10 μg/dl.

▶ This study is corrected for the mother's IQ and the quality of home environment and still finds a relationship between lead and mental function in 2-year-olds. It is hard to divorce the effects of environment and heredity in such a study, and this is a good attempt. One must conclude that lead load has something to do with mental function.

Needleman (1) says it's time we got rid of the lead in the 2 million houses where it still exists. He feels it would be cheaper in the long run to pay unemployed youths to delead the houses than to pay prison costs and institution costs for the lifetime of the children whose brains are injured by the lead paint in ghetto housing. And a note in *The Lancet* (2) about the dangers of lead from storing food in ceramic jars concludes, "The FDA recommends using glass or plastic to store food, especially if it has a high acid content (fruit juice, wine, tomato sauce, vinegar) and not using ceramic pieces that are old, made by amateurs, or purchased abroad."

References

1. Needleman: *Curr Probl Pediatr* 18:697–744, December 1988.
2. *Lancet* 2:1358, Dec 10, 1988.

Neuropsychiatric Symptoms Following Bismuth Intoxication
Weller MPI (Friern Hosp, London)
Postgrad Med J 64:308–310, 1988   13–7

Neurotic symptoms resembling those described in bismuth intoxication occurred in a patient who took a proprietary dyspeptic medication, tripotassium dicitrate bismuthate (De-Nol), over 2 years. Symptoms remitted over 10–12 months after the medication was withdrawn, a period similar to that reported in bismuth intoxication.

Man, 41, with a previously healed duodenal ulcer, took De-Nol intermittently for about 2 years. The estimated dose was 240 mg daily. Progressive numbness and paresthesias occurred in the hands, especially at night, and the patient had restless insomnia and felt uneasy. His concentration was poor, and short-term memory was markedly impaired. The paresthesias were reproduced by rolling the ulnar nerve over the medial humeral epicondyle. Symptoms resolved gradually after replacing the bismuth preparation with calcium and magnesium salts. Dyspepsia remitted rapidly, allowing antacids to be discontinued. The blue line previously noted in an area of gum surrounding a crown faded but remained present.

Prolonged use of bismuth preparations is an organic cause of apparently neurotic complaints. The patient reported feeling irritable and fatigued, and was increasingly uneasy and cognitively disabled. It is possible that an extrinsic factor such as a microorganism sometimes modifies ingested bismuth salts, converting them to a toxic substance.

▶ This reminds one of the so-called "pandemic" or neuropsychiatric symptoms reported in Japan in the 1950s, found to be caused by the use of an intestinal disinfectant, a hydroquinone derivative. When its use was outlawed the symptoms disappeared. The Japanese referred to this condition as SMON because it caused neurologic, mental, gastrointestinal, and ocular symptoms similar to the symptoms caused by long-term ingestion of this bismuth compound.— R.N. DeJong, M.D.

Emergency Department Screening for Unsuspected Carbon Monoxide Exposure
Turnbull TL, Hart RG, Strange GR, Cooper MA, Lindblad R, Watkins JM, Ferraro CM (Univ of Illinois; Mercy Hosp and Med Ctr, Chicago)
Ann Emerg Med 17:478–483, May 1988   13–8

Exposure to carbon monoxide (CO) is the leading toxic cause of death in the United States today. Because CO intoxication may present with subtle and nonspecific symptoms, its diagnosis may easily be missed (Fig 13–2). The frequency of occult CO toxicity is as yet unknown, as is the incidence and clinical significance of asymptomatic CO exposure in the general population. A 2-part study was performed to determine the validity of screening for unsuspected CO exposure in unselected patients in an emergency department.

For the first part of the study, 504 patients in the emergency department during a 15-month study period were prospectively screened with a CO breath analyzer, regardless of complaint. For nonsmokers, CO breath readings greater than 15 parts per million, which correspond to a carboxyhemoglobin (COHgb) level of 3%, were considered abnormal. For smokers, a cutoff of 48 parts per million, which corresponds to a 10% COHgb level, was selected. The second part of the study was a retrospective review of the COHgb levels of 532 patients in the emergency

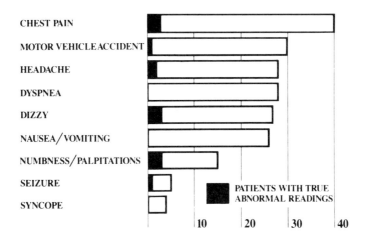

CHEST PAIN

MOTOR VEHICLE ACCIDENT

HEADACHE

DYSPNEA

DIZZY

NAUSEA/VOMITING

NUMBNESS/PALPITATIONS

SEIZURE

SYNCOPE

PATIENTS WITH TRUE ABNORMAL READINGS

10 20 30 40

NUMBER OF PATIENTS WITH COMPLAINT

Fig 13–2.—Patients with chief complaints suggestive of CO exposure. (Courtesy of Turnbull TL, Hart RG, Strange GR, et al: *Ann Emerg Med* 17:478–483, May 1988.)

department who underwent arterial blood gas analyses during the same study period.

Of 504 patients screened by CO breath analysis, 152 had complaints suggestive of CO intoxication, 8 of whom had abnormal CO breath readings. Four of these 8 patients were smokers. Of 532 patients whose blood gas values were retrospectively reviewed, 15 had abnormal CO-Hgb levels, 3 of whom were smokers. In all, only 29 (2.8%) of the 1,038 patients screened by this combined approach had abnormal CO breath readings or abnormal COHgb levels or both. The low yield obtained and the minimal clinical significance of the abnormalities found indicate that routine screening of all patients in the emergency department for unsuspected CO exposure has no practical value.

▶ The authors conclude that screening for unsuspected carbon monoxide exposure in the emergency department is not justifiable. We will just have to go back to the old intraskull computer and try to remember the symptoms of carbon monoxide intoxication before ordering the test.

Extrapyramidal and Other Neurologic Manifestations Associated With Carbon Disulfide Fumigant Exposure
Peters HA, Levine RL, Matthews CG, Chapman LJ (Univ of Wisconsin, Madison)
Arch Neurol 45:537–540, May 1988   13–9

The fumigant most often used to treat corn, wheat, rye, and other grains is a mixture of 20% carbon disulfide and 80% carbon tetrachloride. Among 21 grain storage workers who presented with neurologic symptoms, the 15 elevator grain handlers were most severely affected; 4 malt laboratory workers and 2 grain inspectors also were seen.

The patients exhibited extrapyramidal and cerebellar dysfunction, hearing loss, and peripheral neuropathy. Those most affected had an atypical parkinsonian syndrome, but voice abnormalities were absent. Seven patients had abnormal nerve conduction velocities. Nearly all patients had decreased auditory acuity. Liver function was normal in these patients. The elevator grain handlers reported smelling fumigant residues when they unloaded grain shipments or cleaned the elevator bins. Because carbon disulfide-exposed rats have marked myelin fragmentation in the central nervous system, 4 patients underwent magnetic resonance imaging and exhibited a pattern of central demyelination.

Routine environmental monitoring for neurotoxins is necessary, and less toxic solvents should be used. Workers should be trained in avoiding hazards. Those with evidence of neurotoxicity should be transferred to a work environment free of neurotoxic chemicals and should have periodic neurologic and neuropsychologic assessments.

▶ Here is another toxic cause of atypical parkinsonism with CS_2 as the culprit. The authors note that disulfuram (Antabuse) is metabolized as CS_2 and suggest a study of alcoholic persons treated with Antabuse.

Reye's Syndrome and Aspirin: Evidence for a Dose-Response Effect
Pinsky PF, Hurwitz ES, Schonberger LB, Gunn WJ (Ctr for Infectious Diseases, Atlanta)
JAMA 260:657–661, Aug 5, 1988   13–10

Previous studies indicate a strong association between Reye's syndrome and the use of salicylate in the antecedent respiratory illness or chicken pox. Dose relationships were examined by reviewing data from the Public Health Service Main Study of Reye's Syndrome and Medications. Patients at 70 pediatric tertiary-care centers were included in the study.

Care providers reported directly administering aspirin-containing medication during antecedent illness to 25 of 27 patients and 32 of 140 controls (93% vs. 23%). Patients received greater average and maximal daily doses of aspirin and higher doses on the first 4 days of the antecedent illness. The excess risk associated with increasing doses of aspirin was chiefly caused by doses of 15 to 27 mg/kg daily. The difference in dosage between exposed patients and controls was most marked on days 3 and 4 of the antecedent illness.

Larger doses of aspirin—though doses generally well below the recommended upper limit for antipyretic therapy—are associated with an increased risk of Reye's syndrome. It should be assumed that there is no safe dose of aspirin and that the best means of lowering the risk of Reye's syndrome is to avoid giving aspirin to children and adolescents with chicken pox or respiratory illness.

▶ The last sentence of the abstract says it all.

14 Treatment

The Clinical Spectrum of Alcoholic Pellagra Encephalopathy: A Retrospective Analysis of 22 Cases Studied Pathologically

Serdaru M, Hausser-Hauw C, Laplane D, Buge A, Castaigne P, Goulon M, Lhermitte F, Hauw J-J (Hôpital de la Salpêtrière, Paris; Hôpital Raymond Poincaré, Garches, France)

Brain 111:829–842, August 1988   14–1

Alcoholic pellagra was diagnosed in 22 immoderate drinkers when autopsy showed diffuse chromatolysis of neurons. All but 1 of the patients drank immoderate amounts of wine, and several were undernourished and cachectic. The most frequent clinical features were fluctuating confusion or clouding of consciousness, hypertonus, and startle myoclonus. The hypertonus was of the oppositional type and always involved the limbs. The neck was spared in 10 patients. The electroencephalogram was consistently abnormal.

Eight of 13 patients considered to have "primary onset" disease followed a catastrophic course and died during the first week. Nine others had late onset disease. All of the latter patients and 4 of those who died had received thiamine and pyridoxine but not other B vitamins.

These patients drank mainly red wine, which is a poor source of niacin. The hypertonus resembled the "gegenhalten" or counterfixation described by Kleist in connection with thalamic strokes. Five patients had changes of Wernicke-Korsakoff disease at autopsy, and 8 had evidence of Marchiafava-Bignami disease. All alcoholic persons with undiagnosed encephalopathy should receive multiple vitamin therapy.

▶ The point to this story is don't just give thiamine to the alcoholic patient: give B complex. Turn that intravenous solution to a nice yellow tint. These authors with their careful study have done us a service.

Plasmapheresis in Treatment of Human T-Lymphotropic Virus Type-I Associated Myelopathy

Matsuo H, Nakamura T, Tsujihata M, Kinoshita I, Satoh A, Tomita I, Shirabe S, Shibayama K, Nagataki S (Nagasaki Univ, Nagasaki, Japan)

Lancet 2:1109–1113, Nov 12, 1988   14–2

The pathogenesis of human T-lymphotropic virus type-1 (HTLV-1)-associated myelopathy (HAM) is thought to involve autoimmune mechanisms. Plasma exchange, which removes circulating immune or autoantibody complexes, has brought clinical improvement in some autoimmune diseases. Plasmapheresis was performed 4–6 times in 2 weeks by either plasma separation or passage through an immunoadsorbent column believed capable of selectively adsorbing HTLV-1 antibody in 18 patients with HAM and 3 controls.

Improvement in sensory status, gait, or sphincter function or some combination of these resulted in 11 patients with HAM and lasted 2–4 weeks. Time to walk a specific distance and motor function grade improved; deep tendon reflexes, clonus, and pathologic reflexes did not change. Results were similar with both plasmapheretic methods. The HTLV-1 antibody titers decreased in serum, but not in cerebrospinal fluid. Clinical improvement was not correlated with decreases in antibody titer.

These results suggest a lack of direct association between HTLV-1 antibody and the pathogenesis of HAM. It is likely that plasmapheresis indirectly affects immune mechanisms within the blood-brain barrier.

▶ This disease has been described in several nontropical locations, including Chile and, of course, Japan, and is something of a mystery. That plasmapheresis improved the patients without changing the CSF HTLV-1 antibody levels is peculiar and not understood. The authors speculate that there is something else in the serum, the removal of which benefits the patients. The improvement was not maintained.

Treatment of Narcolepsy With L-Tyrosine
Mouret J, Lemoine P, Sanchez P, Robelin N, Taillard J, Canini F (Hôpital du Vinatier, Bron; Université Claude Bernard, Lyon, France)
Lancet 2:1458–1459, Dec 24–31, 1988   14–3

Some depressed patients have polygraphic abnormalities similar to those described in Parkinson's disease. Their depression and sleep disorder responded rapidly to the dopamine agonist piribedil. If this dopamine-dependent depression (DDD) is due to loss or reduced activity of dopaminergic neurons, surviving neurons would be hyperactive, and tyrosine hydroxylase, which catalyzes conversion of tyrosine to dopa, might not be saturated by substrate. The polysomnographic abnormalities of the Parkinson's disease group were similar to those of a group of patients with narcolepsy. Oral tyrosine therefore was tried in eight narcoleptic patients.

The patients had had narcoleptic symptoms for a month or longer, including daytime sleep attacks and at least five cataleptic episodes a week. The initial dose of tyrosine was 70–80 mg/kg/day in three doses; the final daily dose averaged 100 mg/kg. All patients were free of symptoms within 6 months of the start of treatment. Repeat polygraphic recordings in five patients after a year of treatment confirmed lack of daytime sleep attacks, but nighttime rapid eye movement (REM) latency was unchanged. The stability of REM sleep had improved.

These findings suggest an abnormal dopaminergic system in narcolepsy. Tyrosine may offer a valuable approach to the treatment of this disorder. As in DDD, the dose should be increased if a patient is exposed to physical or mental stress. The addition of vitamin B_6 rapidly counters the benefit from tyrosine.

▶ I find in my vitamin catalog that L-tyrosine is available in 500-mg tablets for about 9¢ each, so this treatment should cost less than $1.00 a day. The authors say all of the patients improved but it took a long time. I trust this study will be done in a blind fashion, and I hope that the authors' optimism is proved. We need a better treatment for narcolepsy.

Double-Blind Controlled Trials of Cronassial in Chronic Neuromuscular Diseases and Ataxia
Bradley WG, Badger GJ, Tandan R, Fillyaw MJ, Young J, Fries TJ, Krusinski PB, Witarsa M, Boerman J, Blair CJ (Univ of Vermont, Burlington)
Neurology 38:1731–1739, November 1988   14–4

Three 1-year double-blind studies compared purified bovine brain gangliosides (Cronassial) in daily intramuscular doses of 40 and 100 mg, with placebo in patients with chronic neuromuscular disorders. Function was assessed each month in 30 patients with Charcot-Marie-Tooth disease, 16 with idiopathic polyneuropathy, and 30 with spinocerebellar degeneration. Twenty-one other patients with various peripheral nerve and spinocerebellar degenerative disorders participated in a 6-month open study of 100 mg Cronassial daily.

The overall findings fail to demonstrate that Cronassial is therapeutically effective. Many measures improved significantly during prolonged placebo administration. Compliance with treatment exceeded 90%. Five of the 37 measures used in the studies were more than 70% likely to detect a 20% difference in the rate of progression of disease.

These and other recent studies of Cronassial indicate that treatment with doses up to 100 mg daily is ineffective in patients with chronic neuromuscular disorders.

▶ Another proposed medication bites the dust in the treatment of these difficult, progressive, and mostly hereditary disorders. The gangliosides do work in equivalent doses in lower animals by increasing peripheral nerve regeneration. One might have expected some effect in the peripheral neuropathy group, but none was shown.

Successful Treatment of Massive Carbamazepine Overdose
Sethna M, Solomon G, Cedarbaum J, Kutt H (Cornell Univ, New York)
Epilepsia 30:71–73, 1989   14–5

An overdose of carbamazepine (CBZ) can be fatal. A patient who experienced near-lethal drug toxicity resulting from delayed CBZ absorption is studied.

Woman, 36, with a long history of complex partial seizures for which she had been treated with CBZ and phenobarbital was admitted with coma, hypotension, and involuntary movements. The patient had become detached and withdrawn 5 hours before admission. On admission, her systolic blood pressure was 80 mm Hg and her heart rate was 60. She had sluggish pupillary and corneal reflexes, and caloric responses were absent. The patient was intubated and given dopamine. Gastric lavage revealed no pill fragments. She was given 130 gm of activated charcoal and a bottle of magnesium citrate. Nine hours after admission, her serum CBZ level was 36.0 mg/L, with a carbamazepine epoxide (CBZ-E) level of 25.3 mg/L. During the first hospital day, her CBZ and CBZ-E levels remained high, and she became increasingly ill. At 36 hours after admission, her CBZ level had dropped to 27.6 mg/L and her CBZ-E level was 16.0 mg/L. However, within hours both levels rose again sharply, suggesting renewed drug absorption. She was given additional activated charcoal. As she had passed no stools since admission, vigorous catharsis was initiated. Within hours, she passed a large stool, then continuous diarrhea developed. Roving eye movements were noted 3 hours after the onset of diarrhea; 2 hours thereafter, she grimaced to pain. She was fully alert within 8 hours after the onset of diarrhea. Her CBZ level 7 hours later was 13.6 mg/L. The patient had a rapid and complete recovery. Although she eventually admitted to a suicide attempt, she was unable to recall how many pills she had swallowed.

Carbamazepine toxicity is best treated by immediate gastric lavage, instillation of activated charcoal, and aggressive intestinal purging until the intoxication is cleared. This approach helps prevent continued absorption of the drug, late exacerbation of symptoms, and a potentially fatal outcome.

▶ My emergency room and dialysis friends knew this was the way to treat carbamazepine overdosage, but I did not. The way to get it out of the body is to grab it with charcoal and rush it through the gut.

Treatment of Focal Dystonias of the Hand With Botulinum Toxin Injections

Cohen LG, Hallett M, Geller BD, Hochberg F (Natl Inst of Neurological and Communicative Disorders and Stroke, Bethesda, Md; Harvard Med School)
J Neurol Neurosurg Psychiatry 52:355–363, March 1989   14–6

Botulinum toxin injection has proved helpful in treating focal dystonias of the eyes, larynx, and neck. This approach was used to treat hand cramps in patients with a diagnosis of writer's or musician's cramp and no apparent peripheral nerve or cervical root abnormality. Nineteen patients with a mean age of 46 years were included. Symptoms had been present for 7 years on the average. Dystonia was a feature in 12 patients. Toxin was injected into the belly of target muscles under electromyographic monitoring of active and passive movements, initially in a dose less than 20 units.

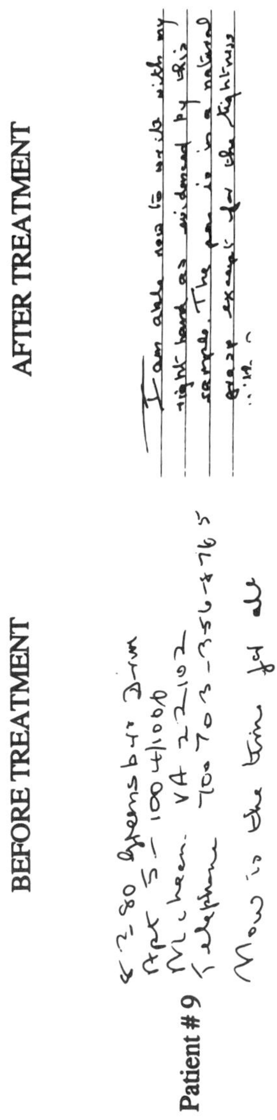

Fig 14–1.—Example of handwriting before and after successful treatment with botulinum toxin in patient with dystonic writer's cramp. The patient had serious difficulties in writing more than 3 to 4 lines because of intense muscle spasms producing pain in the forearm (see interruption in the fifth line of pretreatment writing). After treatment, her handwriting, improved, was smoother, and allowed her to write without experiencing prolonged muscle spasms. (Courtesy of Cohen LG, Hallett M, Geller BD, et al: *J Neurol Neurosurg Psychiatry* 52:355–363, March 1989.)

Subjective functional improvement ensued in 16 patients. Handwriting became more legible in most of the patients with writer's cramp (Fig 14–1), and the musicians were able to play better. Improvement always was accompanied by weakness. Some patients remained improved for as long as 6 months, whereas others required monthly injections of toxin. The only systemic "side effect" was the development of antibodies in 2 patients that precluded a further clinical response.

Botulinum toxin holds promise for use in treating hand cramps. It is necessary in each patient to reach a balance between enough weakness to reduce spasm but not so much as to impede function.

▶ The benefits seem to be unrelated to the weakness produced and last longer than one would expect.

A review on the botulinum toxin treatment of cranial dystonia, blepharospasm, and hemifacial spasm by Kraft and Lang (1) is up to date and comprehensive. They draw their conclusions nòt only from the literature but from their own large series and point out the essentially benign nature of the treatment and the high degree of effectiveness. Eighty percent to 90% achieve excellent relief lasting for an average of 3–4 months.

Reference

1. Kraft, Lang: *Can Med Assoc J* 139:837–844, Nov 1, 1988.

Clinical and Laboratory Characteristics of Focal Laryngeal Dystonia: Study of 110 Cases
Blitzer A, Brin MF, Fahn S, Lovelace RE (Columbia-Presbyterian Med Ctr, New York)
Laryngoscope 98:636–640, June 1988   14–7

Spastic dysphonia is a syndrome that often produces a strained, strangled speech. In a study of 1,280 patients with dystonia, 110 (8.7%) had vocal cord involvement. Of the 110 patients, 73 (66%) had dystonia and 37 (34%) had secondary dystonia. Those patients with primary dystonia were predominantly women; the mean age of onset was 34.6 years. Of the patients in the primary group, 8 (11%) had abductor laryngeal dystonia. In the primary group, the dysphonia was focal in 26 (31%) patients, segmental cranial in 8 (25%), and generalized in 16 (23%). There was a family history of dystonia in 17 (25%) patients with primary dystonia. The dysphonia spread to other parts of the body in 6 (19%) of the 32 patients who had dysphonia as an initial symptom. Electromyography showed that 23% of patients had irregular tremor activity, 17% had enlarged potentials, and 11% had polyphasic potentials.

Patients had previously failed or responded poorly to previous speech or psychotherapy, including biofeedback. Most of the adductor patients had failed therapy or had poor responses to anticholinergics, antiparkinsonian medication, or tranquilizers; 2 abductor patients had a good response to anticholinergics. Botulinum toxin injections were uniformly successful in the 34 patients who were injected, with a 50% to 100% improvement.

Spastic dysphonia must be classified as a dystonia that may be focal or a component of generalized or segmental disease. Electromyographic studies are of value in defining tremor activity. A diagnosis of laryngeal dystonia must be followed by patient counseling because of the possibility that the disease will spread and on the need for follow-up.

▶ This particular neurologic syndrome was believed no so long ago to be hysterical, and it's pleasing to note that it is now universally considered an organic dystonia. The authors find that botulinum toxin is effective, as did Miller, Woodson, and Jankovic (1) a year earlier.

Reference

> 1. Miller, Woodson, Jankovic: *Arch Otolaryngol Head Neck Surg* 113:603–605, 1987.

Controlled Trial of Botulinum Toxin Injections in the Treatment of Spasmodic Torticollis
Gelb DJ, Lowenstein DH, Aminoff MJ (Univ of California, San Francisco)
Neurology 39:80–84, January 1989   14–8

Most drugs used in the treatment of torticollis are beneficial in some patients. A controlled trial of botulinum toxin injections in patients with spasmodic torticollis was done.

Local injections of botulinum toxin were administered to 20 patients. Each patient received 4 sets of injections, consisting of 3 different doses of botulinum toxin and 1 placebo. The sessions were randomly ordered. Subjective improvement to at least 1 dose of botulinum toxin was reported by 80% of the patients. Improvement was substantial in 55%. There was no objective benefit. Side effects were transient and minor, but dysphagia occurred in 4 patients. Some patients stated that the effect of the injection waned despite persistent relaxation or even flaccidity of previously overactive muscles, which suggests a change in the pattern of muscle activity after botulinum toxin administration.

In this series, local injections of botulinum toxin produced subjective improvement in 55% to 80% of patients who had torticollis. The objective benefit was more difficult to assess. Side effects were usually minor and transient, although there were 4 patients with dysphagia. The pattern of muscle activity in torticollis may change after injection; thus, subsequent injection sites may need to be adjusted.

▶ Allowing for difficulty in judging movement disorders in a brief clinical contact, the authors note that the patients' subjective analysis of improvement may be more valid than the objective. They did include a placebo injection, and although no statistical difference between the placebo and the botulinum toxin could be found, the figures tend to support a less than significant benefit.

Patient Evaluations of Low Back Pain Care From Family Physicians and Chiropractors
Cherkin DC, MacCornack FA (Univ of Washington, Seattle; Univ of Northern Colorado, Greeley)
West J Med 150:351–355, March 1989   14–9

TABLE 1.—Patients' Perception of Providers' Concern*

Patients' Perception	Patients of Family Physicians,[†] %	Patients of Chiropractors,[†] %
Amount of time provider spent listening to my description of pain (very satisfied)	28	53
Provider seemed to believe that my pain was real (strongly agree)	38	71
Provider understood my concerns about the cause of my pain (strongly agree)	25	55
Provider's concern about my pain after the office visit (very satisfied)	20	58

*All comparisons are significant at $P < .05$.
†Sample sizes range from 211 to 215 for family physician patients and from 239 to 240 for chiropractor patients.
(Courtesy of Cherkin DC, MacCornack FA: West J Med 150:351–355, March 1989.)

Chiropractors care for a large proportion of patients with low back pain, but little is known about the relative cost or effectiveness of chiropractic vs. allopathic or osteopathic care in the treatment of low back pain. Patients' evaluations of their care from family physicians and chiropractors were compared.

Questionnaires were sent to 268 enrollees in a health maintenance organization who had been treated for low back pain by family physicians and 257 patients who had been cared for by a chiropractor for their low back problems. All patients were asked to rate the care they had received from their respective care providers on a 5-point rating scale.

Sixty-six percent of the chiropractor-treated patients but only 22% of

TABLE 2.—Patients' Perception of Providers' Confidence and Comfort Managing Low Back Pain*

Patients' Perception	Patients of Family Physicians, %	Patients of Chiropractors, %
Provider seemed confident that the diagnosis s/he gave me was correct (strongly agree)	23	60
Provider seemed confident that the treatment s/he recommended would work (strongly agree)	23	61
Provider seemed comfortable dealing with my back pain (strongly agree)	17	59

*All comparisons are significant at $P < .05$. Sample sizes range from 208 to 214 for family physician patients and from 239 to 240 for chiropractor patients.
(Courtesy of Cherkin DC, MacCornack FA: West J Med 150:351–355, March 1989.)

the family physician-treated patients were very satisfied with the care they had received for their low back pain. Patients of chiropractors were also much more likely to have been satisfied with the amount of information provided about the cause of their back pain and to have the perception that their care giver was concerned about them. They were more confident and comfortable in dealing with their problem than were patients of family physicians (Tables 1 and 2). Furthermore, the mean number of days that patients treated by family physicians were unable to perform their normal activities was 39.7, compared with 10.8 days for patients treated by chiropractors. The reasons that patients rated the care received from chiropractors so much higher were not determined. Perhaps some of the specific chiropractic therapies (e.g., spinal manipulation) benefit a good number of patients. However, the findings strongly suggest that the therapeutic effect of the patient-provider interaction itself may greatly influence the outcome of care.

▶ For some reason everybody on whom I have tried the question, "A study was done of patient satisfaction with chiropractors versus physicians in the care of low back pain: who do you think the patients liked the most?" guessed correctly that the chiropractor was perceived as a source of greater satisfaction than the physician. Are we to understand that the chiropractor gives better care for back pain? I am told it is the most common neurologic condition. Maybe we should try to find out what we are not doing or doing wrong.

Clinical Trial of Intensive Muscle Training for Chronic Low Back Pain
Manniche C, Hesselsøe G, Bentzen L, Christensen I, Lundberg E (Univ of Copenhagen)
Lancet 2:1473–1476, Dec 24–31, 1988   14–10

A total of 105 patients with chronic low back pain but no signs of lumbar nerve root compression and no x-ray evidence of spondylolysis or osteomalacia were enrolled in an evaluation of intensive back extensor exercises. The study group (C) performed 30 sessions of dynamic back extensor exercises over 3 months; a placebo group (B) entered a similar program at one fifth exercise intensity. An alternative group (A) used thermotherapy, massage, and mild exercises for 1 month.

Patient responses indicated that the study regimen was superior to both the alternative and placebo programs (Fig 14–2). Pain scores improved significantly with both exercise regimens but not with alternative management.

Intensive back exercises, which can be conducted in groups, are a cost-effective approach to chronic low back pain. It is not clear whether improvement is due to back muscle training or to hyperextension exercises. Clinical and radiologic assessments should precede training. Initially the physiotherapist may deal with 2 or 3 patients, but after some weeks less

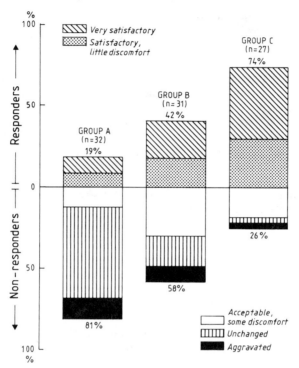

Fig 14–2.—Patients' evaluation after treatment. (Courtesy of Manniche C, Hesselsøe G, Bentzen L, et al: *Lancet* 2:1473–1476, Dec 24–31, 1988.)

supervision will suffice. Theoretically, treatment should probably continue indefinitely.

▶ I am taken with this study. An old friend, a neurologist on the West Coast, tells me we are missing the boat by not manipulating spines as he is doing. Our present treatment of back pain is certainly next to useless. It looks from this study as though intensive exercise as was carried out here is the answer. "Intensive" is a correct characterization. Each one of the exercises in group C was done 100 times per treatment session, with 30 sessions given over a 3-month period. Their results are impressive.

15 Miscellaneous Topics

Effect of Melatonin on Jet Lag After Long Haul Flights

Petrie K, Conaglen JV, Thompson L, Chamberlain K (Waikato Hosp, Hamilton; Air New Zealand, Auckland; Massay Univ, Palmerston North, New Zealand)
Br Med J 298:705–707, March 18, 1989
15–1

Jet lag is a common problem for air travelers who pass through several time zones. It apparently reflects the time needed to resynchronize the body's circadian rhythm to the new night-day cycle. Melatonin, normally secreted by the pineal gland at night in a 24-hour cycle, may act to synchronize several body rhythms. The effects of melatonin were studied in 20 adult volunteers who went through 12 time zones while flying from Auckland to London. The volunteers took 5 mg of melatonin orally in gelatin lactose or a placebo for 3 days before departure, during the flight, and 3 days after arrival. The alternative medication was used on the return trip.

Jet lag retrospective ratings were consistently higher in persons taking placebo than in those taking melatonin (Fig 15–1). Jet lag symptoms were more severe on the westward return journey than on the outward trip traveling east.

Melatonin appears to be a useful remedy for relieving the effects of jet lag experienced after transcontinental flights. However, whether it is necessary to take melatonin before and during the flight or only afterward remains to be determined.

▶ The authors conclude that melatonin may reset the biologic clock and thus make it easier to adjust on arrival. Arendt (1) and Meyer and Theron (2) have

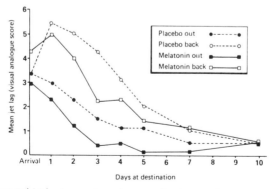

Fig 15–1.–Reported jet lag in experimental groups after journeys from Auckland to London and back, measured on visual analogue scale (*0* = none, *10* = extreme). (Courtesy of Petrie K, Conaglen JV, Thompson L, et al: *Br Med J* 298:705–707, March 18, 1989.)

provided a review of melatonin and the pineal for those interested. Speaking of flying, there have been several recent letters in *The Lancet* about the leg thrombophlebitis that occurs commonly as a result of sitting for long periods on such flights. Various writers have given hints to prevent it. Included are getting up and walking in the aisle regularly, exercising legs in place if that is not possible, forgoing smoking and alcoholic drinks but keeping up fluid intake with nonalcoholic liquids, and perhaps taking an aspirin or two.

References

1. Arendt: *Clin Endocrinol* 29:205–229, 1988.
2. Meyer, Theron: *S Afr Med J* 73:300–302, 1988.

The Use of Extracorporeal Rewarming in a Child Submerged for 66 Minutes
Bolte RG, Black PG, Bowers RS, Thorne JK, Corneli HM (Primary Children's Med Ctr, Salt Lake City)
JAMA 260:377–379, July 15, 1988   15–2

Submersion injury is a significant cause of morbidity and death in children and young adults. Previous reports have described neurologically intact survival after submersion in cold water for as long as 45 minutes. A good neurologic outcome was achieved in a young child who was submerged in cold water for at least 66 minutes.

Girl, 2.5 years, fell into a creek that had a water temperature of about 5C. A sibling saw her fall into the water and immediately told their mother, who searched for the girl for 4–10 minutes before calling emergency personnel. The emergency team arrived within 8 minutes of the call. Sixty-two minutes later, the child was found. She was cyanotic, apneic, and flaccid with fixed, dilated pupils, and no palpable pulse. Cardiopulmonary resuscitation was begun. On arrival to the emergency room, the child's rectal temperature was 22.4C. Core rewarming was begun, but active external rewarming techniques were withheld. About 3 hours after the girls had fallen into the creek, extracorporeal rewarming (ECR) was instituted. The ECR circuit consisted of a membrane oxygenator system with a pediatric heat exchanger. A warming gradient of 10C was maintained between perfusate and core body temperature until a perfusate temperature of 38C was achieved. Medications given while the bypass system was in place included heparin, mannitol, calcium chloride, and sodium bicarbonate. When the child's core temperature reached 25C, a single spontaneous gasp and fine ventricular fibrillation were seen. She opened her eyes spontaneously a few minutes later, and her pupils became reactive. Her neurologic recovery was gradual but steady. One year after the incident, she was functioning at her age level and had a progressively improving tremor.

A coordinated response by the emergency medical team with the hospital-based personnel is essential for such patients.

▶ This child was immersed in very cold water—a runoff from a snow bank near Salt Lake City—and was apparently dead when pulled from the water more than an hour after she fell in. Amazing was the way she recovered neurologic function over a period of many weeks. She had cortical blindness for 7 weeks. Her longest incapacity was a tremor that interfered with fine motor function, but within 12 months after submersion she was functioning at her age level and the tremor was improving. I guess one should never give up.

Clinical Neuropsychiatric and Neuromuscular Manifestations in Systemic Lupus Erythematosus
Omdal R, Mellgren SI, Husby G (Univ Hosp of Tromsø, Norway)
Scand J Rheumatol 17:113–117, 1988   15–3

The importance of neurologic involvement in serum lupus erythematosus (SLE) is widely recognized. Neuropsychiatric disorders are common, and neuromuscular manifestations, less so. The incidence of neuropsychiatric and neuromuscular manifestations from the onset of SLE in 30 patients was sought by retrospective study and clinical neurologic examination in 30 patients.

Neuropsychiatric manifestations were seen in 83% of patients during the course of illness. Migraine was the most commonly found symptom, occurring in 40% of patients, followed by cephalalgia in 20%, vertigo in 20%, and psychiatric disorders in 17%. Amaurosis fugax occurred in 10% of patients as did epileptic fits, which occurred when the disease was most active. Other central nervous system manifestations were less common. The most frequent neuromuscular manifestations were carpal tunnel syndrome and muscular weakness, both occurring in 23% of patients, and myositis, occurring in 10% of patients.

These data confirm the frequency of neuropsychiatric manifestations in SLE; the incidence in this study is higher than that of previous studies. Because there are no specific means of diagnosing SLE in neuromuscular or central nervous system tissue, it is difficult to account for the various neurologic symptoms that frequently occurred with SLE. Further research is necessary to solve the diagnostic, pathogenetic, and therapeutic problems in this area of rheumatology.

▶ It sounds as though the majority of patients in this study had central nervous system involvement if one includes 12 with migraine, 6 with cephalalgia, and 6 with vertigo.

There were 5 with psychiatric disorders, 3 with epilepsy, and others with clear neurologic syndromes in the series. The patients with lupus that I see don't have so many disorders of the central or peripheral nervous system, but that may be only an impression. O'Connor in a recent review (1) of the sensitivity and specificity of diagnostic tests for CNS lupus finds the specificity of all tests to be low but the sensitivity of some, particularly MRI scanning and CSF studies, to be high.

Reference

1. O'Connor: *Can J Neurol Sci* 15:257–260, 1988.

Non-Traumatic Ischaemic Myelopathy: A Review of 25 Cases
Kim SW, Kim RC, Choi BH, Gordon SK (Univ of California, Irvine; VA Med Ctr, Long Beach, Calif)
Paraplegia 26:262–272, August 1988   15–4

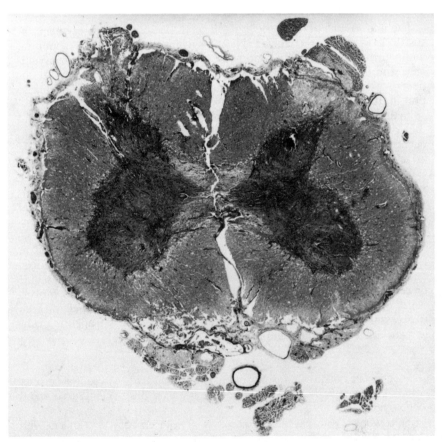

Fig 15–2.—Low-power photomicrograph of spinal cord at L5, showing sharply circumscribed areas of hemorrhagic necrosis that are almost exclusively confined to the gray matter (Masson trichome stain, original magnification, ×14). (Courtesy of Kim SW, Kim RC, Choi BH, et al: *Paraplegia* 26:262–272, August 1988.)

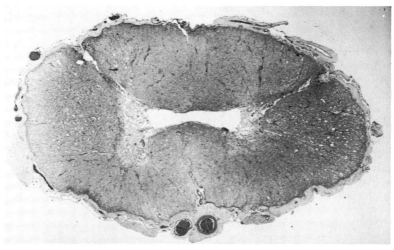

Fig 15–3.—Low-power photomicrograph of spinal cord at L3, showing cavitary necrosis within the gray matter. At this level, the white matter is largely spared (hematoxylin-eosin stain; original magnification, ×16). (Courtesy of Kim SW, Kim RC, Choi BH, et al: *Paraplegia* 26:262–272, August 1988.)

The various ways in which circulatory dysfunction can produce spinal cord damage were examined in a series of 25 men with ischemic myelopathy who were among 1,535 patients admitted to a cord injury service at a VA Center during 1971–1986.

Myelopathy developed in 9 patients after surgical cross-clamping or

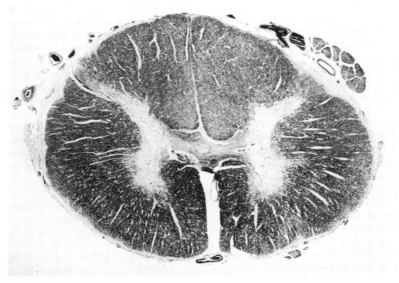

Fig 15–4.—Low-power photomicrograph of spinal cord at L2, showing extensive necrosis of gray matter. Note the sparing of the commissural gray (Kluver-Barrera stain; original magnification, ×18). (Courtesy of Kim SW, Kim RC, Choi BH, et al: *Paraplegia* 26:262–272, August 1988.)

traumatic laceration of the aorta (Fig 15–2). Most of these patients had surgery for aneurysm or traumatic aortic laceration. Four patients had some recovery of function, but in only 1 patient was this significant. Another patient had myelopathy after intercostal artery ligation. Myelopathy developed in 3 patients after aortic aneurysmal dissection (Fig 15–3). Myelopathy followed myocardial infarction or cardiac arrest in 2 other patients (Fig 15–4). Seven patients had spinal vascular disease of unknown origin; the 3 remaining patients had decompression sickness.

Acute spinal cord ischemia secondary to generalized impairment of perfusion tends to damage gray matter the most and to produce a flaccid lower motor neuron type of weakness. Localized impairment of flow may produce cord infarction in the region of a particular vessel. Damage to white matter is more likely to produce an incomplete spastic upper motor neuron type of weakness.

▶ As expected, those with incomplete motor and sensory loss recovered better. Myelopathy following aortic aneurysm dissection had the worst prognosis.

A Case-Control Study of Transient Global Amnesia

Guidotti M, Anzalone N, Morabito A, Landi G (Univ of Milan)
J Neurol Neurosurg Psychiatry 52:320–323, February 1989   15–5

The prevalence of cerebrovascular risk factors and the prognosis of transient global amnesia (TGA) were examined in 30 patients with a first episode of TGA (group 1), 30 with a first transient ischemic attack (TIA; group 2), and 30 with depressive neurosis (group 3). The groups were matched for age and sex.

Most group 1 patients were in good health at the time of the episode, but 90% of them had risk factors for cerebrovascular disease (table).

Cerebrovascular Risk Factors: Odds Ratio and 95% Confidence Limits

	Group 1 (n = 30)	Group 2 (n = 30)	Group 3 (n = 30)	Odds ratio Group 1 vs 2	Odds ratio Group 1 vs 3
Hypertension	14	14	5	1 (– – – – – –) $p = 1$	4·37 (1·37 – 13·93) $p = 0·013$
Smoking	8	8	3	1 (– – – – – –) $p = 1$	3·27 (0·81 – 13·17) $p = 0·1$
Hyperlipidemia	10	9	5	1·16 (0·39 – 3·46) $p = 0·78$	2·5 (0·75 – 8·34) $p = 0·14$
Diabetes mellitus	3	8	1	0·30 (0·07 – 1·23) $p = 0·1$	3·22 (0·35 – 29·53) $p = 0·30$
Cardiopathy	7	11	1	0·52 (0·17 – 1·60) $p = 0·26$	8·8 (1·35 – 57·44) $p = 0·02$

(Courtesy of Guidotti M, Anzalone N, Morabito A, et al: *J Neurol Neurosurg Psychiatry* 52:320–323, February 1989.)

Most attacks occurred during exertion or emotional stress. All patients had normal neurologic findings and all except 2 had normal findings on electroencephalography. The computed tomographic study also was normal in all except 2 patients, and hemodynamically significant stenoses were not seen on Doppler studies. Five patients had TIAs on follow-up. All except 1 of the group 2 patients had cerebrovascular risk factors. Computed tomography examination showed hemispheric lesions in 23% of these patients. Four patients had recurrent TIA and 2 had a stroke during follow-up; none had TGA. About half of the group 3 patients had atherosclerotic risk factors. None of these patients had stroke or TGA during a mean follow-up of about 3 years.

Transient global amnesia is an ischemic event that is triggered not by thromboembolism but by a different, possibly vasospastic, mechanism. The occurrence of TGA in patients without a history of vascular pathology does not necessarily warrant antithrombotic treatment.

▶ It appears we are gradually closing in on this mysterious disorder. These authors compare a group of transient global amnesic patients with a group of TIA patients and a control group of depressed patients in terms of risk factors. The risk factors for the TGA and the TIA groups were similar, but the outlook for the TGA patients was much more benign. They wonder, therefore, whether the TGA cause is vasospasm rather than thromboembolism with both syndromes related to cerebrovascular disease. A TIA of a different sort. Why does it have to be spasm? How about a focal low flow phenomenon without spasm?

Distant Referral of Cutaneous Sensation (Mitempfindung): Observations on Its Normal and Pathological Occurrence

Schott GD (Natl Hosp for Nervous Diseases, London)
Brain 111:1187–1198, October 1988   15–6

The phenomenon in which a scratch or other innocuous stimulus of a small cutaneous area simultaneously produces a painful sensation at a distant but ipsilateral part of the body has long been known as Mitempfindung. A review of the literature shows that the clinical features vary somewhat but occur only among certain healthy persons.

The cutaneous sensation was referred for the first time to a part of the body that was already damaged and painful because of postherpetic neuralgia, neuralgic amyotrophy, or probable postganglionic sensory plexopathy in 4 patients. The phenomenon was transient in 3 of the 4 patients; in other respects, it was typical of Mitempfindung.

Central factors appear to be involved in this phenomenon. The most likely pathway is the spinocervical tract because its axons run ipsilaterally; its cells sometimes are activated by noxious stimuli with input from A-alpha and beta, A-delta and C fibers; and the pathway is variable in human beings.

These data indicate that Mitempfindung may be acquired; its mechanisms remain unknown. Its subjective, evanescent nature, its tendency to occur while the person's attention is focused on something else, and its failure to have any objective signs hinder the study of this curiosity.

▶ This phenomenon is harmless and peculiar. Until I read the article I thought that I was the only person in the world with it, but it has been studied for more than a century.

At one time I charted all of my stimulus and response sites, thinking there must be a clear relationship between the 2 that could be charted to calculate the dermatomal distances. The study is still under way. The phenomenon could be hard wired into the cord, and the authors speculate that it may be carried by the spinocervical pathway. It serves no useful purpose as far as is known but may have, at one time, in our ancestors.

Criteria for Termination of Phase II Chemotherapy for Patients With Progressive or Recurrent Brain Tumor
Friedman HS, Schold SC Jr, Djang WT, Kurtzberg J, Longee DC, Halperin EC, Falletta JM, Coleman RE, Oakes WJ (Duke Univ)
Neurology 39:62–66, January 1989   15–7

Patients with a recurrent or progressive brain tumor ordinarily receive phase II chemotherapy until disease progresses or unacceptable toxicity occurs. In 6 cases regression of primary brain tumor in response to phase II chemotherapy was followed by prolonged stability of disease, prompting termination of therapy.

The patients had progressive tumor in the thalamus, hypothalamus, frontal lobe, or pons when they began phase II chemotherapy. After treatment from 21 to 36 months, contrast-enhancing lesions remained on computed tomography. The 3 patients who underwent positron emission tomography with fluorodeoxyglucose demonstrated hypometabolic lesions. The patients remained well from 24 to more than 57 months after treatment was ended, with no evidence of progressive disease.

Patients with a surgically accessible lesion that is clinically and radiographically stable for 1 year after radiographic evidence of tumor regression from phase II chemotherapy should be considered for histologic analysis and possible resection. If the lesion is not accessible for biopsy or surgery, therapy should be terminated and the patient should be followed closely.

▶ To old timers like me who think of astrocytomas as inevitably fatal, this new concept of control with chemotherapy is exciting and wonderful. No doubt the day will come when these will be as controllable as other forms of cancer are becoming. The sooner the better.

NEUROSURGERY

ROBERT M. CROWELL, M.D.

Introduction

The year 1989 brought a further wealth of new development in neuro-surgery. *DIAGNOSTICS* was again dominated by **magnetic resonance imaging** (MRI), which is helpful for acute intracranial hemorrhage, but the complexity of signals requires additional information from standard computed tomography (Abstract 16–1). Magnetic resonance may be used to study patients with aneurysm clips in place, provided they are nonferromagnetic (Abstract 16–2). Low flip-angle gradient images (GRASS) are extremely helpful in the evaluation of large intracranial aneurysms (Abstract 16–3) and cervical radiculopathy (Abstract 16–4). Magnetic resonance imaging spectroscopy holds great promise for the analysis of metabolic changes in brain tumors (Abstract 16–5). **Biochemical studies** for diagnosis include serum sialic acid for the diagnosis of intracranial tumors (Abstract 16–6), and histopathologic crush preparations, which are helpful for frozen section evaluation (Abstract 16–7).

Electrophysiologic studies have been advanced, including brain stem auditory evoked potentials, which improve results in posterior fossa surgery (Abstract 16–8). Motor action potentials show great promise for intraoperative monitoring (Abstract 16–9). **Other diagnostic techniques** include positron emission tomography, which appears to offer assistance in prognosis for patients with intracranial glioma (Abstract 16–10). Laser-Doppler flowmetry is a new technique for intraoperative measurement of cerebral and tumor regional blood flow (Abstract 16–11).

In **TECHNIQUES,** a number of signal advances occurred in 1989. Histologic studies demonstrate that the Nd:YAG laser may shrink arteriovenous malformations, thus assisting the surgeon (Abstract 17–2). Stereotactic techniques have advanced in dramatic fashion. Stereotactic guidance during open surgery of the brain may assist in the localization of small deep-seated lesions (Abstract 17–3). Lawrence Berkeley Laboratory reports good results in the obliteration of arteriovenous malformations (AVMs) with helium radiosurgery (Abstract 17–4). Postoperative MRI appears to demonstrate obliteration of the lesion, but complications including cerebral infarction in some patients have been reported (Abstract 17–5). The linear accelerator has been adapted for use as a stereotactic radiosurgical device (Abstract 17–6). Results are encouraging to date, and the wide availability of linear accelerator suggests future proliferation. However, the complexity of these methods and their potential risks demand a skilled team including a stereotactic surgeon, physicist, and radiation physician.

Improved open **surgical approaches** include exposure and entry into the cavernous sinus. Tumor removal from this area has been reported with good success (Abstract 17–7), and cavernous aneurysms have also been exposed for surgical obliteration (Abstract 17–8). Several surgeons have described promising supratentorial and infratentorial approaches to the petrous apex for removal of skull base tumors (Abstracts 17–9 and 17–10). With such refined microsurgery, the results are so good as to warrant consideration of surgical attack in the cavernous sinus and clival area, both previously fraught with hazard.

In the area of CNS *TUMORS,* considerable progress has been made. Primary central nervous system lymphoma is becoming increasingly common (Abstract 18–1). A new system of grading astrocytomas has been offered (Abstract 18–2). Extracellular matrix proteins and gene amplification have been identified in intracranial gliomas (Abstracts 18–3 and 18–4). *Magnetic resonance imaging* studies indicate good correlation between MRI patterns and histologic evidence of tumor invasion (Abstract 18–5). Magnetic resonance imaging does not always image pituitary microadenomas, indicating a continuing need for petrosal sinus sampling in some cases (Abstract 18–6). Magnetic resonance imaging may be used to detect cavernous sinus invasion and carotid encasement (Abstract 18–7). Magnetic resonance imaging can predict some histopathologic features (Abstract 18–8). Cranial MRI can be used to detect a host of lesions in central neurofibromatosis (Abstract 18–9). Magnetic resonance and CT appear to have complimentary roles in the evaluation of clival chordomas and chondrosarcomas (Abstract 18–10). Magnetic resonance provides good images of hemorrhagic intracranial neoplasms, but occasionally angiography or even biopsy are needed to clinch the diagnosis (Abstract 18–11). Myelography and CT are superior to MRI for the detection of spinal meningeal carcinomatosis (Abstract 18–12).

As regards *surgery* for tumors, the Sloan-Kettering group reports low mortality and morbidity for total excision of supratentorial gliomas, bolstering the philosophy of total excision (Abstract 18–13). On the other hand, Lunsford and colleagues report excellent results with stereotactic biopsy of malignant gliomas followed by radiotherapy without cytoreductive surgery (Abstract 18–14). Thus, both the aggressive and conservative philosophies of management of gliomas continue to find adherents and supportive data. Surgical management of intraorbital meningiomas has been discussed (Abstract 18–15), and radiation has been recommended for many of these cases. Results of transsphenoidal microsurgery for somatotropic pituitary adenomas are excellent, and postoperative radiation is warranted only in selected instances (Abstract 18–16). Trigeminal schwannoma can often be excised largely or wholly with good clinical outcome (Abstract 18–18). Epidermoid tumors may also be excised with good results, though in certain critical locations adherent capsule should be left behind to avoid injury to the delicate neural structures (Abstract 18–19).

Adjunctive therapy of tumors has also been advanced. Preoperative irradiation of highly vascular cerebellopontine angle neurinomas has been advocated, with conversion of extremely hemorrhagic tumors into more manageable lesions (Abstract 18–20). Malignant melanoma treated with radiotherapy in the brain yields poor results (Abstract 18–21). Interstitial brachytherapy for metastatic brain tumors has posted encouraging but as yet inconclusive results (Abstract 18–22). Systemic interferon-γ was ineffective in the treatment of recurrent glioma (Abstract 18–23). Adoptive immunotherapy is promising for the treatment of recurrent glioblastoma (Abstracts 18–24 and 18–25). Experimental studies show that opening the blood-brain barrier may assist in delivery of immunotherapy to brain tumors. Preoperative treatment of acromegaly with a long-acting somatostatin analogue has been shown to shrink pituitary macroadenomas (Abstract 18–27).

Management methods for *VASCULAR* diseases are in rapid evolution. In the area of *ischemia,* the most dramatic changes have to do with the decrease in the performance of carotid endarterectomies, with a dramatic 22% decline in 1986 (Abstract 19–1). Scientifically established indications for this procedure must await conclusion of appropriately controlled clinical trials. In the meantime, it is probably best to restrict utilization of the procedure to symptomatic patients with hemodynamically significant lesions operated by surgeons with morbidity and mortality less than 4%. In a related study, 53 patients at the University of Iowa aged 70 years or more underwent carotid endarterectomy with excellent surgical outcome and no perioperative mortality (Abstract 19–2). The Mayo Clinic reports radiation-associated atheromatous disease of the internal carotid artery (Abstract 19–3). For many surgeons the difficulties of endarterectomy in this group may well warrant a medical treatment program. Long-term studies indicate that carotid endarterectomy protects against late ipsilateral stroke, but myocardial infarction is a major cause of premature death in these individuals (Abstract 19–4).

Regarding cerebral *aneurysms,* MRI of acute subarachnoid hemorrhage discloses the extent of bleeding and often the site and source of hemorrhage (Abstract 19–5). Intra-arterial digital subtraction angiography may provide definitive diagnosis of intracranial aneurysm even down to lesions as small as 1–2 mm (Abstract 19–6). Early surgery gives rather satisfactory results, as reported by the University of Iowa group (Abstract 19–7). Suzuki and colleagues recommend an interhemispheric approach for wide exposure of carotid ophthalmic aneurysms (Abstract 19–8). Solomon and Stein describe various surgical approaches to aneurysms of the vertebral and basilar arteries (Abstract 19–9). Spetzler and colleagues have successfully treated large and giant aneurysms of the basilar artery with circulatory arrest and barbiturate protection (Abstract 19–10). Endaneurysmorrhaphy has been recommended in the treatment of giant middle cerebral artery aneurysms (Abstract 19–11). In a controlled trial, there is convincing evidence that nimodipine improves the outcome of poor-grade aneurysm patients (Abstract 19–12). The weight of evidence appears to favor utilization of this agent for patients who have undergone subarachnoid hemorrhage, and the drug is now commercially available. Intrathecal thrombolytic therapy appears effective and safe in a primate model of cerebrovascular vasospasm (Abstract 19–13).

For *arteriovenous malformations,* MRI shows relationships to vessels, and parenchymal abnormalities (Abstract 19–14). Stable xenon CT estimates CBF around AVMs (Abstract 19–15). Höllerhage (Abstract 19–16) in a series of 53 patients operated for AVM reports 29 excellent results, 20 good results, and 4 moderate disabilities. Micro-AVMs (less than 1 cm) are described by Willinsky (Abstract 19–17). The group at Henry Ford Hospital (Abstract 19–18) reports successful removal of six AVMs of the basal ganglia. For surgery of malformations of the vein of

Galen, the Mayo Clinic group reported 3 catastrophic bleeding problems, possibly related to perfusion breakthrough (Abstract 19–19).

SPINE NEUROSURGERY has advanced in several aspects. Regarding *spinal degeneration,* anterior cervical diskectomy without fusion was quite safe and neurologic improvement occurred in many cases (Abstract 20–1). Cervical laminoplasty has been recommended for enlargement of the spinal canal in cases of cervical spondylosis and ossification of the posterior longitudinal ligament (Abstracts 20–2 and 20–3). For *thoracic* herniated disk, a transthoracic approach has been used from T4 through T12 with good results (Abstract 20–4). In the *lumbar* spine, experience with extreme lateral disk herniation was favorable in a large series (Abstract 20–5). Complications in lumbar disk surgery are relatively frequent (13.75%), but serious complications are quite uncommon (Abstract 20–6). Among 100 percutaneous diskectomies, 87 patients were believed to have had a successful outcome (Abstract 20–7). For evaluation of the postsurgical lumbar spine, gadolinium-enhanced MRI discriminates epidural scar from retained disk (Abstracts 20–8 and 20–9).

Spinal tumors are demonstrated by MRI, often providing histologic diagnosis (Abstract 20–10). Extramedullary hematopoiesis in thalassemia may cause spinal cord compression (Abstract 20–11). For tumors of the thoracic and lumbar spine, one-stage posterolateral decompression and stabilization is effective and relatively safe (Abstract 20–12).

In the management of *syringomyelia,* syringosubarachnoid shunting led to 29 good to excellent results in 40 cases (Abstract 20–13). Good results were also reported in 5 cases subjected to suboccipital craniectomy and duraplasty (Abstract 20–14).

In the *TRAUMA* field, a review of boxing-related injuries in the U.S. Army from 1983 to 1985 discloses one death, one new blindness, and 67 hospitalizations, raising the question of the propriety of boxing in the Army (Abstract 21–1). A population-based study indicates that skull fractures are correlated with severity of deficit and mortality (Abstract 21–2). There is disproportionate severe memory deficit in relation to other intellectual functions after closed head injury (Abstract 21–3). Subcranial surgery for frontobasal-midfaced fracture gives cosmetically rewarding results and a very low complication rate (Abstract 21–4). Transfrontal microsurgical decompression for optic nerve injury gives good results in selected cases (Abstract 21–5). There is solid evidence supporting barbiturates in the control of elevated intracranial pressure after head injury (Abstract 21–6). Hypertonic saline enhances cerebral perfusion in multiple injury patients (Abstract 21–7).

In *spine trauma,* isolated T2 fractures are rather stable and well managed with external immobilization (Abstract 21–8). Surgery and immobilization is preferred for cervical spine fracture and fracture dislocation (Abstract 21–9). For thoracolumbar spinal injuries, a three-column concept is proposed (Abstract 21–10). Nonsurgical therapy for thoracolumbar burst fractures without neurologic deficit leads to excellent outcome (Abstract 21–11). Surgical intervention improves outcome for thoracolumbar spinal fractures with deficit (Abstract 21–12). In a controlled study, there was no benefit for surgery in cases of acute penetrating spinal injury (Abstract 21–13). For gunshot injuries of the conus medullaris and cauda equina, good results were obtained with laminectomy (Abstract 21–14). In vertebral artery trauma, open surgical ligation of the vertebral artery has often been successful, but this can now be accomplished with balloon catheter in stable patients (Abstract 21–15). Compartment syndromes in the limbs must be diagnosed on clinical grounds and promptly decompressed (Abstract 21–16).

In *PEDIATRIC NEUROSURGERY,* gadolinium-enhanced MR imaging identifies and sizes CNS tumors (Abstract 22–1). For juvenile pilocytic astrocytoma, radiation therapy should be offered for patients aged more than 3 years with incomplete resection (Abstract 22–2). Flow cytometry can predict prognosis for medulloblastoma (Abstract 22–5). Suprasellar germinomas of childhood are best treated with subtotal resection and radiation therapy (Abstract 22–6). Dysembryoplastic neuro-epithelial tumors have slow progression and a substantial chance for surgical cure (Abstract 22–7). For pineal region tumors in children, open biopsy is suggested with low morbidity (Abstract 22–8). Preirradiation chemotherapy for pediatric tumors permits delay of radiotherapy until the child's brain can tolerate radiation (Abstract 22–9). Radiation itself can lead to growth hormone deficiency but is not the reason for growth retardation (Abstract 22–10). Radiotherapy can actually cause intracranial tumors (Abstract 22–11). Among *vascular* lesions, cerebral aneurysms in childhood are more common in the posterior fossa and are frequently of giant size (Abstract 22–12). Serial angiography in Moyamoya disease demonstrates a gradual shift of flow to the posterior circulation (Abstract 22–14). For *hydrocephalus,* ventriculopleural shunts may be performed with low morbidity when an antisiphon device is utilized (Abstract 22–15). Differentiation between shunt malfunction and "slit ventricle syndrome" may be assisted by radionuclide patency scans (Abstract 22–16). In pediatric *trauma,* MRI after head injury shows changes that correlate with the clinical findings (Abstract 22–17). Preliminary experience with brachial plexus exploration for injury in children is encouraging, but results are inconclusive (Abstract 22–18).

Regarding *INFECTION,* ESR and WBC are better indicators than In-WBC scanning in the detection of spinal osteomyelitis (Abstract 23–1). The introduction of CT scanning has provided the most significant recent advance in the management of brain abscess, leading to a drop in mortality from 40% to 4% (Abstract 23–2). An infected spine may be managed by drainage and immediate posterior stabilization (Abstract 23–3). Creutzfeldt-Jakob disease may be transmitted by cadaver dura graft (Abstract 23–4).

In *FUNCTIONAL* neurosurgery, recurrent glycerol injection into the trigeminal cistern has unfortunately led to frequent painful dysesthesias (Abstract 24–1). Long-term follow-up data after microvascular decompression indicates a powerful beneficial effect on trigeminal neuralgia (Abstract 24–2). A magnetic field of epileptic spikes agrees nicely with operative localization in complex partial epilepsies (Abstract 24–3). Although corpus callosum section may reduce seizure disturbances for patients with intractable epilepsy, there is a significant complication rate (Abstract 24–4). Olivier has achieved remarkable effectiveness in controlling temporal lobe epilepsy by surgery (Abstract 24–5). Psychologic disorders are not increased by surgical treatment of seizures (Abstract 24–6). Magnetic resonance imaging provides quantitative evaluation of resection of the temporal lobe for epilepsy (Abstract 24–7). Modified leukotomy still has a place in psychiatric therapy and should remain available as a measure of last resort (Abstract 24–8). Stereotactic thalamotomy can improve neurologic status in patients with cerebral palsy (Abstract 24–9). A careful American investigation indicates modest improvement in patients undergoing adrenal medullary transplantation for parkinsonism (Abstract 24–10).

In *NERVE* surgery, ultrasonography can image peripheral nerve tumors (Abstract 25–1). Tumors of the vagus nerve generally present as an asymptomatic mass in the neck (Abstract 25–2). Extensive clinical nerve transfer may be the best treatment for simultaneous injury to median and ulnar nerve in the forearm (Abstract 25–3). For the management of facial palsy, a combination of techniques may be required (Abstract 24–5).

Remarkable advances in *NEUROSCIENCE* have enormous implications for neurosurgery. Axons appear to be guided biochemically by extracellular signals to the appropriate targets (Abstract 26–1). Cerebral evolution is best understood in relation to the radial unit hypothesis of cortical parcellation (Abstract 26–2). Different synaptic boutons have different likelihoods of transmitter release, giving rise to a new model of synaptic transmission (Abstract 26–3). Multiple postsynaptic receptors modulate the same ion channels in the synapse (Abstract 26–4). Hippocampal neurons produce nerve growth factor that maintains cholinergic projections to the hippocampus, a remarkable trophic feedback loop (Abstract 26–5). Muscarinic systems appear to be important in long-term potentiation (Abstract 26–7). Medial temporal lobe neurons appear to encode individual words and faces (Abstract 26–8). Amyloid protein precursor messenger RNAs appear to have differential expression in Alzheimer's disease (Abstract 26–9).

In *MISCELLANEOUS* investigations, CSF rhinorrhea seems best evaluated by CT with intrathecal metrizamide (Abstract 27–1) and may sometimes be repaired by fibrin glue (Abstract 27–2). Modern neuroanesthesia can prevent malignant hyperthermia in susceptible patients (Abstract 27–3). Shunting procedures are often effective in treatment of benign intracranial hypertension (Abstract 27–4). Craniotomy is associated with intracranial hemorrhage postoperatively in 0.8%, and postoperative hypertension appears to be an important factor (Abstract 27–5). Decisions to limit care raise troubling legal and moral ramifications (Abstract 27–6).

Robert M. Crowell, M.D.

16 Diagnostics*

Introduction

In 1989, there were remarkable advances in *magnetic resonance imaging* (MRI) as this diagnostic technique gains further dominance for cranial and spinal imaging. Zimmerman and colleagues (Abstract 16–1) have contributed useful studies regarding intensity changes on sequential MR scans after acute intracranial hemorrhage. The studies suggest that the complex nature of the intensity changes immediately after hemorrhage makes precise diagnosis difficult, and CT scanning remains the procedure of choice in the initial diagnosis of acute hemorrhage.

Romner and colleagues (Abstract 16–2) have studied MRI and aneurysm clips. Many clinicians have feared clip movement with MRI, but nonferromagnetic aneurysm clips like the Yasargil Phynox, Sugita Elgiloy, and Variangle McFadden clips do not move in the MR field. In addition, these nonferromagnetic clips cause only limited image artifact.

Large intracranial aneurysms are beautifully imaged with low flip angle gradient refocused imaging (GRASS). These studies provide anatomical and physiologic data not obtained with routine MR, for example, differentiation of thrombus from flow artifact (Abstract 16–3). According to Hedberg and co-workers (Abstract 16–4), GRASS MR imaging is also valuable in the evaluation of cervical radiculopathy. Heindel and colleagues (Abstract 16–5) have reported interesting metabolic changes in brain tumors detected by MRI spectroscopy, and the method holds great promise for differential diagnosis in the future.

Biochemical and histopathologic studies for diagnosis were also advanced. According to Marth and colleagues (Abstract 16–6), serum levels of sialoglycoproteins are increased in patients with intracranial tumors. Sialic acid appears to be a marker for the differentiation between benign and malignant intracranial tumors. Crush preparations obtained from stereotactic needle biopsy provide a valuable adjunct to the examination of frozen sections (Abstract 16–7). Examination of crush preparations may even permit a diagnosis in cases that cannot be diagnosed on frozen section.

Electrophysiologic studies have also been improved. According to the group at Duke University, intraoperative brain stem auditory evoked potentials led to a decrease in postoperative morbidity in patients undergoing microvascular decompression (Abstract 16–8). Motor action potentials (MAPs) show great promise for intraoperative monitoring (Abstract 16–9). Experimental studies have shown alterations in MAP proportional to spinal cord mechanical distortion.

---

*Unless otherwise noted, all comments in the Neurosurgry section are those of Robert M. Crowell, M.D.

Other diagnostic techniques were also improved. Positron emission tomography appears to offer assistance in prognosis for patients with intracranial glioma (Abstract 16–10). Laser Doppler flowmetry is a new technique for the intraoperative measurement of cerebral and tumor blood flow on a real-time regional basis (Abstract 16–11).

Magnetic Resonance Imaging

Acute Intracranial Hemorrhage: Intensity Changes on Sequential MR Scans at 0.5 T

Zimmerman RD, Heier LA, Snow RB, Liu DPC, Kelly AB, Deck MDF (Cornell Univ, New York)
AJR 150:651–661, March 1988   16–1

The intensity of hematomas on nuclear magnetic resonance (NMR) images is dependent on several factors, including the time from ictus and the pulse sequences used. Recent NMR studies of intracranial hemorrhage during the acute and resolving phases indicated that the field strength of the magnetic resonance (MR) imager also affects the intensity of hematomas on MR scans, i.e., acute hemorrhage may be more easily detected at ultralow (0.02 tesla [T]) or high (1.5 T) field strengths than at intermediate (0.1–0.6 T) field strengths. To further elucidate the MR findings in acute hemorrhage, 37 patients with hemorrhages confirmed with computed tomography were studied prospectively with a 0.5-T MR imager within 1 week of acute hemorrhagic ictus. Special attention was given to the precise relationship between the intensity of the lesion and the time from ictus.

Twelve patients underwent serial scanning, and 12 patients had multiple hematomas in different intracranial compartments, for a total of 57 hematomas. The intensity of the hemorrhages was compared qualitatively with that of white matter on T_1-weighted spin-echo (SE) images with a short repetition time (TR) of 500 msec and short echo time (TE) of 32 msec (SE, 500/32), a long TR and intermediate TE (SE, 2,000/60), and a long TR and long TE (SE, 2,000/120).

There was significant variation among patients, particularly between days 3 and 7 postictus. Hematomas studied between 12 and 24 hours after hemorrhage were mildly hyperintense on short TR/short TE scans and markedly hyperintense on long TR/intermediate TE and long TR/long TE scans. During the next 1–2 days, hematomas became isointense to mildly hypointense on short TR scans and markedly hypointense on long TR scans. On day 4 after ictus, hematomas became markedly hyperintense on short TR scans. On days 5 and 6, hematomas became again hyperintense on long TR scans. By the end of the first week after ictus, hematomas were hyperintense on all pulse sequences (Fig 16–1).

The complex nature of the intensity changes immediately after an acute intracranial hemorrhage, and the difficulty in distinguishing these changes from those seen in other lesions suggest that computed tomography is still the procedure of choice in the initial diagnosis of acute intra-

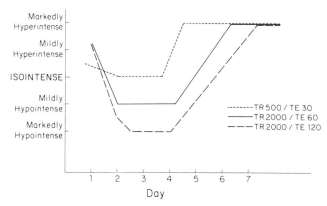

Fig 16–1.—Mean intensities only are plotted for spin-echo (SE) 500/32 and SE 2,000/60–120 scans. Data on patients in whom multiple episodes of hemorrhage were present have been eliminated to simplify curves. (Courtesy of Zimmerman RD, Heier LA, Snow RB, et al: *AJR* 150:651–661, March 1988.)

cranial hemorrhage. However, MR is useful for providing additional data once a diagnosis has been made on computed tomography.

▶ It is gratifying for a neurosurgeon to see that even neuroradiologists find MR signal changes confusing after acute intracranial hemorrhage. From the practical standpoint, I applaud the authors' recommendation that computed tomography is still the procedure of choice in the initial diagnosis of acute intracranial hemorrhage.

Magnetic Resonance Imaging and Aneurysm Clips: Magnetic Properties and Image Artifacts
Romner B, Olsson M, Ljunggren B, Holtås S, Säveland H, Brandt L, Persson B
(Univ Hosp, Lund, Sweden)
J Neurosurg 70:426–431, March 1989   16–2

Special treatment of aneurysm usually involves occlusion of the neck of the ruptured aneurysm by a metal clip. Metal clips cause pronounced beam-hardening artifacts on computed tomography (CT). Furthermore, CT may provide insufficient information on more subtle white-matter lesions of the brain. Magnetic resonance imaging (MRI) can visualize white-matter abnormalities, but there is concern that ferromagnetic and nonferromagnetic clips may pose hazards. The magnetic properties of various aneurysm clips were investigated to determine which could be used safely, and clip-induced MRI artifacts were studied using a geometric phantom.

The 12 different aneurysm clips studied were individually put into nonmagnetic plastic tubes and magnetized by an electromagnet with a magnetic field strength of 0.2 tesla for approximately 0.1 second. Magnetic remanence was measured 3 times with a sensitive flux-gate magnetometer, with demagnetization and remagnetization before each reading. Clip movement resulting from magnetic forces was investigated by placing clips on a cardboard sheet and exposing them to the magnetic field of a 0.3-tesla MR imager.

A geometric pattern was used to study image artifacts caused by the clips. The effects of metal clips on an MRI were measured at 2 distances, and the phantom was scanned in axial, coronal, and sagittal projections.

Nonferromagnetic aneurysm clips such as the Yasargil Phynox, Sugita Elgiloy, and Vari-Angle McFadden clips apparently did not contraindicate MRI studies using a FONAR β-3000M imager. There was no clip movement when the phantom was introduced into the MR imager. Image artifacts caused by the clips were limited. Ferromagnetic clips showed the most pronounced image distortion in the phantom study (Fig 16–2).

Patients harboring nonferromagnetic aneurysm clips can safely and ef-

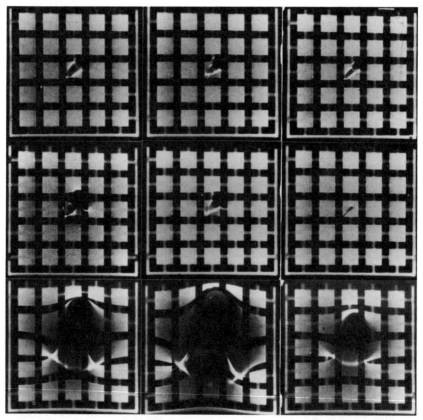

Fig 16–2.—Standard spin-echo axial magnetic resonance images of the geometric phantom with different aneurysm clips. The direction of the main magnetic field is parallel to the slices. The ferromagnetic clips show the most severe image distortion. **Upper row** (from *left* to *right*), Sugita Elgiloy, Yaşargil Phynox, and Vari-Angle McFadden. **Center row,** Sugita gold-plated, Yaşargil 316, and siver clip. **Lower row,** Mayfield, Heifetz 17-7PH, and Scoville. (Courtesy of Romner B, Olsson M, Ljunggren B, et al: *J Neurosurg* 70:426–431, March 1989.)

fectively be examined with medium-field MRI. This technique may yield information not available with any other type of radiologic study.

▶ Mayfield, Scoville, Heifetz 17–7PH, and Drake clips cause severe MRI distortion and may be dangerous because of possible displacement. Patients with these clips should not be subjected to MRI scanning. Other nonferromagnetic clips cause less distortion, and there is no danger of clip displacement during MRI performance. In selecting clips for surgery, neurosurgeons should be aware of these differences. In recommending MRI, the physician must be aware of the clip type and its potential hazard.

MR Evaluation of Large Intracranial Aneurysms Using Cine Low Flip Angle Gradient-Refocused Imaging
Tsuruda JS, Halbach VV, Higashida RT, Mark AS, Hieshima GB, Norman D
(Univ of California, San Francisco)
AJR 151:153–162, July 1988   16–3

Evaluation of intracranial aneurysms by magnetic resonance (MR) imaging has several known advantages over both angiography and contrast-enhanced computed tomography (CT). However, with slow flow or even-echo rephasing, it may be difficult to distinguish flowing blood from thrombus. Cine MR using gradient-recalled acquisition in the steady state (GRASS) was recently approved to evaluate dynamic cardiac function in normal and diseased hearts.

To determine whether cine MR using GRASS with routine MR and angiography is useful in assessing large and giant intracranial aneurysms, 8 women (mean age, 53) and 5 men (mean age, 35) with angiographically confirmed intracranial aneurysms were evaluated. Eight patients had giant intracranial aneurysms from 2.6 to 4.7 cm in cross-sectional diameter, 4 had large aneurysms from 1.6 to 2.6 cm in diameter, and 1 had an aneurysm 0.9 cm in diameter. Eight patients underwent transvascular occlusion with a detachable balloon solidified with a hydrophilic polymer.

Cine MR provided anatomical and physiologic data not obtained with routine MR, CT, or angiography. Cine MR clearly differentiated thrombus from flow artifacts, and documented turbulence and the effect of pulsatile motion on the surrounding parenchyma. After transvascular embolization, cine MR was superior to routine MR in differentiating between flowing blood and the occlusion balloons within the aneurysm. However, cine MR was not reliable for evaluating the adjacent parenchymal abnormalities. Other current limitations of cine MR included partial volume artifacts and less than optimal spatial resolution.

▶ Gradient echo studies with MR are confirmed to have improved visualization of large intracranial aneurysms. This should not be confused with MR angiography, a technique now in development, which is likely to provide even more information regarding intracranial vascular structures.

Gradient Echo (GRASS) MR Imaging in Cervical Radiculopathy
Hedberg MC, Drayer BP, Flom RA, Hodak JA, Bird CR (St Joseph's Hosp and Med Ctr, Phoenix)
AJR 150:683–689, March 1988   16–4

Myelography and computed tomography (CT) are now routinely used to diagnose degenerative spondylosis and herniated disks, but complications and patient discomfort from intrathecal injection of contrast medium and subsequent imaging often result. Magnetic resonance (MR) imaging of the cervical spine is therefore being used more frequently. However, CT and myelography are still performed after MR imaging and before surgery to confirm the precise anatomy of the involved area. The newly developed limited flip angle (LFA) technique used in MR imaging may obviate the need for such follow-up examinations.

During a 4-month study period, 130 patients with known or suspected cervical radiculopathy were evaluated by LFA gradient echo MR imaging. The LFA images were obtained with a gradient recalled acquisition in the steady state (GRASS) pulse sequence and a flow compensation regimen to eliminate signal loss from motion-induced temporal and spatial phase shift. Magnetic resonance images were obtained in the axial plane of all 130 patients, and in the sagittal plane of 75 patients.

The quality of the LFA images was excellent in 95 cases, good in 33 cases, and poor in 2 cases. Imaging contrast and relative relaxation time weighting in GRASS imaging are related not only to the operator-selected repetition time (TR) and echo time (TE) as with spin-echo imaging but also to pulse flip angle. A 10- or 15-degree flip angle with a TR of 75 msec and a TE of 12.3 msec provided better image contrast of the spinal cord against surrounding subarachnoid space than a 30-degree flip angle. Both axial and sagittal LFA images were important in detecting extradural defects and distinguishing a herniated disk from an osteophyte. For the 13 patients who underwent surgical exploration at 30 sites, correlation between surgical findings and MR images was excellent.

It appears that LFA gradient echo imaging should be the initial procedure of choice in the evaluation of suspected cervical radiculopathy.

▶ It is suggested that GRASS is highly helpful in the evaluation of cervical radiculopathy. Others have found the method less useful, and cervical myelography is still widely used for this evaluation. Further data will be required to establish this point.

Combined ¹H-MR Imaging and Localized ³¹P-Spectroscopy of Intracranial Tumors in 43 Patients
Heindel W, Bunke J, Glathe S, Steinbrich W, Mollevanger L (Univ of Cologne; Philips Med Systems, Hamburg, West Germany; Best, The Netherlands)
J Comput Assist Tomogr 12:907–916, November–December 1988   16–5

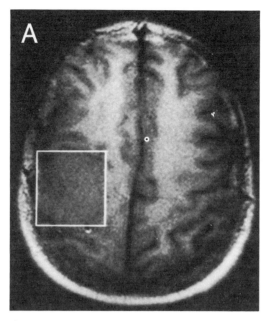

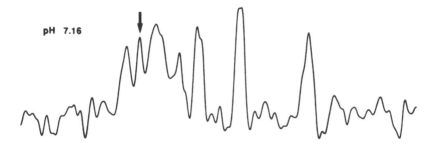

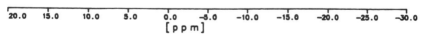

Fig. 16–3.—Man aged 46 years with meningioma of the convexity. **A,** [1]H-MR (SE, 250/30) image for centering the volume of interest (45 × 45 × 50 mm) on the tumor. **B,** ^{31}P-MRS of the tumor shows a drastic decrease of phosphocreatine (PCr) below the level of adenosinetriphosphate and a reduction of phosphodiesters. Intracellular pH calculated from the chemical shift of inorganic phosphate *(arrow)* versus PCr is shifted to the alkaline range. (Courtesy of Heindel W, Bunke J, Glathe S, et al: *J Comput Assist Tomogr* 12:907–916, November–December 1988.)

The findings of magnetic resonance (MR) imaging were correlated with those of radiophosphorus MR spectroscopy in 35 normal volunteers and 43 patients with brain tumors. Three patients with inoperable tumors had follow-up spectroscopy. Histologic material was available in 35 tumor cases. Both hydrogen 1 imaging (^{1}H-MR) and phosphorus 31 spectroscopy (^{31}P-MRS) were carried out using a 1.5-tesla whole-body MR system.

The ^{31}P spectra of meningiomas differed most obviously from normal brain tissue, with a markedly reduced phosphocreatine peak (Fig 16–3). Tissue acidosis was not seen in tumor tissue, in contrast to ischemic infarction. Gliomas exhibited less marked spectral changes. In cases of metastasis, the quality of the spectra was reduced by the small tumor volume. In low-grade astrocytomas, the ^{31}P spectrum could not be distinguished from that of the normal hemisphere. Follow-up studies showed metabolic change in 1 patient when imaging methods indicated no change.

It is feasible to routinely perform in vivo MR spectroscopy in a clinical environment. Volume-selective ^{31}P-MRS may be combined with conventional MR imaging of the head in an examination time of 60–90 minutes at most. The differential diagnosis of larger brain tumors may be possible, as well as assessment of the results of treatment.

▶ These results suggest that MRI spectroscopy may be useful in the differential diagnosis of intracranial tumors. To date, however, the method has only crude spatial resolution and specificity is low. Future refinements could change all that, and the possibility of combining spectroscopy with other markers of malignancy, for example, sialic acid (see Abstract 16–6), appears to hold great promise for the future of noninvasive, histologically specific diagnosis.

Brief Notes on MRI

MRI AND HEMORRHAGE DETECTION

Magnetic resonance imaging demonstrates chronic subdural hematoma as hyperintense on T_1 and T_2 weighted images. The T_1 values may be isointense or hypointense in occasional cases (Hosoda K et al: *J Neurosurg* 67:677–683, 1987).

The presence of mixed subacute and chronic hemorrhage suggested by mixed high and low signal intensity components on MR may be characteristic of cavernous hemangiomas of the spinal cord (Fontaine S et al: *Radiology* 166:839–841, 1988).

Magnetic resonance imaging has successfully imaged an intrachiasmatic hemorrhage (Moffit B et al: *J Comput Assist Tomogr* 12:535–536, 1988).

MRI AND ARTERIES

Magnetic resonance imaging for the carotid bifurcation with GRASS and other techniques still has significant drawbacks lowering its utilization (Masaryk TJ et al: *Radiology* 166:461–466, 1988).

Magnetic resonance imaging can demonstrate the tortuous vertebral artery as the cause of hemifacial spasm (Tash RR et al: *J Comput Assist Tomogr* 12:492–494, 1988).

Magnetic resonance imaging was especially useful in diagnosis of symptomatic vertebrobasilar dolichoectasia (Giang DW et al: *Neuroradiology* 30:518–523, 1988).

MRI AND TUMORS

Studies of 160 cases show that T_1, T_2, and proton density values are so variable in brain tumors as to preclude reliable histologic diagnosis (Just M, Thelen N: *Radiology* 169:779–785, 1988).

Gadolinium MR appears to be the method of choice for depiction of intraparenchymal metastases (Zsze G et al: *Radiology* 168:187–194, 1988).

Magnetic resonance imaging demonstrates intracranial mass lesions with greater precision than CT and may lead to radiation therapy without biopsy (Robinson DA et al: *J Comput Assist Tomogr* 12:275–279, 1988).

Magnetic resonance imaging of cerebellar pontine angle tumors reveal that differentiation by special characteristics is more reliable than differentiation by signal intensity differences (Press GA, Hesselink JR: *AJR* 150:1371–1381, 1988).

In comparison of CT and MRI with gadolinium, the latter was clearly superior in diagnosis and preoperative evaluation of acoustic neuroma (Stack JP et al: *Br J Radiol* 61:800–805, 1988).

Gadolinium improved sensitivity of MR imaging for benign extra-axial tumors especially in cases of residual or recurrent acoustic neuromas (Haughton VM et al: *Radiology* 166:829–833, 1988).

Magnetic resonance imaging precisely images jugular foramen neurinomas (Matsushima T et al: *Acta Neurochir (Wien)* 96:83–87, 1989).

Computed tomography and MR provide complimentary data on tuberous sclerosis (Altman NR et al: *Radiology* 167:527–532, 1988).

Gadolinium MR assists in the imaging of leptomeningeal lymphoma (Bers DH et al: *J Comput Assist Tomogr* 12:499–500, 1988).

MRI AND TRAUMA

Magnetic resonance imaging is highly sensitive for the diagnosis of trauma to the corpus callosum, which is associated with primary brain stem injury, diffuse axial injury, and intraventricular hemorrhage (Gentry LI et al: *AJNR* 9:1129–1138, 1988).

Magnetic resonance is recommended for documenting brain contusions during the subacute and chronic stages of head injuries (Hesselink JR et al: *AJNR* 9:269–278, 1988).

OTHER MRI STUDIES

Magnetic resonance imaging with gadolinium is more sensitive than enhanced CT for detecting acute cerebral infarction (Imakita S et al: *Neuroradiology* 30:372–378, 1988).

S. Murayama and co-workers (*J Comput Tomogr* 12:251–252, 1988) report that eosinic granuloma of the skull shows bright signal on T_2 in MRI.

Magnetic resonance imaging shows diffuse edema in the brain in cases of pseudotumor cerebri (Moser FG et al: *AJR* 150:903–909, 1988).

Magnetic resonance imaging showed reversal of brain shrinkage after 5 weeks of abstinence in 9 alcohol-dependent patients (Schroth G et al: *Neuroradiology* 30:385–389, 1988).

Magnetic resonance images combined with plain films offer an accurate noninvasive test for cervical radiculopathy and myelopathy (Brown BM et al: *AJR* 151:1205–1212, 1988).

S.W. Atlas and associates (*AJR* 151:1025–1030, 1988) report that spin-echo provides more information than short inversion time–inversion recovery sequences for imaging of the orbit.

Spectroscopy can be used for the noninvasive quantitative measurement of deoxyhemoglobin in brain (Chance B et al: *Proc Natl Acad Sci USA* 85:4971–4975, 1988).

Biochemical Studies

Sialic Acid as a Marker for Differentiation Between Benign and Malignant Intracranial Tumors
Marth E, Flaschka G, Stiegler S, Möse JR (Univ of Graz, Austria)
Clin Chim Acta 176:251–257, September 1988   16–6

Serum levels of sialoglycoproteins are increased in various neoplastic disorders. The authors measured the level of the sialic acid N-acetylneuraminic acid in 136 patients with intracranial tumors, both enzymatically and by high-performance liquid chromatography.

Both methods were 90% specific if infectious inflammation could be ruled out. The determination was 72.6% sensitive, with a cutoff level of 2.75 mmol/ml. A shift in distribution maxima was seen between benign and malignant lesions (Fig 16–4). Except for neuromas and benign malformations, patients with tumors had sialic acid levels significantly different from those in controls without neoplasms. Although 97% of benign tumors were below the cutoff level, 71% of malignant tumors were above.

Serum sialic acid is a specific marker of malignant disease in patients with central nervous system tumors. However, the possibility of inflammation due to infection always must be excluded.

▶ Serum levels of sialic acid appear to be a remarkably helpful marker for differentiation between benign and malignant intracranial tumors. As shown in Figure 16–4, the malignant tumors certainly have a higher mean level of sialic acid in the serum. On the other hand, there remains a troublesome overlap of benign and malignant tumors in the intermediate range. Moreover, the mean values do not differ greatly for primary brain tumors of benign and malignant variety. Nonetheless, this sort of effort is to be commended. One may look to the future when a combination of noninvasive imaging studies plus biochemical studies such as this may provide the clinician with specific diagnosis without biopsy.

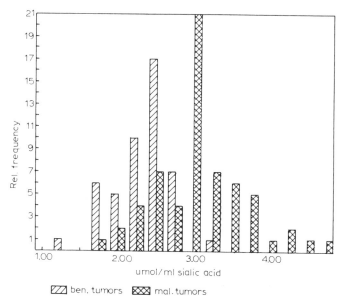

ben. tumors   mal. tumors

Fig 16–4.—Comparison of the relative frequency of benign and malignant tumors. (Courtesy of Marth E, Flaschka G, Stiegler S, et al: *Clin Chim Acta* 176:251–257, September 1988.)

Cytology of Neuroectodermal Tumors of the Brain in Crush Preparations: A Review of 56 Cases of Deep-Seated Tumors Sampled by CT-Guided Stereotactic Needle Biopsy
Nguyen G-K, Johnson ES, Mielke BW (Univ of Alberta, Edmonton)
Acta Cytol 33:67–73, January–February 1989   16–7

The advent of computed tomography (CT)-guided stereotactic needle biopsy has greatly facilitated the clinical assessment of patients with brain tumors. However, the size of the specimens procured by stereotactic needle biopsy is small, making pathologic examination of the specimens as frozen sections difficult. Crush preparations of brain tissue were made as a supplement to frozen sections for the rapid intraoperative diagnosis of specimens sampled by stereotactic needle biopsy.

Fifty-six brain tumors of neuroectodermal origin were sampled. Crush preparations prepared from tiny tissue fragments showed distinctive cytologic characteristics of different tumor types in 77% of the cases. The tumors included low- and high-grade astrocytomas (Fig 16–5), primary and recurrent oligodendroglioma, ependymoma, choroid plexus tumors, and medulloblastoma. The cytologic features of the different types of neuroectodermal brain tumors in crush preparations were described.

Cytologic examination of crush preparations from CT-guided needle biopsies of the brain is a valuable adjunct to the examination of frozen sections of specimens obtained by CT-guided stereotactic needle biopsy.

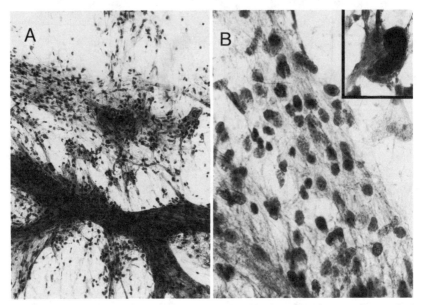

Fig 16–5.—High-grade astrocytoma. **A,** large branching blood vessels with surrounding neoplastic astrocytes and a large cluster of tumor cells. **B,** pleomorphic tumor cells in a fibrillary background. **Inset,** a bizarre multinucleated giant tumor cell. Hematoxylin and eosin; original magnification, **A**= ×100, **B** = ×400. (Courtesy of Nguyen G-K, Johnson ES, Mielke BW: *Acta Cytol* 33:67–73, January–February 1989.)

Examination of crush preparations may even permit a diagnosis in cases in which frozen sections do not.

▶ This report indicates an excellent correlation of crush preparations with final histologic diagnoses. Among 56 brain tumors so sampled, only 2 had substantial differences between the 2 tests that caused reconsideration of treatment; crush preparations gave a diagnosis of gliosis in 2 instances, which were felt to be grade II astrocytomas on final diagnosis. Crush preparations appear valuable in the stereotactic biopsy of intracranial tumors.

Brief Notes on Chemical Studies

LN-1 is a new immunoperoxidase marker for microglia (Miles JM, Chan SM: *J Neuropathol Exp Neurol* 47:579–587, 1988).

Electrophysiologic Studies

Intraoperative Brainstem Auditory Evoked Potentials: Significant Decrease in Postoperative Morbidity
Radtke RA, Erwin CW, Wilkins RH (Duke Univ)
Neurology 39:187–191, February 1989   16–8

Evoked potentials are often used for intraoperative monitoring of neural tissue under surgical threat. However, there is a lack of unequivocal evidence showing its efficacy in preventing neural injury. A retrospective comparison was made of the auditory morbidity of posterior fossa microvascular decompressive surgery before and after the introduction of intraoperative brain stem auditory evoked potentials (BAEPs).

The nonmonitored group was composed of 151 patients undergoing 152 retromastoid craniectomies for microvascular decompression or partial sensory rhizotomy from 1975 to 1983. After 1983, intraoperative BAEPs were used during this procedure in 67 patients undergoing 70 operations. A single surgeon performed all of the operations. The monitored and nonmonitored groups were comparable in age, sex, and indications for surgery. Among nonmonitored patients, auditory morbidity did not decline with the increasing experience of the surgeon. Of the nonmonitored patients, 10 (6.6%) had a profound hearing loss. In the monitored group, none of the patients had a profound hearing loss (Fig 16–6).

The introduction of intraoperative BAEPs resulted in a significant decline in morbidity. None of the monitored patients suffered a profound hearing loss, whereas 6.6% of nonmonitored patients did.

▶ The authors report decline in operative morbidity since the introduction of BAEPs during posterior fossa operations for trigeminal pain. Although statistically this is certainly borne out by the data presented, it is worth knowing that both false positive and false negative evoked response changes have been noted in other reports, that is to say, even a stable evoked response during surgery may not assure a good clinical outcome, nor does distortion of the response necessarily imply postoperative deficit.

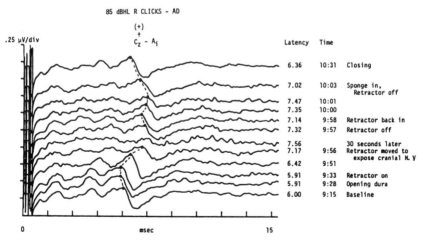

Fig 16–6.—The serial BAEPs displayed demonstrate an abrupt shift and apparent loss of wave V at 9:56 when the cerebellar retractor was moved to better expose the trigeminal nerve. Return of wave V (although later and decreased in amplitude) is seen less than 1 minute after removal of the retractor. Subsequent replacement of the retractor did not result in significant BAEP changes, and the patient had normal postoperative hearing. (Rate 31/sec, 2,000 trials/average, LF = 150 Hz, HF = 3,000 Hz.) (Courtesy of Radtke RA, Erwin CW, Wilkins RH: *Neurology* 39:187–191, February 1989.)

Monitoring of Motor Action Potentials After Stimulation of the Spinal Cord

Machida M, Weinstein SL, Yamada T, Kimura J, Itagaki T, Usui T (Nihon Univ, Tokyo; Univ of Iowa)

J Bone Joint Surg 70-A:911–918, July 1988   16–9

Neurologic deficits secondary to spinal surgery for scoliosis have increased as more complex operations such as segmental spinal instrumentation have come into use. The effects of progressive spinal distraction on motor action potentials recorded from the cat hind leg on cord stimulation were examined. The recording electrode was in the epidural space cephalad to the level of distraction. An apparatus similar to Harrington instrumentation was applied to the spinous processes in 1-mm increments.

The amplitude of the motor action potential varied substantially. Potentials were elicited by stimulation caudad but not cephalad to a pyra-

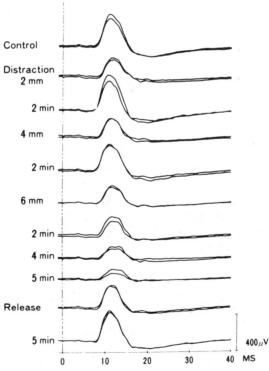

(Distraction between Th. 7 and Th. 8)

Fig 16−7.—Changes in the motor action potential with incremental distraction and after the release of distraction in 1 cat. The amplitude of the motor action potential returned to the baseline value when distraction was limited to 4 mm, but it decreased progressively after 6 mm of distraction. The motor action potential returned to the baseline level within 5 minutes after the release of distraction. (Courtesy of Machida M, Weinstein SL, Yamada T, et al: *J Bone Joint Surg* 70-A:911–918, July 1988.)

midal tract transection. Potential amplitude declined with 4 mm of distraction and more markedly with 6 mm of distraction (Fig 16–7). The spinal evoked potential and motor action potential responded similarly to distraction in a majority of the animals studied.

That these findings are directly applicable to scoliosis surgery remains to be shown. It is likely, however, that cord dysfunction can best be detected at a stage when it is reversible if the motor action potential and spinal evoked potential are monitored simultaneously.

▶ This report provides preliminary data correlating changes in motor action potentials during surgery to long-term neurologic deficit in experimental animals. Further data will be required in this setting in order to establish electrophysiologic guidelines for irreversibility. There seems great hope for this method, however, in terms of intraoperative monitoring of clinically relevant spinal cord function.

Brief Notes on Electrical Studies

Halothane, enflurane, and isoflurane in nitrous oxide have substantial effects on somatosensory evoked potentials (Pataj KS: *Anesthesiology* 70:207–212, 1989).

Normal brain stem auditory evoked potentials have been reported with abnormal latency-intensity studies in some patients with acoustic neuromas (Legatt AD et al: *Arch Neurol* 45:1326–1330, 1988).

Other Diagnostic Techniques

Positron Emission Tomography in Patients With Glioma: A Predictor of Prognosis
Alavi JB, Alavi A, Chawluk J, Kushner M, Powe J, Hickey W, Reivich M (Univ of Pennsylvania)
Cancer 62:1074–1078, Sept 15, 1988   16–10

Adult patients with primary malignant brain tumors have a poor prognosis. Prognostic criteria include patient age, performance status, pathologic grade, and tumor size according to computed tomography scans. These criteria are useful for predicting survival in patients with low-grade tumors, but more precise prognostic criteria for the intermediate-grade and high-grade malignancies are needed. Positron emission tomography (PET) was used to determine whether the glucose metabolic state of a malignant brain tumor would provide additional prognostic information.

The study was done in 29 patients aged 20–73 years with confirmed supratentorial primary brain tumors; 27 had a histologic diagnosis of malignant glioma. All had had computerized axial tomography or magnetic resonance imaging to confirm diagnosis.

Positron emission tomography was performed using 18-F-fluorodeoxyglucose administered in the fasting state. Patients underwent PET scanning from several days before operation to 7 years after diagnosis. Eight (28%) patients had PET scans before radiation therapy; 21 (72%)

were studied after radiation therapy. Sixteen patients had both radiation therapy and chemotherapy before scanning. The follow-up period after PET scanning ranged from 6 to 84 months, with a median follow-up of 24 months for the 9 surviving patients.

The glucose metabolic state of the tumor was increased in 16 patients and normal or decreased in 13. Nine of 23 patients with hypometabolic high-grade tumors had an estimated median survival time of 19 months after PET scanning, compared with a median 7 months' survival for the 14 patients with hypermetabolic high-grade tumors. At 1 year after PET, only 29% of the 16 patients with hypermetabolic lesions were still alive, compared with 78% of the 13 patients with hypometabolic lesions.

The differences in 1-year survival were most pronounced for treated patients: 4 of the 6 patients with low-grade hypometabolic tumors had previously had radiation therapy and were still alive 12 months after PET scanning (Fig 16–8). Median survival had not yet been reached at 40 months. Thus patients with hypometabolic malignant brain tumors survived significantly longer than those with hypermetabolic lesions.

It appears that glucose metabolic studies provide an independent measure of the aggressiveness of a brain tumor that supplements pathologic grading.

▶ This excellent study suggests another indication for PET scanning: The metabolic characteristics of gliomas studied with this method correlate with out-

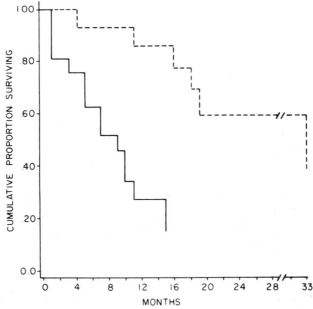

Fig 16–8.—Survival from the time of PET scan, all patients. *Solid line,* survival curve of those with hypermetabolic tumors; *broken line,* those with hypometabolic tumors. (Courtesy of Alavi JB, Alavi A, Chawluk J, et al: *Cancer* 62:1074–1078, Sept 15, 1988.)

come. If these observations can be confirmed, the method may likewise be useful in classifying patients before randomization for various treatment modalities.

Intraoperative Measurement of Cerebral and Tumor Blood Flow With Laser-Doppler Flowmetry
Arbit E, DiResta GR, Bedford RF, Shah NK, Galicich JH (Mem Sloan-Kettering Cancer Ctr, New York)
Neurosurgery 24:166–170, February 1989   16–11

Cerebral tumor circulation has important diagnostic and therapeutic implications, but knowledge in this area has been limited by the lack of rapid, noninvasive methods for measuring cerebral blood flow (CBF). Laser-Doppler flowmetry (LDF) is an optically based modality for measuring velocity or volume of liquid flow that holds the promise of satisfying many of the requirements for studying blood flow in cerebral tumors. Blood flow responses in brain and brain tumor to changes in blood pressure and arterial blood gas were evaluated intraoperatively.

Experiments using a rat brain preparation was done first to establish the correlation and calibration factor relating LDF output to units of absolute flow. Then, regional CBF was measured in chosen areas of normal brain and cerebral tumor in 12 patients. In the rat brain, the 2 methods were highly correlated, but the form of the relationship was not linear (Fig 16–9). In the patients, most tumors retained the ability to compensate for increased pCO_2. Blood flow in brain tumor was lower than in normal brain tissue except in meningiomas and metastatic melanoma. Tumor response to blood pressure varied: 1 group showed an autoregulatory capacity, another behaved passively, and a third had no response.

Blood flow is reduced in most cerebral tumors, and most tumors retain

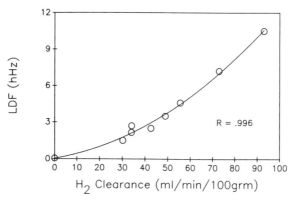

Fig 16–9.—Correlation between LDF and hydrogen clearance techniques, as measured in rat brain. (Courtesy of Arbit E, DiResta GR, Bedford RF, et al: *Neurosurgery* 24:166–170, February 1989.)

the normal response to changes in arterial blood gas. However, the responses vary.

▶ This important communication introduces laser-Doppler flowmetry into the neurosurgical operating room. The technique provides continuous determination of local cerebral blood flow and doubtless will find application for monitoring in the operating room and, as an implanted probe, in the neurosurgical ICU where continuous CBF monitoring may be of extraordinary value.

Brief Notes on Other Diagnostic Techniques

PET

Positron emission tomography fluorodeoxyglucose studies aid in distinguishing tumor metabolism from normal brain and radiation injury (Valk PE et al: *J Neurosurg* 69:830–838, 1988).

Positron emission tomography studies show that, after chemotherapy, glucose consumption and blood volume decreased in tumor tissue (Ogawa T et al: *J Comput Assist Tomogr* 12:290–297, 1988).

A task force on clinical PET concluded that PET studies provide (1) localization of an epileptogenic focus for surgical management, (2) diagnostic and prognostic information in the management of gliomas, and (3) specific distinction of recurrent tumor from radiation necrosis (*J Nucl Med* 29:1136–1143, 1988).

Doppler Ultrasonography

Transcranial Doppler is useful in the evaluation of brain death (Newell DW et al: *Neurosurgery* 24:509–513, 1989).

Transcranial Doppler sonography may be used as an additional method for the diagnosis of brain death (Vanvelthoven V, Caloiauw L: *Acta Neurochir (Wien)* 95:57–60, 1988).

Carbon dioxide reactivity of blood flow in human basilar artery may be estimated with the transcranial Doppler method (Ogawa F et al: *Ultrasound Med Biol* 14:479–483, 1988).

Blood flow velocity in middle cerebral artery showed a variable correlation to rCBF during carotid endarterectomy (Halsey JH et al: *Stroke* 20:53–58, 1988–1989).

A multigate pulse Doppler system produces results comparable with B-mode combined with single-gate Doppler (VanMarode T et al: *Ultrasound Med Biol* 14:459–464, 1988).

Changes in Doppler wave forms can predict pressure reduction across internal carotid artery stenosis (Siloesen H, Schroeder T: *Ultrasound Med Biol* 14:649–655, 1988).

M. L. Robinson and associates (*AJR* 151:1045–1049, 1988) report that peak systolic velocity in the internal carotid artery on duplex sonography is as good as any other criterion and is more easily measured, whereas combined parameters offer no statistical advantage.

Intraoperative color Doppler flow imaging is useful in AVM surgery for loculization of residual lesion and confirmation of complete resection (Rubin JM et al: *Radiology* 170:217–222, 1989).

17 Techniques

Introduction

In 1989, the field of **instrumentation** was advanced in several ways. Careful quantitative experimental investigations of self-retaining brain retractors established thresholds for time and regional cerebral perfusion pressure for the development of brain retractor injury (Abstract 17–1). Histologic studies have shown that the Nd:YAG laser may shrink arteriovenous malformations with thrombosis, but the instrument must be used with great caution (Abstract 17–2).

Stereotaxy progressed in dramatic fashion. As discussed by Sedan and colleagues (Abstract 17–3), stereotaxic guidance during open surgery of the brain may assist in the localization of small deep-seated lesions. Charged particle stereotactic radiosurgery is expanding dramatically. The group at Lawrence Berkeley Laboratory reported good results in the obliteration of intracranial AVMs with helium radiosurgery (Abstract 17–4). In postoperative studies, magnetic resonance imaging (MRI) appears to demonstrate obliteration of the lesions, with progressive loss of signal void. The technique is not without hazard, however; complications including cerebral infarction have been reported, with some patients showing benefit from steroid therapy (Abstract 17–5). Winston and Lutz have adapted the linear accelerator for use as a stereotactic radiosurgical device (Abstract 17–6). To date, results are too scanty to indicate the efficacy and safety of this approach, but certainly the wide availability of linear accelerators suggests that this method is likely to proliferate. It is clear that the complexity of the technique will require a dedicated and skilled team of stereotaxic surgeon, physicist, and radiation physician to obtain optimal results.

Several improved **surgical approaches** were described in 1989. The cavernous sinus has increasingly been entered with satisfactory outcomes. Al-Mefty and Smith have described removal of tumors invading the cavernous sinus (Abstract 17–7), and the group at Henry Ford Hospital has reported direct surgical management of aneurysms in the cavernous sinus (Abstract 17–8). Approaches to the petroclival area have been advanced. Samii has described a promising presigmoid approach that offers supratentorial and intratentorial access without ligation of the lateral sinus (Abstract 17–9). The method of Al-Mefty and colleagues is quite similar, but the transverse sinus is preserved (Abstract 17–10). George and colleagues have reported a lateral approach to the anterior foramen magnum, obtained by transposition of the vertebral artery and division of the sigmoid sinus (Abstract 17–11).

Robert M. Crowell, M.D.

211

Instrumentation

The Risk of Ischaemic Brain Damage During the Use of Self-Retaining Brain Retractors

Rosenørn J (Copenhagen County Hosp, Glostrup, Denmark)
Acta Neurol Scand 79(suppl):9–30, 1989   17–1

During microneurosurgery, self-retaining brain retractors are indispensable, permitting the surgeon to work in a confined space unhindered by an assistant's hands. Hand-held retractors are less stable and sometimes produce an undesirable and unnecessarily high brain retractor pressure. All retractors produce a certain pressure on the surface of the brain. This brain retractor pressure is transmitted to the adjacent brain tissue, thus decreasing the regional perfusion pressure (rCPP) with the risk of ischemic brain damage developing. Thresholds in cerebral ischemia are still debated. A series of studies was done to determine the limitations of the use of self-retaining brain retractors.

First, animal studies with male Wistar rats were done to measure regional cerebral blood flow (rCBF) changes during brain retractor pressure provided by lead weights. The weights were applied for different periods on the parietal cortex after craniotomy. To measure rCBF, autoradiography with carbon 14 iodoantipyrine was used. The thresholds of rCBF, rCPP, and time were 20–25 ml/100 gm/min, 20 mm Hg, and 7–10 minutes, respectively. Patients without neurologic deficits and in whom preoperative computed tomographic scans did not show signs of infarction were then studied. During surgery, hypotension was induced in 20 patients and mannitol was administered in 6. Twenty-three patients were followed up for 3 months. The thresholds of rCPP and time were 10 mm Hg and 6–8 minutes, respectively. Other researchers have reported a rCBF threshold of 10–13 ml/100 gm/min.

Except for the differences in the thresholds of rCBF and rCPP, the results obtained in the rat studies were comparable to those obtained in the human studies. The time threshold of cerebral ischemia appeared to be fairly equal in rats and humans. Intermittent brain retractor pressure was recommended if these thresholds are reached. The most easily handled retractors—those with a flat profile—did not reduce the rCBF more than other types of retractors.

▶ This nice study illustrates with scientific validation what all surgeons know to be true: brain retraction can injure the brain. The threshold of 6–8 minutes of critical retraction pressure has the important practical implication that one should release brain retraction intermittently to minimize brain retraction injury.

Acute Effect of the Nd:YAG Laser on the Cerebral Arteriovenous Malformation: A Histological Study

Zuccarello M, Mandybur TI, Tew JM Jr, Tobler WD (Univ of Cincinnati; Mayfield Neurological Inst, Cincinnati)
Neurosurgery 24:328–333, March 1989   17–2

Several reports have attested to the beneficial role of the Nd:YAG laser in achieving hemostasis during surgery. Acute changes caused by laser irradiation in the vessels of exercised cerebral arteriovenous malformations (AVMs) were described.

Ten patients with single cerebral AVMs that were surgically removed comprised the study population. The Nd:YAG laser was used as a primary adjunct to resection in these patients. It was used as a focused beam to treat surface and deep, penetrating blood vessels to produce occlusion. The surgeons were careful to avoid exposing adjacent brain and blood vessels in normal tissue. Every specimen was resected as a nidus. Blade resection of normal brain tissue was never done.

The immediate sequelae of occlusion in AVM vessels with the laser was predictable, consisting of shrinkage of collagen; the elastic laminae and the basement membrane were swollen and homogenized to enhance luminal stenosis. A mild shrinking in the media was also noted. Histologic assessment of the brain tissue confined to the resected AVM showed no signs of acute damage. Resection was accomplished safely in all 10 cases, with no morbidity or increased neurologic deficits attributable to the use of the laser technique.

▶ Zuccarello and colleagues have demonstrated successful application of Nd:YAG laser to resect arteriovenous malformations. The tissue absorption characteristics of this laser suggest that it might be useful for resecting AVMs, and the observed changes in the collagen matrix of vascular channels offer a reasonable explanation of the beneficial effects in this type of surgery. It is important to note that, although damage to the cerebral cortex was rare in this study, the Nd:YAG laser is not innocuous and can cause serious injury to nervous tissue, thus warranting use of the device only by neurosurgeons trained in its application.

Stereotaxy

Stereotaxic Guidance During Open Surgery of the Brain
Sedan R, Peragut JC, Farnarier P, Derome P, Fabrizi A (Hôpital de la Timone, Marseille, France)
Neurochirurgie 34:97–101, 1988   17–3

Stereotactic guidance was first introduced in 1955 as an aid in localizing certain deep-seated arteriovenous aneurysms. Since then, other investigators have expanded its use to ablation of angiomas and astrocytomas.

A technique was developed in which stereotactic guidance is used before operation to pinpoint small superficial or small deep-seated intracerebral lesions. A preoperative computed tomographic (CT) scout view is enlarged to the size of a plain film radiograph taken during the stereotactic procedure. Superimposing the CT scan over the radiograph allows the precise definition of the lesion on the grid, which then lines up with the center of the lesion in vivo. Using the CT scan, the shortest distance between the center of the lesion and the cranium can be calculated. This procedure makes it possible to drill only a very tiny incision in the skull and eliminates the need for shaving the patient's head. The technique was used in 21 patients with small superficial lesions and in 16 patients with deep-seated small lesions.

Fourteen of the 21 patients with small superficial cerebral lesions first underwent stereotactic guidance to obtain a biopsy. The same incision made in the skull for the biopsy was used again to complete ablation of the lesion. In all 14 patients, the lesions were found immediately, and total macroscopic ablation of the lesion could be accomplished in 12 cases. Ten lesions were located in areas that control speech or mobility. Only 2 of these 10 patients had marked postoperative speech impairment. Biopsy was not performed in the other 7 patients with small superficial lesions, and stereotactic guidance was used for primary operation. Five of these patients had lesions in areas involving speech and mobility. In all 7 patients, the lesions were found immediately without any problems, and total ablation could be accomplished without any postoperative neurologic sequelae.

In the 16 patients with deep-seated small lesions, stereotactic guidance was performed about 48 hours before operation to localize the lesion. A catheter placed at the point of the lesion was left in place until operation. In 8 patients with small tumors, total macroscopic ablation was accomplished without the development of new postoperative neurologic deficits. Postoperative aphasia developed in only 1 of 3 patients with cerebral aneurysms. All 5 patients with an angioma in the left quadrant had some postoperative speech impairment, which resolved in less than 15 days in 3 cases, and in about 2 months in 1 patient. The authors now use preoperative stereotactic guidance routinely.

▶ It should not be forgotten that stereotactic technique can be of great value for pinpointing lesions during open surgical operations. This French experience documents 37 uses of this approach. It is particularly useful for deep small lesions and may also be utilized for lesions whose gross characteristics make them difficult to discern from nearby normal structures. The Brown-Roberts-Wells stereotactic frame is nicely adaptable for this particular application.

In *IEEE Transactions on Biomedical Engineering,* Y. S. Kwoh and associates describe a robot with improved absolute positioning accuracy for CT-guided stereotaxic brain surgery (1).

Reference

1. Kwoh YS et al: *IEEE Trans Biomed Eng* 35:153–160, 1988.

Intracranial Vascular Malformations: Imaging of Charged-Particle Radiosurgery: Part I. Results of Therapy

Marks MP, Delapaz RL, Fabrikant JI, Frankel KA, Phillips MH, Levy RP, Enzmann DR (Stanford Univ; Univ of California, Berkeley)
Radiology 168:447–455, August 1988   17–4

There are 4 types of vascular malformations: arteriovenous malformations (AVMs), venous angiomas, cavernous hemangiomas, and capillary telangiectases. Arteriovenous malformations, which carry a high risk for hemorrhage, have been treated with surgery, embolization, or radiosurgery. Evaluation of results from the latter method can be obtained from

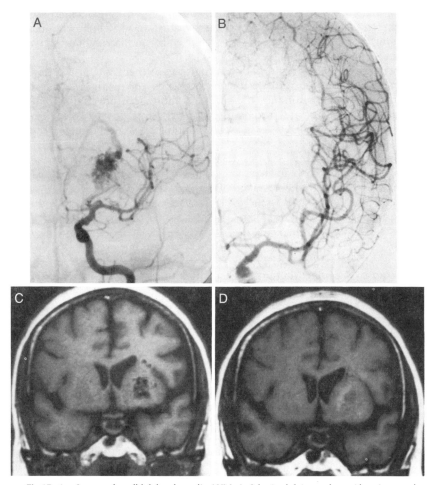

Fig 17–1.—Images of small left basal ganglia AVM. **A,** Selective left internal carotid angiogram obtained before therapy. **B,** Same view obtained 18 months after therapy demonstrates complete obliteration of the AVM. **C,** T$_1$-weighted coronal MR image obtained before therapy demonstrates signal flow voids in the AVM. **D,** T$_1$-weighted coronal MR image obtained 18 months after therapy (obtained simultaneously with **B**) demonstrates replacement of signal flow voids with intermediate signal, indicating thrombosis of the AVM. (Courtesy of Marks MP, Delapaz RL, Fabrikant JI, et al: *Radiology* 168:447–455, August 1988.)

angiography, computerized tomography (CT), or magnetic resonance imaging (MRI).

Twenty patients with high-flow AVMs and 4 with slow-flow lesions were evaluated before and after radiosurgery. Angiograms and MRI scans showed that 18 of 20 (90%) AVMs were significantly reduced in size, whereas 10% had no size change. Arteriovenous malformations smaller than 8 cm^3 were more likely to show complete resolution. Using CT did not accurately delineate the boundaries of the AVM after radiosurgery: CT scans showed persistent contrast enhancement, even when the AVM appeared completely resolved on angiograms.

In 5 patients who underwent MRI and angiography at similar times, complete resolution was visible on angiograms, and MRI showed loss of the flow void in the AVM. This was replaced by an intermediate signal in T_1- and T_2-weighted images (Fig 17–1).

There is a latency period between the time of therapy and the time of complete obliteration of the lesion. In this series, the mean time was 14.9 months. Magnetic resonance imaging was more accurate than CT in revealing hemorrhage after radiosurgery. The technique of choice for examining patients with AVMs is a combination of MRI and angiography.

▶ This important report indicates that MRI can demonstrate thrombosis of AVMs (see Fig 17–1). In addition, the authors point out that there is a delay of more than a year before obliteration of the lesion can be seen after radiosurgical treatment. According to this report, however, only 5 of the patients subjected to radiosurgery showed complete obliteration, thus indicating a continuing potential for hemorrhage.

Intracranial Vascular Malformations: Imaging of Charged-Particle Radiosurgery. Part II. Complications
Marks MP, Delapaz RL, Fabrikant JI, Frankel KA, Phillips MH, Levy RP, Enzmann DR (Stanford Univ; Univ of California, Berkeley)
Radiology 168:457–462, August 1988   17–5

In 7 of 24 patients with cerebral arteriovenous malformations (AVMs) who were treated with helium-ion Bragg-peak radiosurgery, new or worsening neurologic symptoms and radiologic abnormalities developed 4–28 months after treatment. All had received 20–45 Gy over 1–3 days. Five patients had been treated for high-flow AVMs, 1 patient was thought to have a left pons malformation, and 1 patient had a right frontoparietal cryptic malformation. Of the 7 patients with late complications, 5 underwent computed tomography (CT), 5 were examined with magnetic resonance imaging (MRI), and 4 underwent angiography.

Five patients had similar patterns of abnormal white matter involvement on CT and MR images, with the abnormalities centered in the radiation field. Their symptoms were similar to those previously described as late-delayed reactions. One patient had gray matter changes with abnormal enhancement in the thalamus and hypothalamus outside the radiation field. In this patient there was also angiographic evidence of vasculopathic changes in the vessels of the anterior cerebral artery circulation. One patient had signs of rapid-onset vascular occlusive disease in large vessels in the region of radiation exposure.

The data reported are only the preliminary findings in this study population. A longer follow-up is needed to make valid statistical comparisons between untreated and treated cerebral arteriovenous malformations.

▶ This important communication documents some complications after charged-particle radiosurgery of intracranial vascular malformations. The authors point out that more than a third of patients with this type of therapy had symptoms and neurologic signs in relation to vasogenic edema, vasculopathic changes, or large vessel occlusion. Though some of the changes are certainly reversible, particularly the vasogenic edema, the vasculopathic changes may be permanent. Steroid therapy may be helpful. Magnetic resonance imaging follow-up appears to be quite helpful. One patient in this group had a cryptic malformation, and Steiner (1) had evidence of poor results in this category of patients with gamma radiation treatment. Although stereotactic radiosurgery is quite promising in the treatment of intracranial vascular malformations, it must be kept in mind that significant complications can result from this treatment.

At the 1989 Annual Meeting of the Congress of Neurological Surgeons, Neil Martin, M.D., presented data suggesting substantial complications of proton radiosurgery, including symptomatic radionecrosis and recurrent SAH from AVM.

After incomplete adenoma removal and acromegaly, the results of proton and conventional radiation therapy are similar; because proton has a tendency for more serious side effects, conventional radiation is recommended (2).

References

1. Steiner L in Wilson CB, Stein BM (eds): Intracranial arteriovenous malformations. Baltimore, Williams & Wilkins Co, 1984, pp 295–313.
2. Ludecke DK et al: *Acta Neurochir (Wien)* 96:32–38, 1989.

Linear Accelerator as a Neurosurgical Tool for Stereotactic Radiosurgery
Winston KR, Lutz W (Harvard Univ)
Neurosurgery 22:454–464, March 1988   17–6

A stereotactic apparatus and a 6-MeV linear accelerator having a special collimator have been adapted to deliver large doses of radiation to precise volumes of about 0.6–10.0 ml within the brain (Fig 17–2). The 20-mm collimator allows treatment of a nearly spherical volume of 2.1 ml. Dosage outside the treatment field declines to 80% of the dose prescribed for the periphery of the lesion over 1.8 mm, and to 50% over the next 3.4 mm. A localizer box was designed for angiographic localization. Localization with computed tomography also is possible. Treatment is with an arcing beam of photon radiation with the turntable in each of 4

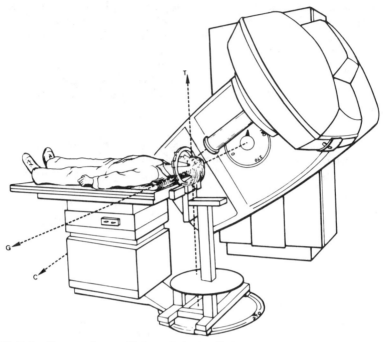

Fig 7–2.—Linear accelerator with Brown-Roberts-Wells floor stand mounted to plate overlying the bearing that supports the turntable (treatment couch). The collimator approaches within a few centimeters of the patient's head. *Dotted lines* indicate axes of rotation of the gantry *(G)*, the turntable *(T)*, and the collimator *(C)*. These 3 axes intersect at the center of the patient's lesion (see text). (Courtesy of Winston KR, Lutz W: *Neurosurgery* 22:454–464, March 1988.)

positions. Alignment first is verified by exposing a steel sphere simulating the patient's lesion

The system has been extensively tested for accuracy in alignment and distribution of radiation. There is no concern over dose homogeneity within the treated lesion. The localization error for angiography was substantially less than that for computed tomographic scanning, resulting in a smaller treatment error.

The system appears to be dependable and precise. Verification of alignment for each patient is essential because of the potentially catastrophic results of error.

▶ Winston and Lutz have designed and validated a lovely system for stereotactic radiosurgery utilizing relatively inexpensive, readily available instrumentation. Although results with this particular approach are as yet limited, it is expected that the excellent results for obliteration of arteriovenous malformation by the Gamma unit (1) can be reproduced with this technology. It is attractive to think that many health care institutions can replicate this instrumentation for widespread utilization; however, to emulate the work of Winston and Lutz, continuous active participation by stereotactic neurosurgeons and experienced radiation physicists will be essential for the safe and effective implementation of this substantial advance.

Stereotactic radiosurgery with the linear accelerator caused total obliteration of AVM in 27 of 41 patients (65.8%) at 24 months (2). These results are not as good as Steiner's with Gamma knife (85% total obliteration at 2 years). The very precise methodology of Winston and Lutz may also produce excellent results, but more data are needed.

References

1. Steiner LN in Wilson CB, Stein BM: *Intracranial Arteriovenous Malformations.* Baltimore, Williams & Wilkins Co, 1984, pp 295–313.
2. Betti OO et al: *Neurosurgery* 24:311–321, 1989.

Surgical Approaches

Surgery of Tumors Invading the Cavernous Sinus
Al-Mefty O, Smith RR (Univ of Mississippi, Jackson)
Surg Neurol 30:370–381, November 1988   17–7

The risk of injuring neurovascular structures in the cavernous sinus frequently precludes total removal of tumors at the cranial base. However, a direct operative approach is indicated when a lesion can thereby be removed. A variety of lesions are effectively dealt with via the supraorbital-pterional approach. The internal carotid is controlled proximally and the anterior clinoid and optic canal are removed before entry into the sinus. Typically the sinus is entered laterally through the triangle of Parkinson (Fig 17–3). Entry via the superior surface of the sinus is an alternative. The tumor is dissected by bipolar coagulation.

Eighteen benign tumors involving the cavernous sinus were removed surgically at 2 centers in 1983–1988. Magnetic resonance imaging was the best way of demonstrating tumor invasion and its relation to the intracavernous carotid artery. One patient with postoperative vasospasm died consequent to hypothalamic infarction. Four patients had cranial

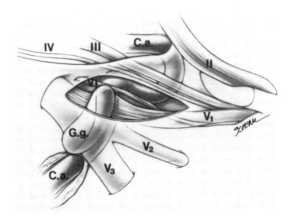

Fig 17–3.—Cavernous sinus entry through the lateral wall. V_1, V_2, V_3, divisions of the trigeminal nerves; *II, III, IV, VI,* cranial nerves; *C.a.,* carotid artery; *G.g.,* Gasserian ganglion. (Courtesy of Al-Mefty O, Smith RR: *Surg Neurol* 30:370–381, November 1988.)

nerve palsy, and 1 had hemiplegia. All but 1 of the 17 surviving patients were considered to have a good outcome.

Direct surgery can be done on tumors involving the cavernous sinus space with acceptable morbidity and mortality. Microsurgical technique helps in dissecting and preserving neural and vascular structures at this site.

▶ The authors present another impressive series of intracavernous tumor resections. Technical steps permitting this difficult dissection are outlined. Some remarkable total removals with good results are described. However, 2 of the cases were known to be partial removals, and among the apparent total removals, histologic persistence and eventual recurrence, of course, is still a possibility. Moreover, 1 patient died, 1 was hemiplegic, and 4 had worsened cranial nerve palsies among the 18 patients with benign tumor. In considering such surgery, one certainly must weigh carefully the presenting symptomatology, the age of the patient, and the risk of radical surgery. It is important to keep in mind that, despite gross total removal of tumors in this location, recurrence of meningioma in the paraclinoid region is unfortunately quite common. Thus it will remain an attractive possibility in many such cases to perform substantial subtotal resection, in some cases supplemented by postoperative radiation therapy. It is possible to accomplish this program with a very low risk and attack the tumor again at some later time should symptomatic recurrence come about.

Surgical Management of Aneurysms in the Cavernous Sinus
Diaz FG, Ohaegbulam S, Dujovny M, Ausman JI (Henry Ford Hosp, Detroit)
Acta Neurochir (Wien) 91:25–28, 1988   17–8

Aneurysms of the internal carotid artery (ICA) in the cavernous sinus region produce a symptom complex known as the superior orbital fissure syndrome. Surgical treatment of these aneurysms was long considered contraindicated because the ICA in the cavernous sinus region is close to several cranial nerves, and because of the high risk for hemorrhage associated with entering the cavernous sinus.

During an 8.5-year study period, 32 patients with aneurysms in the cavernous sinus region underwent operation through an intradural pterional approach. Twenty-two patients had aneurysms contained entirely within the cavernous sinus, and 10 had aneurysms arising from the ICA in the cavernous sinus but extending into the subarachnoid space. All 22 patients with pure intracavernous lesions had superior orbital fissure syndrome.

In 6 patients, complete dissection of the ICA and the aneurysm was not possible because of the aneurysm's size. Therefore, the aneurysm was trapped by ligating the ICA in the neck and in its supraclinoid portion distal to the aneurysm, and an extracranial-intracranial anastomosis to a proximal branch of the middle cerebral artery was performed at the same time. One patient died of massive cerebral infarction after an aneurysm-trapping procedure. One patient died of intraoperative hemorrhage. In 2 patients moderate hemiparesis developed; it resolved within the first 6 postoperative weeks. Two patients with severe preoperative visual impairment progressed to complete loss of vision after operation. The remaining patients had complete resolution of their preoperative symptoms and have remained well at follow-up.

▶ This communication presents an aggressive direct attack on aneurysms in the cavernous sinus. The results indicate that, although most (26 of 32) could be completely dissected and obliterated, nonetheless there were substantial complications, including 2 deaths. An alternative to this approach is carotid ligation, with or without extracranial-intracranial bypass graft (1). One is impressed with the low risk of bypass and balloon catheter occlusion of the internal carotid artery, but further data will be required to establish clearly the superiority of any treatment method.

Reference

1. Spetzler RF et al: *J Neurosurg* 53:22–27, 1980.

The Combined Supra-Infratentorial Pre-Sigmoid Sinus Avenue to the Petro-Clival Region: Surgical Technique and Clinical Applications
Samii M, Ammirati M (Nordstadt-Krankenhaus, Hannover, West Germany)
Acta Neurochir (Wien) 95:6–12, 1988
17–9

The surgical approach to tumors at the petroclival region is hindered by the deep location and proximity to vital neurovascular structures. The presence of cranial nerves III through XII, often distorted by the tumor, raises the potential for significant morbidity. A modification of the combined supratentorial and infratentorial approach was designed that allows for preservation of the transverse sinus while maintaining or improving surgical exposure.

Technique.—The surgical approach involves a temporal craniotomy, a suboccipital craniectomy, an extensive mastoidectomy, and petrous pyramid drilling without entry into the bony labyrinth, the middle ear, or the Fallopian canal. The dura is incised supratentorially over the posterior temporal lobe and infratentorially in front of the sigmoid sinus, and the temporal lobe is retracted superiorly and the cerebellum and sigmoid sinus, medially.

This approach was used in 9 patients: 2 had petroclival meningiomas, 4 had foramen jugulare neurinomas, and 3 had glomus jugulare tumors. None of the patients died, and total tumor removal was accomplished in all of them. All patients remained independent after the surgery.

The combined supratentorial and infratentorial approach anterior to the sigmoid sinus is a very short distance to the petroclival area, offers multiangled exposure, and preserves the dural sinuses. The approach does not impair hearing, and it minimizes temporal lobe retraction. It was found to be especially useful in patients with large tumors.

▶ This report describes a very logical development by Professor Samii for surgery of certain skull base lesions. In essence, the supra-infratentorial approach previously was the best available to certain lesions near the petrous apex, but ligation of the lateral sinus was required. The present presigmoid avenue has clear advantages: (1) the avenue of attack is shorter, and (2) the sigmoid sinus and lateral sinus are preserved. This technique has been utilized for Samii for some extraordinary tumor resections as documented by figures in the article. Surely such excisions could be accomplished only by the most masterful neurosurgeons, but additionally the new technique appears to provide substantial help for the surgeon. In addition to application for tumors, we have used this approach for dealing with vertebral basilar aneurysms in the pontine area.

Petrosal Approach for Petroclival Meningiomas
Al-Mefty O, Fox JL, Smith RR (Univ of Mississippi, Jackson; Georgetown Univ; King Faisal Specialist Hosp, Riyadh, Saudi Arabia)
Neurosurgery 22:510–517, March 1988   17–10

Eight of 13 consecutive cases of petroclival meningioma were treated using a new petrosal approach that requires minimal cerebellar and temporal lobe retraction and shortens the operative distance to the clivus. All neural and otologic structures are preserved, as are the transverse and sigmoid sinuses and the basal occipital veins. The vascular supply of the tumor is intercepted early in the course of surgery.

Technique.—An incision is made starting at the zygoma in front of the ear of the supine patient and descending behind the mastoid process. Bur holes are made on either side of the transverse sinus to elevate a bone flap. The temporal bone is drilled, using an operating microscope, to perform a complete mastoidectomy. Incisions are made along the floor of the temporal fossa and to the jugular bulb to retract the posterior temporal lobe, preserving the vein of Labbe. The tumor then is resected, taking great care to avoid the seventh and eighth nerves and the inferior cerebellar arteries (Fig 17–4). The tumor capsule then is dissected free, and the area of tumor insertion is vaporized extensively with the laser. Any tumor extensions are removed before closing the dura and turning the periosteum over the petrous bone to avoid spinal fluid leakage.

Tumor was completely removed in all but 2 of the 13 patients. No deaths occurred during an average follow-up of 26 months. Function improved in several patients, but in 2 cases the facial nerve was disrupted at operation. One patient required reexploration for cerebrospinal fluid leakage. Five patients had evidence of pulmonary embolism.

The petrosal approach is an effective and relatively safe means of removing petroclival meningiomas. The high rate of pulmonary embolism is a problem in these cases.

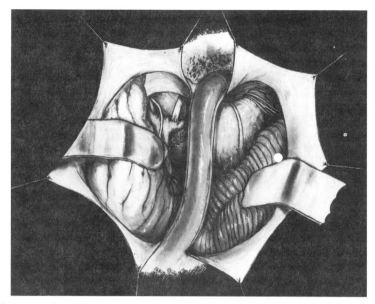

Fig 17–4.—The supratentorial extension of the tumor has been removed, and the tentorium has been split open. The relationship of the tumor to the cranial nerves (third through eleventh) and to the brain stem is demonstrated. (Courtesy of Al-Mefty O, Fox JL, Smith RR: *Neurosurgery* 22:510–517, March 1988.)

▶ The authors describe in nice detail a very useful adaptation of the infratemporal, transmastoid, and suboccipital routes into a single approach to meningiomas of the petrous apex. Dural incision immediately next to the transverse and sigmoid sinuses, as modified by the authors, assists in this exposure. Careful skeletalization of the vein of Labbe permits substantial temporal lobe retraction with preservation of this critical structure. Extensive drilling of the retrolabyrinthine petrous bone, which requires intimate knowledge of temporal bone anatomy, gives improved access while preserving intratemporal structures such as the facial nerve. The excellent surgical results are the proof of the pudding. In some cases with huge tumors of this sort, especially in older patients, a subtotal resection, often with postoperative radiation, may be a safer approach.

Lateral Approach to the Anterior Portion of the Foramen Magnum: Application to Surgical Removal of 14 Benign Tumors: Technical Note
George B, Dematons C, Cophignon J (Hôpital Lariboisière, Paris)
Surg Neurol 29:484–490, June 1988   17–11

The anterior approach to tumors in the anterior foramen magnum involves a deep, narrow field and a risk of infectious complications. Posterior approaches are limited by the medulla covering the tumor. A lateral extension of the posterior approach retains its advantages while reducing manipulation of the medulla. This method requires control of the vertebral artery in all cases (Fig 17–5) and of the sigmoid sinus at the jugular

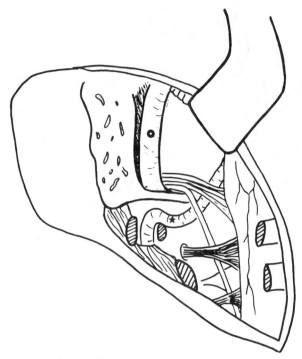

Fig 17–5.—Exposure of the vertebral artery and sigmoid sinus. After laminectomy of C1 and C2 and opening of the transverse foramen of C1, the vertebral artery *(black star)* is controlled. Through partial resection of the mastoid process, the sigmoid sinus *(white star on black field)* is exposed. (Courtesy of George B, Dematons C, Cophignon J: *Surg Neurol* 29:484–490, June 1988.)

foramen in some cases. A more lateral exposure is possible through transposition of the vertebral artery, and an even more lateral approach is the division of the sigmoid sinus at the junction of its vertical and horizontal portions.

A lateral approach to the anterior foramen magnum was used in 14 cases during the past 4 years. Ten patients had meningiomas, and 4 had neurinomas. Tumor was limited to the foramen magnum in 7 cases. A majority of tumors were located anterolaterally in the foramen magnum. The sigmoid sinus was exposed in 11 cases. Three patients died, 1 at reoperation. The lower cranial nerves were resected in all cases with normal preoperative function. Two patients required ventriculoatrial shunting for postoperative hydrocephalus.

Lateral extension of the posterior approach does not prolong surgery excessively in patients with tumors in the anterior part of the foramen magnum. When working anterior to the neural axis, retraction and damage of the spinal cord or medulla are avoided.

▶ This nice technical paper describes a method of visualization of the anterior rim of foramen magnum by mobilization of the vertebral artery and ligation of the sigmoid sinus. These adjuncts may be necessary in some few cases. However, in most cases of foramen magnum meningioma, the tumor is eccentric enough to permit satisfactory lateral visualization through a suboccipital craniectomy and C1 removal. Radical removal of a portion of the condyle with a high-speed drill (1) facilitates this approach. Of great importance to the surgeon is the preoperative axial MR examination, which shows quite clearly any eccentricity of the lesion. Occasionally gadolinium contrast will be needed to demonstrate the tumor satisfactorily for this determination.

Reference

1. Heros RC: *J Neurosurg* 64:559–562, 1986.

18 Tumors

Introduction

The basic *biology* of intracranial neoplasms was enriched in 1989. According to Hochberg and colleagues, primary central nervous system lymphoma is becoming more common in nonimmunosuppressed persons, and it will soon be the most frequent neurologic neoplasm because of increases in both sporadic occurrence and in the AIDS population (Abstract 18–1). The Mayo Clinic group has proposed a simple and reproducible method of grading of astrocytomas based on neuropathologic criteria (Abstract 18–2), but the classification of Borger and Vogel involving differentiation of glioblastoma and anaplastic astrocytoma has gained a wide acceptance by neuro-oncologists (1). Extracellular matrix proteins containing gliofibrillary acidic protein appear to play an important role in the growth of gliomas (Abstract 18–3). Studies of gene amplification in gliomas indicate that cells of different morphology may contain the same genetic alteration (Abstract 18–4).

Magnetic resonance imaging (MRI) continues to expand knowledge of intracranial neoplasms. Correlations of MRI done postmortem with neuropathological findings indicates good correlation between the histologic findings and the MRI patterns (Abstract 18–5). In a study of adrenocorticotropic hormone–producing pituitary adenomas, 3 were seen only after contrast enhancement on MRI and 3 were not imaged, indicating persistent need for petrosal sinus sampling in these patients (Abstract 18–6). Magnetic resonance imaging is not a very sensitive means of detecting cavernous sinus invasion, but unilateral carotid encasement within the sinus was a specific sign of invasion (Abstract 18–7). Magnetic resonance histopathologic correlation in meningiomas demonstrated a clear-cut histologic basis for the varied MRI appearance (Abstract 18–8). This type of data suggests that in the future MRI may help predict preoperatively important surgical features of a tumor, including vascularity, suckability, and the like. Magnetic resonance imaging is useful in the imaging of intracranial neurofibromatosis, especially with gadolinium enhancement (Abstract 18–9). Magnetic resonance imaging and computed tomography (CT) appear to be complimentary in the evaluation of clival chordomas and chondrosarcomas, and CT is probably better for long-term follow-up (Abstract 18–10). Magnetic resonance can image hemorrhage from intracranial neoplasms, but often the identification of the source of bleeding will require angiography or even biopsy (Abstract 18–11). In the detection of spinal meningeal carcinomatosis, a careful comparative study shows that CT with myelography is superior to MRI (Abstract 18–12).

Regarding *surgery:* the aggressive posture of total excision of gliomas receives support from the communication from Sloan-Kettering Center describing low mortality and morbidity for this approach (Abstract 18–13). To the contrary, the Pittsburgh group reports long survival after stereotaxic biopsy and radiation for malignant gliomas without major mass effect (Abstract 18–14). Thus the aggressive and conservative schools of glioma management continue to find adherents and supportive data. Intraorbital meningiomas have been treated both surgically and with radiation therapy (Abstract 18–15). Somatotropin pituitary adenomas treated with microsurgery had excellent results in 214 cases (Abstract 18–16). Even large pituitary adenomas appear to do better after transsphenoidal surgery as compared with transfrontal surgery (Abstract 18–17). Trigeminal schwannoma can be largely or wholly excised with good results (Abstract 18–18). Excellent results can be obtained with surgical excision of intracranial epidermoid tumors, but again in some cases capsule will have to be left adherent to delicate structures (Abstract 18–19).

In *adjunctive therapy,* preoperative irradiation of highly vascular cerebellar pontine angle neurinoma converted 3 extremely difficult vascular tumors into surgically excisable lesions (Abstract 18–20). Radiation therapy for central nervous system involvement in malignant melanoma does not alter the very poor outlook for these patients (Abstract 18–21). Interstitial brachytherapy for metastatic brain tumors appears to be well tolerated, but whether it has a beneficial effect on the lesions remains unknown (Abstract 18–22). Systemic interferon-γ therapy for recurrent gliomas is ineffective (Abstract 18–23). Intralesional infusion of lymphokine-activated killer cells and interleuken-2 and adoptive immunotherapy have low risk and appear to be promising treatments for recurrent glioma (Abstracts 18–24 and 18–25). In the experimental laboratory setting, blood-brain barrier disruption appears to be a promising method to enhance delivery of monoclonal antibody to the area of intracranial tumor (Abstract 18–26). Preoperative treatment of acromegaly with long-acting somatostatin analogues leads to shrinkage of invasive pituitary macroadenomas and improves surgical remission rate (Abstract 18–27).

Robert M. Crowell, M.D.

Reference

1. Borger, Vogel: *Surgical Pathology of the Nervous System and Its Coverings,* ed 2. New York, John Wiley & Sons, 1982.

Biology

Primary Central Nervous System Lymphoma

Hochberg FH, Miller DC (Massachusetts Gen Hosp, Boston; Univ of Medicine and Dentistry of New Jersey)
J Neurosurg 68:835–853, 1988   18–1

Primary lymphoma of the CNS accounts for fewer than 1% of all primary brain tumors and recently has increased in frequency among nonimmunosuppressed persons. It soon will be the most frequent neurologic neoplasm because of increases in both sporadic occurrence and among the AIDS population. Patients with inherited disorders such as severe combined immunodeficiency and Wiskott-Aldrich syndrome and those with acquired immune system disease are disposed to development of CNS lymphoma, in addition to transplant recipients. The role of Epstein-Barr virus remains uncertain.

Clinical data on 96 cases were reviewed; pathologic material was available in 61 instances. The most frequent presentation of non-Hodgkin's lymphoma is with solitary or multiple intracranial tumor masses. Diffuse meningeal or periventricular lesions, uveal or vitreous deposits, and localized intradural spinal masses also are encountered. Both contrast computed tomography and magnetic resonance imaging (MRI) delineate the number and extent of lesions of non-Hodgkin's lymphoma in the brain parenchyma. However, subarachnoid and vitreal lesions are not demonstrated. Primary spinal lesions are best demonstrated with myelography, but MRI also may be useful. Non-Hodgkin's lymphoma of the CNS most often consists of histiocytic cells or large immunoblastic cells with B-cell surface markers. Multiple areas of the neuraxis, multiple intracranial sites, and the eye may be involved without obvious systemic lymphoma. Very few cases of T-cell non-Hodgkin's lymphoma of the CNS have been reported.

Untreated patients with non-Hodgkin's lymphoma of the CNS live only 1.5 months on average. Age is not an important factor in survival, but immunocytoma has a better prognosis than lymphoblastoma or immunoblastoma. Various radiotherapeutic regimens have been utilized, and they seem to increase survival times. Adjuvant chemotherapy trials are under way at several centers. Studies in virology may be fruitful. In addition, antibodies against non-Hodgkin's lymphoma may be used to carry substances to the tumor in vivo.

▶ Because of the dramatic increase in the frequency of these tumors, all clinical neuroscientists must be familiar with their presentation and management. Although the diagnosis may be suspected on clinical and radiographic grounds, in most cases histologic specimens, either from cerebrospinal fluid or stereotaxic biopsy, will be required to confirm the specific diagnosis. The outlook is dismal despite treatment, and therefore it is appropriate that a number of trials are under way with combined radiation therapy and chemotherapy to control this devastating type of intracranial tumor.

Grading of Astrocytomas: A Simple and Reproducible Method
Daumas-Duport C, Scheithauer B, O'Fallon J, Kelly P (Mayo Clinic, Rochester, Minn)
Cancer 62:2152–2165, Nov 15, 1988   18–2

A simple grading system for gliomas of "ordinary" cell types is based on the presence or absence of nuclear atypia, mitoses, endothelial proliferation, and necrosis. Grade 1 lesions meet none of these criteria, whereas grade 2 tumors meet 1 criterion, grade 3 lesions meet 2, and grade 4 lesions meet 3 or 4 criteria.

The grading system was applied to 287 ordinary astrocytomas treated with radiotherapy. In ordinary astrocytoma cases, each of the four histologic criteria and the resultant grade were correlated closely with survival during a 15-year follow-up. Median survival ranged from 4 years in grade 2 cases to 0.7 years in grade 4 cases. Grade was the preeminent prognostic factor, The Kernohan grading system, in contrast, accurately distinguished only 2, not 4 major grades of disease. Two independent observers graded 94% of lesions the same in a double-blind trial. Reproducibility was 81% for low-grade lesions and 96% for grade 3 and grade 4 tumors.

This simple reproducible grading system for ordinary astrocytomas will allow comparison of clinical and therapeutic data from different centers. Use of a binary system limits subjectivity in grading, but strict histologic definitions of the features in question is important.

▶ Neuropathologic grading of astrocytomas has often seemed an inspired art of the neuropathologist. For many years the Kernohan system was predominant, but clarity was a problem, particularly in the differentiation of grade 2 from grade 3 lesions. More recently, there has been widespread utilization of a 3-level grading system, namely, astrocytoma, anaplastic astrocytoma, and glioblastoma. But precise definition of the distinctions in these 3 grades has remained elusive. Thus the present report supplies a highly specific and evidently easily reproducible system for grading primary brain tumors. Whether this system is adopted generally will remain to be seen; however, its usefulness in comparing results from various centers is very attractive.

Products of Cells Cultured From Gliomas: VII. Extracellular Matrix Proteins of Gliomas Which Contain Glial Fibrillary Acidic Protein
McKeever PE, Fligiel SEG, Varani J, Castle RL, Hood TW (Univ of Michigan; Wayne State Univ, Detroit)
Lab Invest 60:286–295, February 1989   18–3

Proteins of the extracellular matrix (ECM) are needed for cellular attachment and structural integrity of the tissue. These proteins may be involved in the growth of neoplasms. In gliomas, a distinct aspect of tumor progression is diminution of glial and increase of ECM expression with increased malignancy. These changes include reductions in glial fibrillary acid protein (GFAP) and rises in fibronectin. Changes in GFAP and fibronectin occur in situ and in vitro, but their cause is not known. A study was done to examine a spectrum of ECM components expressed by GFAP+ glioma cell cultures.

Extracellular matrix components of GFAP+ lines U251 and UM6 were studied by silver stain, morphometry, immunofluorescence, enzyme-linked immunosorbent assay, and biosynthetic labeling. Both lines expressed laminin, type IV collagen, extracellular fibrils of silver-reducing collagen, and a pattern of reactivity with lectins similar to that with previously studied GFAP− gliomas. Both GFAP+ glioma proteins expressed less collagen and more laminin than GFAP− gliomas. Sparse collagen of GFAP+ gliomas was found to aggregate as extracellular masses. Individual UM6 cells simultaneously expressed GFAP and mesenchymal ECM components. There were qualitative similarities of ECM expression among GFAP+ and GFAP− gliomas, suggesting a common lineage of these cell types and universal expression of 2 epithelial components of ECM, laminin, and type IV collagen among cultured gliomas. A diversity of quantity and type of ECM proteins of GFAP+ gliomas with the U251 line most restricted in its expression of ECM components and with UM6 manifesting markers of epithelial and mesenchymal lineage was seen, suggesting a capacity for regulation of phenotypic expression of ECM beyond that explained simply by the presence of 2 cell types of different lineage (Fig 18−1).

▶ The extracellular matrix currently is receiving great attention in relation to tu-

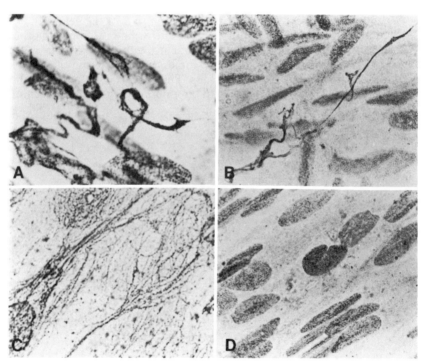

Fig 18−1.—Collagen of UM6 and U251 GFAP + gliomas and fibroblasts localized by Tibor Pap silver stain in fields selected for abundant fibrils. Sparse, thick bundles of collagen produced by UM6 (**A**) and by U251 (**B**) stain intensely in contrast to the ubiquitous fine lace work of fibrils produced by fibroblasts (**C**). Oval and spindle-shaped nuclei are in plane of focus below fibrils. **D**, UM6 stained after pretreatment with collagenase. **A** and **C**, original magnification, ×1,900; **B** and **D**, original magnification, ×1,240. (Courtesy of McKeever PE, Fligiel SEG, Varani J, et al: *Lab Invest* 60:286−295, February 1989.)

mor biology. It is clear that extracellular components such as laminin, type 4 collagen, and extracellular fibronectin are important in determining the growth patterns of neoplasms. A body of information is growing on the pathophysiology of the matrix, its cellular elaboration, and genetic control of the entire process. Enhanced understanding of these aspects will likely be helpful in diagnosis and management of intracranial tumors.

Gene Amplification in Malignant Human Gliomas: Clinical and Histopathologic Aspects

Bigner SH, Burger PC, Wong AJ, Werner MH, Hamilton SR, Muhlbaier LH, Vogelstein B, Bigner DD (Duke Univ; Johns Hopkins Univ)
J Neuropathol Exp Neurol 47:191–205, May 1988   18–4

Gene amplification occurs in up to half of malignant human gliomas. Sixty-four tumors were genetically characterized to relate amplification of the epidermal growth factor receptor (EGFR), N-*myc*, c-*myc*, and *gli* genes to the histopathologic features. Expression of EGFR protein was estimated immunohistochemically.

Twenty-eight tumors exhibited amplification of 1 of the genes studies; 24 had an amplified EGFR gene. Only 4 patients had received radiotherapy before tumor resection. Among patients with glioblastoma multiforme and gliosarcoma, those whose tumors contained amplified genes survived slightly longer than the others (Fig 18–2). Prominent lymphocytic infiltrates were more prevalent in tumors without amplification.

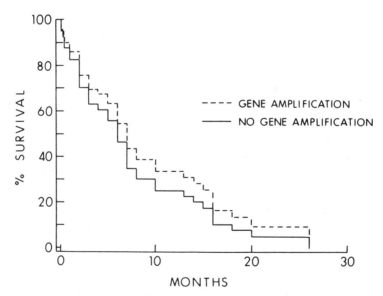

Fig 18–2.—Mortality distributions for patients whose tumors contain gene amplification (- - -) and for patients without demonstrable gene amplification in their tumors (——) are similar. (Courtesy of Bigner SH, Burger PC, Wong AJ, et al: *J Neuropathol Exp Neurol* 47:191–205, May 1988.)

There were no other apparent histopathologic differences. In situ hybridization of tumors with amplification using an EGFR messenger ribonucleic acid probe showed intense labeling of neoplastic cells only, including fibrillary and protoplasmic astrocytes, gemistocytes, anaplastic cells, and multinucleated giant cells.

Glioma cells of differing morphology in the same tumor may contain the same genetic alteration. Gene amplification cannot be predicted by the histologic features of gliomas.

▶ This interesting communication demonstrates that glioma cells of different morphology within the same tumor may contain the same generic alteration of amplification. Systematic further investigation of gene defects may well help unravel the mystery of glioma.

Levy and Litham (1) studied quantitative immunohistochemistry in situ for anterior pituitary hormone mRNA species in human pituitary adenomas. Among 21 tumors, evidence of activitation of more than 1 anterior pituitary hormone existed in 16, which only showed a pattern of activitation or amplification of gene expression. From these data it is not possible to postulate isolated deregulation of a single second messenger transduction pathway.

Reference

1. Levy A, Litham SL: *Acta Endocrinol (Copenh)* 119:397–404, 1988.

Brief Notes on Tumor Biology

PRIMARY CNS LYMPHOMA

Incidence of primary brain lymphoma (unrelated to AIDS and immunocompromise) appears to be rising in the United States (Eby NL et al: *Cancer* 62:2461–2465, 1988).

Primary lymphoma of the CNS has been reported in children with AIDS (Epstein LG et al: *Pediatrics* 82:355–363, 1988).

Lymphocytic lymphoma may appear as a primary meningeal deposit (Nguyand, Nathwani BN: *Am J Surg Pathol* 13:67–70, 1989).

Dexamethasone, high-dose cytarabine, and cisplatin give encouraging results with brain lymphoma (McLaughlin P et al: *J Natl Cancer Inst* 80:1408–1413, 1988).

A patient with histologically proven lymphoma is symptom free 79 months after craniotomy (Trapella G et al: *Ital J Neurol Sci* 9:275–278, 1988).

In primary central nervous system lymphoma, favorable factors are age less than 60, Karnovsky score greater than 70, strictly hemispheric mass, radiation dose between 4,000 and 5,000 cGy, and chemotherapy, as well as complete tumor resection (Pollack IF et al: *Cancer* 63:939–947, 1989).

ACOUSTIC NEUROMA

Acoustic neuromas arise in vestibular ganglion cells, which exhibit features of immaturity in humans. In species in which acoustic neuroma has never been reported, these abnormalities are not seen (Viala P et al: *Sem Hop Paris* 64:2319–2320, 1988).

Meningiomas

In flow cytometry of meningiomas, DNA index and proliferative index were correlated with brain invasion, associated edema, and recurrence (Crone KR et al: *Neurosurgery* 23:720–724, 1988).

Epidermal growth factor receptors and somatostatin receptors are found together in meningiomas but in an inverse relationship in gliomas (Renbi JC et al: *Am J Pathol* 134:337–344, 1989).

Epidermal growth factor receptor in meningiomas is expressed predominantly on endothelial cells (Shiurba RA et al: *Cancer* 62:2139–2144, 1988).

Epidermal growth factor receptors are found in meningiomas, but levels are low in anaplastic lesions and undetected in angiomatous lesions (Grimaux M et al: *Rev Neurol [Paris]* 144:96–103, 1988).

Cytogenetic analysis of multiple meningiomas excludes cell migration and points to a different origin for each tumor as a pathogenic factor (Buttig et al: *Surg Neurol* 31:255–260, 1989).

In meningiomas, CD-8 subtype lymphocytes were present in 70%, CD-4 positive T lymphocytes were present in 1 benign meningioma, and HLA DR antigen was present in 60%. The presence of these cells raises questions about lymphocytic infiltration in relation to prognosis (Rossi ML et al: *J Clin Pathol* 41:314–319, 1988).

Immunohistochemical studies suggest that meningiomas express both epithelial and glial markers, angioplastic meningiomas and peripheral hemangiopericytomas both express only glial markers, and the markers are unreliable in differentiating meningioma from acoustic schwannoma (Winek RR et al: *Am J Surg Pathol* 13:251–261, 1989).

In patients aged more than 60 years undergoing surgery for meningioma, morbidity was 48% with neurologic decline in 31% and serious disability in 15% at 3 months. Best outcomes occurred with little preoperative disability and convexity lesions (Awad IA et al: *Neurosurgery* 24:557–560, 1989).

Prolactinoma

CV 205–502 appears to be a safe and effective oral alternative to other dopamine agonists in the treatment of hyperprolactinemia (Vance ML et al: *J Clin Endocrinol Metab* 68:336–338, 1989).

The natural history of untreated hyperprolactinemia is rather benign, with progression unlikely and clinical and radiographic improvement possible (Schlecke J et al: *J Clin Endocrinol Metab* 68:412–418, 1989).

Neurofibromatosis

Somatomedin C may be a pathogenetic factor in the development of neurofibromatosis (Hansson AJ et al: *Scand J Plast Reconstr Surg* 22:7–13, 1988).

In situ hybridization assists in the study of cellular differentiation and expression of matrix genes in type I neurofibromatosis (Peltonen J et al: *Lab Invest* 59:760–771, 1988).

A case of familial multiple neurilemoma has been reported and may be a forme fruste of Recklinghausen's disease (Yamazaki F et al: *Arch Orthop Trauma Surg* 107:256–258, 1988).

RECEPTORS AND MARKERS

Messenger RNAs for platelet-derived growth factor and their receptors have been isolated from gliomas, thus demonstrating an autocrine (self-stimulating) loop for these tumors (Nister M et al: *Cancer Res* 48:3910–3918, 1988).

Immunocytochemical determinations show widespread distribution of glial fibrillary acidic protein and vimentin and cast doubt upon the concept of VM as a marker for dedifferentiation (Izukawa D, Lach B: *Can J Neurol Sci* 15:114–118, 1988).

Immunohistochemical studies suggest apolipoprotein E may be a marker for glial tumors and an indicator of astrocytic tumor cell differentiation (Murakami M et al: *J Clin Invest* 82:177–188, 1988).

NEOVASCULARIZATION

Studies in a rabbit brain model of tumor growth correlates proliferation of blood vessels in the tumor with breakdown of the blood-brain barrier (Zagzag D et al: *Ann J Pathol* 131:361–372, 1988).

VX-2 carcinoma was implanted in the rabbit brain, and tumor angiogenesis correlated with logarithmic intracerebral tumor growth (Zagzag D et al: *Am J Pathol* 131:361–372, 1988).

Intercapillary distances are less in the proliferating area of human glioma (Yoshii Y, Sugiyama K: *Cancer Res* 48:2938–2941, 1988).

OTHER BASIC TUMORS STUDIES

W. J. Bodell and associates (*Cancer Res* 48:4489–4492, 1988) report differences in DNA alkylation products formed in sensitive and resistant human glioma cells.

M.C. Kuppner and co-workers report immunohistologic and functional analysis of lymphoid infiltrates in human glioblastomas (*Cancer Res* 48:6926–6932, 1988).

Transforming growth factor beta-1 is a potent inducer of plasminogen activator inhibitor type 1 in human glioblastoma (Helseth E et al: *APMIS* 96:845–849, 1988).

Specific binding of atrial natriuretic peptide increases cyclic GMP levels in human astrocytoma cells (Lyall F et al: *J Endocrinol* 117:315–321, 1988).

When BUDR was used to label cells in DNA synthesis, low labeling indices were noted for teratomas, craniopharyngiomas, and dermoid tumors. Elevated DNA synthesis was present for immature teratoma, embryonal carcinoma, choriocarcinoma, and some cases of chordoma (Cho KG et al: *Cancer* 62:740–748, 1988).

Immunohistochemical and electron microscopic studies suggest that both oligodendrogliomas and oligoastrocytomas arise from a common progenitor cell (Sarkar C et al: *Cancer* 61:1862–1866, 1988).

Magnetic Resonance Imaging

Human Cerebral Gliomas: Correlation of Postmortem MR Imaging and Neuropathologic Findings
Johnson PC, Hunt SJ, Drayer BP (Barrow Neurological Inst, Phoenix)
Radiology 170:211–217, January 1989   18–5

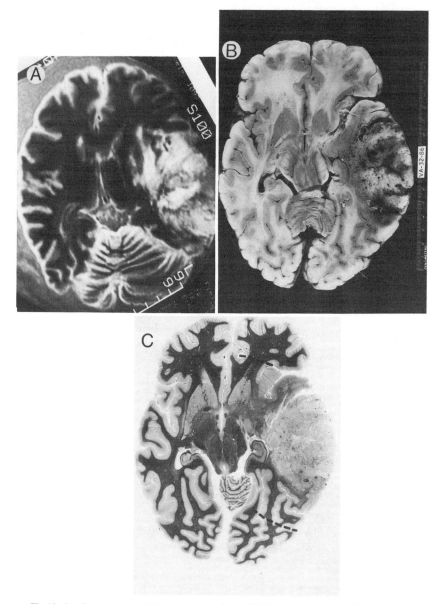

Fig 18–3.—A, postmortem MR image (spin-echo, 2,000/80) of an untreated glioblastoma multi-forme shows a markedly variegated signal hyperintensity in the left temporal and parietal lobes because of interspersed hemorrhage and necrosis. **B,** gross section was obtained slightly off from the plane of the MR image, but both the variegated character of the tumor and tumor extent are strongly correlated with the MR imaging appearance. **C,** gross section (Weil stain). The *dashed lines* demonstrate the limit of the tumor corona. The MR image (**A**) shows less extensive abnormality; however, angulation of the section is different. (Courtesy of Johnson PC, Hunt SJ, Drayer BP: *Radiology* 170:211–217, January 1989.)

Computed tomography (CT) cannot be used to depict precisely the limits of tumors with an outer rim of isolated tumor cells infiltrating otherwise intact brain tissue. This is a major impediment in planning treatment for patients with glioblastoma multiforme and other astrocytic neoplasms. The value of magnetic resonance (MR) imaging in such cases was assessed.

Findings from T_2-weighted MR images of postmortem, in vitro human brain glioma specimens were correlated with histologic findings from whole-brain sections. Six of the patients had not been treated, 2 were in remission after surgery and radiation therapy, and 10 had recurrent disease. Findings from MR imaging generally correlated well with the histologic extent of untreated tumors in white matter. The heterogeneous appearance of glioblastomas multiforme distinguished them from less malignant gliomas. Magnetic resonance images overestimated the extent of tumors in remission because of the extensive surrounding edema and radiation necrosis (Fig 18–3).

In this study MR imaging findings were well correlated with histologic findings from whole-brain sections. Knowledge of a patient's disease stage was also found to be important in interpreting MR images of astrocytoma.

▶ Careful correlation of MRI and tumor histology can be helpful in a number of ways. First it is important for clinicians to know the precise meaning of various signals detected on the imaging studies. For example, recent imaging studies indicate that gadolinium positivity is not correlated precisely with solid tumor but may instead indicate a more nonspecific set of changes within and around the tumor. The present study adds to our knowledge of the correlation of various MRI signal changes and various abnormalities within gliomas. Another type of valuable by-product of such studies may be related to preoperative assessment of operability and operative risks. For example, Russel Patterson and colleagues at Cornell have some data indicating that preoperative MRI may help in assessing the firmness of sellar tumors, suggesting the relative operability of such lesions via the transsphenoidal route. These studies provide a substantial advance in the sophistication of our utilization of modern imaging techniques for preoperative evaluation.

Gadolinium DTPA Enhanced MR Imaging of ACTH-Secreting Microadenomas of the Pituitary Gland

Doppman JL, Frank JA, Dwyer AJ, Oldfield EH, Miller DL, Nieman LK, Chrousos GP, Cutler GB Jr, Loriaux DL (Natl Insts of Health, Bethesda, Md; Georgetown Univ)
J Comput Assist Tomogr 12:728–735, September–October 1988   18–6

Adrenocorticotropic hormone (ACTH)-secreting pituitary gland adenomas can be diagnosed by sampling the inferior petrosal sinuses for ACTH levels before and after corticotropin-releasing hormone administration. However, petrosal sinus sampling is invasive and expensive. Re-

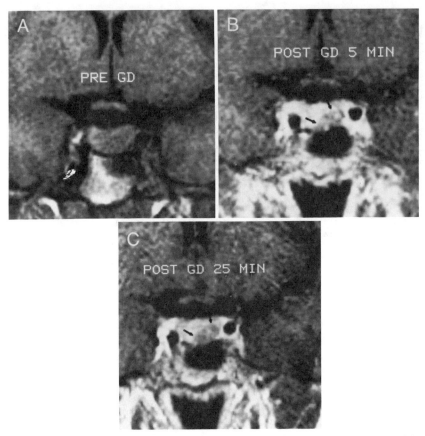

Fig 18–4.—Pre-Gd T_1-weighted (spin-echo, 500/20) coronal image shows an 8-mm oval area of decreased signal in left lower quadrant of pituitary gland (a), much more apparent on 5-minute post-Gd scan (b; *arrows*). Enhancement of normal pituitary gland persists on 25-minute post-Gd scan (c; *arrows*) but by 50 min returned to appearance (a). (Courtesy of Doppman JL, Frank JA, Dwyer AJ, et al: *J Comput Assist Tomogr* 12:728–735, September–October 1988.)

portedly, nuclear magnetic resonance (MR) imaging using an intermediate-field strength magnet (0.5 tesla [T]) and image enhancement with the paramagnetic contrast agent gadolinium diethylenetriamine penta-acetic acid (Gd-DTPA) significantly improves detection of pituitary gland adenomas. Also, a high-field strength (1.5 T) magnet has correctly identified more than 90% of pituitary adenomas without need for a contrast agent. A 1.5-T magnet was used with Gd-DTPA to diagnose suspected pituitary microadenomas in 8 women aged 22–50 years with biochemically confirmed Cushing's disease and negative contrast-enhanced coronal computed tomographic (CT) findings. All underwent MR scanning before and after intravenous Gd-DTPA administration; transsphenoidal exploration was done, and the surgical findings were correlated with the findings on MR imaging.

Three (38%) of the 8 patients did not have microadenomas detected either at surgery or on MR, with or without Gd-DTPA enhancement. All 3 patients were cured by hemihypophysectomy according to the findings of postoperative petrosal sinus ACTH sampling. The other 5 patients had adenomas detected at surgery. The microadenomas in 2 of these 5 patients appeared as hypointense foci with Gd-DTPA enhancement but were not detected on unenhanced scans. The microadenomas in the other 3 patients were seen on both the unenhanced and the enhanced MR scans (Fig 18–4).

▶ These data suggest gadolinium MRI can be used to diagnose most microadenomas, but cavernous sinus sampling is still necessary to detect those missed on gadolinium MRI.

MR Imaging of Cavernous Sinus Involvement by Pituitary Adenomas
Scotti G, Yu C-Y, Dillon WP, Norman D, Colombo N, Newton TH, De Groot J, Wilson CB (Univ of California, San Francisco; Univ of Milan, Italy; Cheng-Kung Univ, Tainan, Taiwan; Ospedale Niguarda Ca Granda, Milan)
AJR 151:799–806, October 1988   18–7

Pituitary adenomas frequently involve the cavernous sinuses to varying degree. The value of magnetic resonance imaging (MRI) in assessing cavernous sinus involvement was examined in a review of 74 patients and a

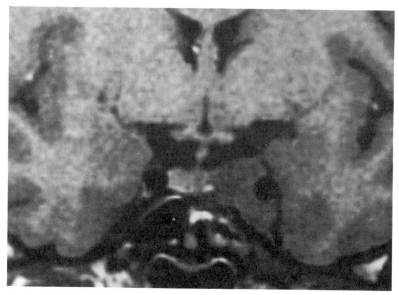

Fig 18–5.—Fourteen-millimeter nonsecreting recurrent pituitary adenoma, with surgically proved invasion of left cavernous sinus. Left carotid artery is surrounded by tumor, and there is lateral bowing of lateral dural reflection as well as marked enlargement of medial and superior compartments by this tumor, which has signal intensity significantly lower than that of adjacent pituitary and temporal lobe. (Courtesy of Scotti G, Yu C-Y, Dillon WP, et al: *AJR* 151:799–806, October 1988.)

prospective analysis of 30 others with pituitary adenoma. Both sagittal and coronal MRI are recorded.

Asymmetric cavernous sinus signal intensity was noted in only 2 of 13 invasive microadenomas in the retrospective series. Ten of 11 invasive macroadenomas produced sinus asymmetry. The cavernous segment of the carotid artery was displaced only in macroadenomas. In macroadenomas with cavernous sinus invasion, unilateral involvement of the sinus and occasional carotid encasement were observed (Fig 18–5). Encasement occurred only with invasive tumors. In the prospective series, the cavernous sinuses were asymmetrically enlarged in 5 of 9 patients with proved sinus invasion and in 3 others. Absence of the medial wall of the sinus was a poor predictor of invasion. There were 4 false negative MRI studies and 3 false positive scans.

Magnetic resonance imaging is not a very sensitive means of detecting cavernous sinus invasion by pituitary adenoma. Unilateral carotid encasement within the sinus is a specific sign of sinus invasion. The finding of normal compressed pituitary between the tumor and cavernous sinus or bilateral carotid displacement helps exclude cavernous sinus invasion.

▶ Magnetic resonance imaging is evidently not very sensitive for the detection of cavernous sinus invasion. One wonders how sensitive surgical transsphenoidal exploration is in making this diagnosis. On the other hand, pathologic evidence of invasion of the dura by pituitary adenoma is unexpectedly common and may have no clear bearing on clinical outcome. Long-term follow-up data relating clinical outcome to these various observations will be needed to establish their predictive utility.

Meningiomas: MR and Histopathologic Features
Elster AD, Challa VR, Gilbert TH, Richardson DN, Contento JC (Wake Forest Univ, Winston-Salem, NC)
Radiology 170:857–862, March 1989   18–8

Several studies have been published on the magnetic resonance (MR) appearance of intracranial meningiomas. Later researchers have noted appreciable variability in signal characteristics, with more than half of the tumors becoming significantly hypointense or hyperintense to brain on certain pulse sequences. The pathologic basis of this MR signal heterogenicity was explored.

The MR appearances of 40 biopsy-proved meningiomas were blindly evaluated and correlated with their predominant histologic pattern: fibroblastic, transitional, syncytial, angioblastic, or mixed. T_1-weighted images were not especially useful in discriminating pathologic subtype because most tumors were isointense with or hypointense to cortex, irrespective of histologic type. Signal intensity and features on T_2-weighted images were found to correlate strongly with histopathologic findings in more than 75% of cases (Fig 18–6). Meningiomas significantly hypointense to cortex on T_2-weighted images consisted of mostly fibroblastic or

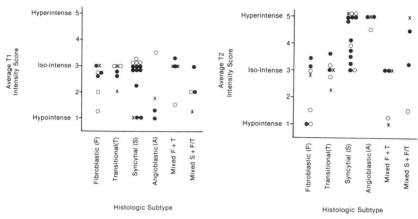

Fig 18–6.—Average T_1 (**right**) and T_2 (**left**) intensity scores as a function of histologic subtype. Each point represents the average score of the 4 readers for each tumor. *Shaded circles* represent images obtained at 0.15 tesla (T); *crosses*, images obtained at 0.35 T or 0.5 T; *open circles*, images obtained at 1.5 T. (Courtesy of Elster AD, Challa VR, Gilbert TH, et al: *Radiology* 170:857–862, March 1989.)

transitional elements, whereas markedly hyperintense meningiomas demonstrated predominance of syncytial or angioblastic elements. Examining secondary features visible at MR imaging resulted in a more specific histologic prediction in more than half of the remaining isointense tumors.

The varied MR appearance of meningiomas has a clear histologic basis. Crude prediction of pathologic subtype was concluded to be possible in more than 75% of the cases.

▶ Subtypes of meningioma have specific MR signatures. This is of interest to the histopathologist, but of more interest to the surgeon is the correlation with vascularity and firmness of the tumor, 2 characteristics that significantly affect the difficulty of surgery. Perhaps MR-surgical correlation will lead to recognition of tumor vascularity and texture preoperatively and thus to improved estimate of risk.

Cranial MR Imaging in Neurofibromatosis
Bognanno JR, Edwards MK, Lee TA, Dunn DW, Roos KL, Klatte EC (Indiana Univ, Indianapolis)
AJR 151:381–388, August 1988   18–9

Medical records and magnetic resonance (MR) images of 53 patients with a tentative diagnosis of neurofibromatosis were reviewed to determine the nature, extent, and number of intracranial abnormalities. Of these 53 patients, 30 were neurologically asymptomatic and 23 had clinical or previous findings on computed tomography (CT) consistent with intracranial or cranial nerve abnormalities. Recent cranial CT scans were available for 40 of the 53 patients.

Parenchymal central nervous system or extra-axial intracranial lesions

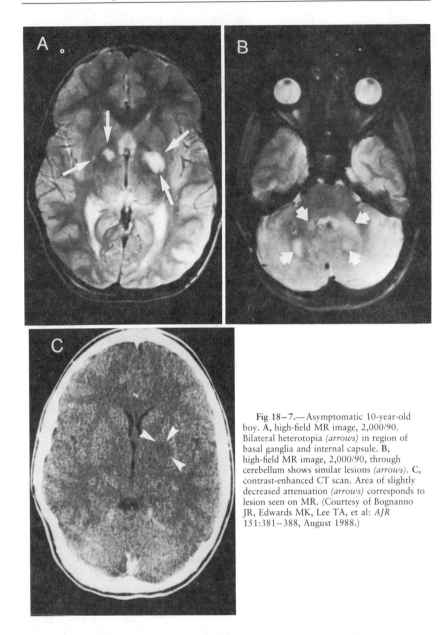

Fig 18–7.—Asymptomatic 10-year-old boy. **A,** high-field MR image, 2,000/90. Bilateral heterotopia *(arrows)* in region of basal ganglia and internal capsule. **B,** high-field MR image, 2,000/90, through cerebellum shows similar lesions *(arrows)*. **C,** contrast-enhanced CT scan. Area of slightly decreased attenuation *(arrows)* corresponds to lesion seen on MR. (Courtesy of Bognanno JR, Edwards MK, Lee TA, et al: *AJR* 151:381–388, August 1988.)

were detected by MR screening in 46 of the 53 patients. The other 7 patients had normal scans. Thirty-two patients had single lesions, and 14 had multiple lesions. Small focal areas of increased signal on T_2-weighted scans within the brain, found in 23 patients, appeared to be focal areas of heterotopic or possibly dysplastic tissue. The areas were located primarily in the basal ganglia and internal capsule with other lesions seen in the midbrain, cerebellum, and subcortical white matter. Computed tomography and T_1-weighted MR images revealed few or no abnormalities in corresponding locations (Fig 18–7). Eight patients had chiasmal gliomas, 2 had optic nerve gliomas, 9 had parenchymal gliomas, 2 had ischemic changes, and 1 had a colloid cyst. Extra-axial lesions included acoustic neuromas in 5 patients, meningiomas in 4, trigeminal neurofibromas in 1, and dysplasia of the sphenoid wing in 2. Twenty-three of the 30 asymptomatic patients had lesions on MR scanning; therefore a baseline screening MR study in all patients with neurofibromatosis is highly recommended.

▶ Magnetic resonance imaging is an excellent method of imaging known disease and detecting lesions in asymptomatic patients with neurofibromatosis (NF). A screening MR study is recommended for patients with NF.

The Role of MR and CT in Evaluating Clival Chordomas and Chondrosarcomas

Oot RF, Melville GE, New PFJ, Austin-Seymour M, Munzenrider J, Pile-Spellman J, Spagnoli M, Shoukimas GM, Momose KJ, Carroll R, Davis KR (Massachusetts Gen Hosp, Boston; Harvard Med School)
AJR 151:567–575, September 1988   18–10

Chordomas are rare, slow-growing, but locally aggressive tumors arising from remnants of the notochord. Total surgical resection is generally impossible. Tumor volume and its relationship to adjacent neural structures must be accurately defined before radiation therapy and in following up patients' treatment responses. The relative abilities of magnetic resonance (MR) imaging and computed tomography (CT) in providing this information were determined.

Sixteen patients with chordomas and 9 with chondrosarcomas of the clivus underwent CT and MR imaging examination before or after treatment with proton beam irradiation. In all cases, the tumor was detected and its gross margins identified with both CT and MR imaging. No reliable diagnostic features enabling differentiation between the 2 tumors could be identified.

In general, MR imaging was better at defining the exact position of the brain stem and optic chiasm relative to the tumor, and it also often provided superior information about tumor extension into the nasopharynx and cavernous sinus. Computed tomography was always better than MR imaging at showing tumoral calcification and defining the exact anatomy of the bone destruction. Magnetic resonance imaging was generally better than CT at showing the position of the cavernous internal carotid artery relative to the tumor and frequently provided superior visualization of the vertebral and basilar arteries. Magnetic resonance imaging was also very valuable in planning irradiation therapy for patients in whom bone-induced artifact obscured the interface between the neural axis and the tumor in the CT image or in whom the tumor had suprasellar extension

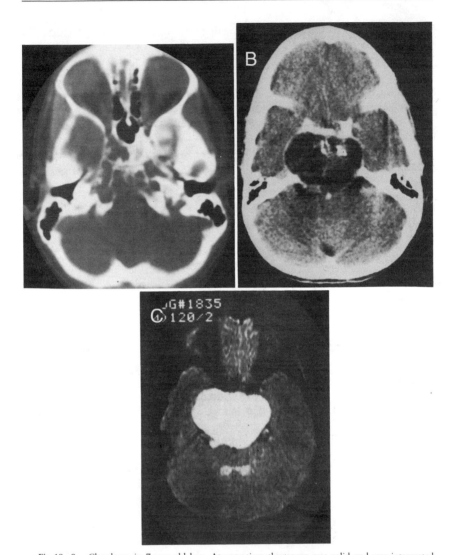

Fig 18–8.—Chordoma in 7-year-old boy. At operation, the tumor was solid and was interpreted pathologically as chordoma, with some features suggestive of a cartilaginous component. Tumor did not invade dura. **A** and **B,** axial postcontrast CT scans show that tumor is of low density, associated with extensive bone destruction. **C,** axial spin-echo, 2,000/(60),120 MR image shows that tumor has very prolonged T_2 relaxation time and homogeneous appearance. (Courtesy of Oot RF, Melville GE, New PFJ, et al: *AJR* 151:567–575, September 1988.)

and was likely to compress the optic chiasm and tracts. The high occurrence of clinically asymptomatic signal intensity changes in MR examinations of previously treated patients seems to limit the differential diagnostic value of these data (Fig 18–8).

In this assessment of the relative capabilities of MR imaging and CT in depicting tumor volume and its relationship to adjacent neural structures, information provided by CT and MR images often proved complementary in planning proton beam therapy. Computed tomography appears to be the technique of choice for routine follow-up of previously treated patients because of its greater availability and lower cost.

▶ This study indicates that MR and CT are both needed for evaluation of clival tumors. Computed tomography appeared to be more valuable for routine follow-up because of the availability and lower cost. Unfortunately, gadolinium MRI was not utilized in this study. Chordomas and chondrosarcomas are highly positive in gadolinium enhancement, which may well turn out to be the best way of following these lesions postoperatively.

MR Imaging of Hemorrhagic Intracranial Neoplasms
Destian S, Sze G, Krol G, Zimmerman RD, Deck MDF (Cornell Univ; Mem Sloan-Kettering Cancer Ctr, New York)
AJNR 9:1115–1122, November–December 1988   18–11

An attempt to distinguish between hemorrhagic tumor and pure hemorrhage was made in a study of 30 patients with bleeding intracranial neoplasms who had both magnetic resonance imaging (MRI) and computed tomographic (CT) studies. Twenty-four patients had metastatic tumors, most frequently melanoma. Computed tomographic scans were obtained with and without contrast. Six patients with metastatic tumor had follow-up studies.

Initial lesions were isointense or mildly hypointense on short repetition time (TR) sequences and hypointense on long TR sequences (table); subsequently, hyperintensity was evident on both short and long TR sequences. Stage III lesions had a well-defined black rim on long TR sequences. Some patients had mixed patterns. Stage I lesions contained fresh hemorrhage on histologic study; as the stage advanced the hemorrhage became organized. However, the intensity pattern did not always reflect the clinical age of hemorrhage.

Magnetic resonance imaging should help determine the cause of intracranial hemorrhage at any specific site. If hemorrhage evolves slowly or

---

Signal Intensity Patterns of Hemorrhagic Neoplasms Compared With Described Evolution of Pure Hemorrhage

Hemorrhagic Neoplasm		Signal Intensity		Pure Hemorrhage	
Stage	Age	Short TR	Long TR	Stage	Age
1	Variable	Iso, Hypo	Hypo	Acute	2–5 days
2	Variable	Iso→Hyper	Iso→Hyper	Subacute	5–14 days
3	Variable	Hyper	Hyper with black rim	Chronic	2 wk–mos
M	Variable	Variable	Variable		

(Courtesy of Destian S, Sze G, Krol G, et al: *AJNR* 9:1115–1122, November–December 1988.)

develops hyperintensity as it evolves, underlying tumor should be suspected. A pattern of mixed-signal intensity is also suggestive of neoplasm. If a hemosiderin rim develops, tumor should not be ruled out.

▶ This report characterizes hemorrhagic features on MRI for intracranial neoplasms. Some of the fetuses are helpful in comparing hemorrhagic neoplasm with pure hemorrhage, but even the data provided by this study cannot uniquely define the origin of hemorrhage in each patient. It is of value to the clinician to use this data and in certain cases repeat the studies after a suitable interval has elapsed. When angioma or aneurysm is a significant consideration, angiography, and even repeat angiography, may be important in pursuing the evaluation. In a small number of cases, in order to clinch the diagnosis and protect against future deterioration, craniotomy and removal of the lesion may be the best approach.

MR of Cranial and Spinal Meningeal Carcinomatosis: Comparison With CT and Myelography
Krol G, Sze G, Malkin M, Walker R (Mem Sloan-Kettering Cancer Ctr, New York)
AJR 151:583–588, September 1988   18–12

Neoplastic involvement of the leptomeningeal membranes can result from neoplasms arising in the central nervous system or can occur as a metastatic process originating from a distant primary tumor. Computed tomography (CT) of the cranium without and with contrast and complete myelography with water-soluble contrast medium are used in the conventional radiographic evaluation of the extent of disease. Because magnetic resonance (MR) imaging has shown superiority over other imaging techniques in the assessment of numerous cranial and spinal abnormalities, the contribution of MR imaging to the diagnostic assessment of patients with meningeal carcinomatosis was studied.

Thirty-nine patients with histologically proved primary neoplasms, focal neurologic deficits, and positive cytologic findings in the cerebrospinal fluid underwent enhanced cranial CT and MR imaging assessment or complete myelography and MR imaging of the spine. Fifty-six percent of the patients had intracranial anomalies on CT, including abnormal enhancement of subarachnoid space and ventricular walls, ventricular dilation, obliteration of cortical sulci, and enhancing nodules in the subarachnoid cisterns and lumen of the lateral ventricles. The degree of ventricular enlargement and the intraventricular tumor deposits were equally well visualized with CT and MR imaging, but involvement of ventricular walls, tentorium, subarachnoid cisterns, or subarachnoid space interpreted as abnormal enhancement on CT was not readily appreciated on T_1- and T_2-weighted spin-echo sequences. The findings in 44% of the CT scans and 65% of the MR images were believed to be normal.

Myelographic findings were highly correlated with clinical diagnosis;

none of the observations on myelograms were false negative. Myelography demonstrated nodular filling defects in the subarachnoid space, thickening and crowding of roots of the cauda equina, irregularity of individual roots, and scalloping of the subarachnoid membranes, all of which were not well depicted by MR imaging, which showed a definite abnormality of the subarachnoid space in only 27% of the patients with positive myelographic findings. In 44%, interpretation of MR images of the spine was false negative.

The technique of choice for assessing the central nervous system for presence and extent of neoplastic involvement of the leptomeninges remains contrast-enhanced CT and complete myelography with water-soluble contrast material. Nonenhanced MR imaging of the head and spine is much less sensitive in depicting such changes, although the use of gadolinium holds promise.

▶ This communication indicates that myelography is superior to MRI in the detection of spinal meningeal carcinomatosis. However, recent experiments suggest that MRI with gadolinium is even more sensitive, and in an earlier study, Sze and associates found that gadolinium MRI was extremely effective in depicting intradural extramedullary disease of the spine down to 3-mm nodules (1). Further experiments with this technique will be needed to establish this point.

Reference

    1. Sze G et al: *AJR* 150:911–921, 1988.

Brief Notes on Tumor Imaging

GLIOMAS

H. T. Whelan and co-workers (*Pediatr Neurol* 4:279–283, 1988) studied CT and MRI with pathologic confirmation in a canine glioma model. They found that gadolinium enhancement corresponds to areas of pathologically proved tumor infiltration. Autopsy findings were correlated better with MRI than with CT.

Evolution of gliomatosis cerebri into glioblastoma multiforme was documented by magnetic resonance and computed tomography (Romero SJ et al: *J Comput Assist Tomogr* 12:253–257, 1988).

In 3 surgically proven cases, gangliocytomas show hyperdensity on CT without enhancement and mixed signal on T_1-weighted MR images and decreased signal on T_2-weighted images (Altman NR: *AJNR* 9:917–921, 1988).

Glioblastoma multiforme may masquerade as a pleomorphic xanthoastrocytoma (Gaskill SJ et al: *Childs Nerv Syst* 4:237–240, 1988).

ADENOMAS

Among 24 surgically verified cases of microadenoma of the pituitary gland, 18 cases were confirmed with MRI, which proved to be the most sensitive and effective diagnostic tool (Wichmann W et al: *Fortschr Rontg* 149:239–244, 1988).

With gadolinium MRI, pituitary adenomas were imaged in 10 of 12 patients found to have lesions at surgery (Dwyer AF et al: *Radiology* 163:421–426, 1987).

Thin-section MRI of the sella for ACTH-secreting adenomas has a sensitivity of 71% and specificity of 87% (Peck WW et al: *AJR* 152:145–151, 1989).

Pituitary adenomas and intrasellar meningiomas may be associated with non-visualization of diaphragma sellae and elevated prolactin level (Michael AS, Paige ML: *J Comput Assist Tomogr* 12:944–946, 1988).

Computed tomographic scans were used to correctly identify 13 of 16 somatotroph adenomas (Marcovitz S et al: *AJNR* 9:19–22, 1988).

MENINGIOMAS

For juxtasellar meningiomas, high-resolution MR was considered superior to CT and often predicted the results of angiography (Yeakley JW et al: *AJNR* 9:279–285, 1988).

Fine-needle aspiration cytology may accurately diagnose recurrent ectopic meningioma (Gonzalez-Campora R et al: *Acta Cytol* 33:85–87, 1989).

OTHER PARASELLAR DIAGNOSTICS

Magnetic resonance can image hypothalamic hamartomas (Beningfield SJ et al: *Br J Radiol* 61:1177–1180, 1988).

Computed tomography and MR may diagnose craniopharyngioma presenting as a nasopharyngeal mass (Benitez WI et al: *J Comput Assist Tomogr* 12:1068–1072, 1988).

Computed tomography and MRI have depicted a single instance of multicystic acoustic neuroma (Drapkin AJ, Rose WS: *Acta Radiol* 30:7–9, 1989).

Visual evoked potentials are often more sensitive than conventional methods for evaluation of visual function in patients with nonfunctioning chromophobe adenomas (Holder GE, Bullock PR: *J Neurol Neurosurg Psychiatry* 52:31–37, 1989).

Intracavernous sinus catheterization and venous sampling is extremely useful in the diagnosis of ACTH-secreting microadenomas (Marola B et al: *World J Surg* 12:445–448, 1988).

Selective bilateral simultaneous catheterization of the inferior petrosal sinus permits sampling of petrosal venous blood, and CRF stimulates prolactin secretion from ACTH-producing macroadenomas in Cushing's disease (Schulte HM et al: *Clin Endocrinol* 28:289–295, 1988).

Among myelograms in 34 children with posterior fossa medulloblastomas, 15 patients had intraspinal spread (Stanley P, Suminski N: *Am J Pediatr Hematol Oncol* 10:283–287, 1988). Three patients with positive myelograms had negative CSF, and only 1 patient had symptoms referable to the spine.

Surgery

Morbidity and Mortality of Craniotomy for Excision of Supratentorial Gliomas
Fadul C, Wood J, Thaler H, Galicich J, Patterson RH Jr, Posner JB (New York Hosp–Cornell Univ Med College)
Neurology 38:1374–1379, September 1988   18–13

Although surgery is important in the management of supratentorial gliomas, some believe that operative morbidity outweighs any potential

Most Common Neurologic Complication After Complete or
Partial Resection

	Superficial tumors				Deep midline or bilateral tumors†	
	Complete resection		Incomplete resection*			
Complication	#	%	#	%	#	%
Hemorrhage						
NYH	0/22	(0)	6/69	(8.7)	0/18	(0)
MSKCC	0/45	(0)	0/40	(0)	4/19	(21.1)
Total	0/67	(0)	6/109	(5.5)	4/37	(10.8)
			$p = 0.84$			
Herniation						
NYH	0/22	(0)	8/69	(11.6)	1/18	(5.6)
MSKCC	0/45	(0)	0/40	(0)	1/19	(5.3)
Total	0/67	(0)	8/109	(7.3)	2/37	(5.4)
			$p = 0.025$			
Neurologic deterioration						
NYH	3/22	(13.6)	19/69	(27.5)	6/18	(33.3)
MSKCC	9/45	(20.0)	11/40	(27.5)	8/19	(42.1)
Total	12/67	(17.9)	30/109	(27.5)	14/37	(37.8)
			NS			

*Biopsy and partial resection.
†All resections were incomplete.
(Courtesy of Fadul C, Wood J, Thaler H, et al: *Neurology* 38:1374–1379, September 1988.)

benefit. In order to determine whether such patients should undergo resection and to what extent, the short-term morbidity and mortality of 104 supratentorial glioma patients who underwent surgery was assessed prospectively. The results obtained on 109 patients at another center were also reviewed.

Total mortality was 3.3%. Total morbidity was 31.7%. Significant worsening of neurologic function occurred in 19.7% of these patients. Complications were more frequent in those patients with preoperative disabilities. Patients undergoing complete resection had fewer acute neurologic complications (table) than those with less extensive resections. Deep-midline lesions had a higher rate of complications and mortality; bilateral lesions had a higher rate of hemorrhage and hydrocephalus. There was a significantly higher surgical mortality risk for patients aged more than 55 years and for those receiving high daily doses of dexamethasone. Reoperation had no greater risks than initial operation.

These results suggest that complete resection should be performed for supratentorial glioma. This procedure is no riskier than lesser surgical procedures. However, there is a 20% risk of worsening as a result of the operation.

▶ This report provides further support for the superiority of total gross excision of gliomas. Patients with complete resection had fewer acute neurologic complications. The investigators noted a higher rate of complications for deep midline lesions, bilateral lesions, older patients, and those receiving high-dose steroid therapy. This stratification may be helpful to clinicians in case selection.

In a related study, gross total resection of recurrent malignant astrocytoma was carried out in 15 cases without complications; glioblastoma cases maintained Karnovsky scale unchanged for a mean of 13 weeks and anaplastic astrocytoma for 37.2 weeks (1).

Reference

1. Vick NA et al: *Arch Neurol* 39:430–432, 1989.

Survival After Stereotactic Biopsy of Malignant Gliomas
Coffey RJ, Lunsford LD, Taylor FH (Univ of Pittsburgh)
Neurosurgery 22:465–473, March 1988   18–14

Although patients with malignant gliomas who are treated with cytoreductive surgery and irradiation now survive longer, surgical resection is not always the most appropriate first line of treatment for all such patients. This group includes patients with tumors in functionally important or inaccessible areas of the brain, those with small tumors and minimal neurologic deficits, and patients whose medical condition precludes major surgery under general anesthesia. In such patients the diagnosis of malignant glioma is best established by stereotactic biopsy.

To assess the role of stereotactic biopsy in the diagnosis of malignant glioma and to evaluate the outcome of various nonsurgical treatment modalities, records of all patients treated for malignant glioma during a 5-year period were reviewed. Of 91 such patients with malignant gliomas diagnosed by stereotactic biopsy, 64 had glioblastoma multiforme (GBM) and 27 had anaplastic astrocytoma (AA).

After stereotactic biopsy, each patient received 1 or more of the following treatments: supportive care only, adequate radiation therapy (RT), palliative RT only, chemotherapy, iodine 125 boost interstitial irradiation, or tumor resection.

Tumors involving deep or midline cerebral structures occurred in 64% of the patients with GBM and in 33% of those with AA. The median survival for 19 of the 64 patients with GBM who had only supportive care or palliative RT was 8.8 weeks, whereas the other 45 patients with GBM with adequate therapy had a median survival of 29.5 weeks (Fig 18–9). The median survival for 3 of the 27 patients with AAs with only supportive care or palliative RT was 11.1 weeks, whereas the other 24 patients, who had adequate therapy, survived for an average of 74 weeks. Treatment after biopsy, tumor location, histologic findings, and the patient's age at presentation were all statistically important predictors of survival. Stereotactic biopsy followed by RT and nonoperative adjuvant therapy prolongs survival and preserves neurologic function in patients with malignant gliomas who are not candidates for surgical intervention.

GBM : TREATMENT PRESCRIBED

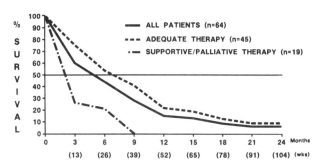

Fig 18–9.—The effect of treatment prescribed on Kaplan-Meier survival curves in 64 patients with GBM. Survival curves are shown for all 64 patients (median survival, 21 weeks), for 19 patients prescribed supportive care or palliative RT (median survival, 8.8 weeks), and for 45 patients prescribed adequate therapy (median survival, 29.5 weeks). The latter 2 curves are significantly different ($P = .0005$, Breslow and Mantel-Cox). (Courtesy of Coffey RJ, Lunsford LD, Taylor FH: *Neurosurgery* 22:465–473, March 1988.)

▶ This very important study challenges the widely held concept of cytoreductive surgery for gliomas. The authors present data which suggest that tumor resection beyond biopsy does not affect outcome in patients without significant midline shift. The results support a conservative approach to intracranial gliomas, with diagnosis by stereotactic biopsy followed by adequate radiation therapy.

These data are at odds with reports emphasizing the advantage of glioma resection as regards both function and survival (1–2). Because of the small numbers in the several studies, firm conclusions cannot be drawn, and we must wait for further data, hopefully uniformly classified by the method of Burger and colleagues.

References

1. Jelsma R, Bucy PC: *Arch Neurol* 20:161, 1969.
2. Ciric: *Neurosurg* 1988.

Intraorbital Meningiomas: Surgical Management and Role of Radiation Therapy
Ito M, Ishizawa A, Miyaoka M, Sato K, Ishii S (Juntendo Univ, Tokyo)
Surg Neurol 29:448–453, June 1988   18–15

Primary optic nerve meningioma may be difficult to remove without sacrificing the central retinal artery. Secondary orbital meningiomas also present a challenge. Eleven cases of intraorbital meningioma were encountered between 1978 and 1985, seven of primary and four of secondary orbital meningioma. Two patients were of pediatric age. All patients with primary orbital tumors presented with progressive visual disorder. Proptosis was more evident in the secondary cases. The operating microscope was used for intraorbital and intracranial procedures.

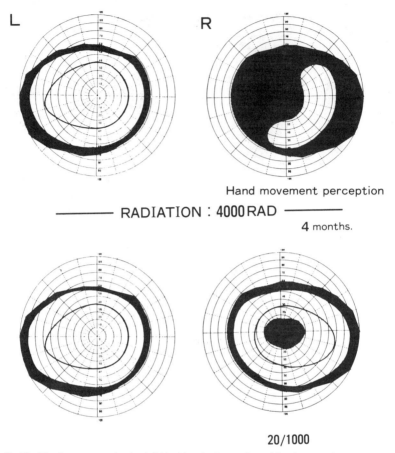

L   R

Hand movement perception

———— RADIATION : 4000 RAD ————

4 months.

20/1000

Fig 18–10.—Improvement in visual field and acuity in a patient with primary optic nerve meningioma after radiation at a dose of 40 Gy. **Upper panel,** preradiation state, and **lower panel,** postradiation state. (Courtesy of Ito M, Ishizawa A, Miyaoka M, et al: *Surg Neurol* 29:448–453, June 1988.)

Radiotherapy proved to be a useful adjunct to surgery in treating some of these patients (Fig 18–10). Two patients received radiotherapy after partial removal of intracranial or intraorbital meningioma so that the tumor would not recur.

A combined surgical and, where indicated, radiotherapeutic approach is useful in the management of primary and secondary intraorbital meningiomas. However, controlled studies have not been done to document the effectiveness of radiotherapy in delaying or preventing tumor recurrence.

▶ The authors present an aggressive surgical approach to the management of intraorbital meningioma. Among 11 cases, only 1 had total excision with improvement of the visual situation. Three other cases treated with radiation showed improvement. Radiation was offered in a total of 5 cases. The precise role of both surgery and radiation in these cases has yet to be defined. An additional point not examined in this presentation is the importance of the cosmetic aspect and preservation of the extraocular motions.

In a related study, 38 cases of optic nerve sheath meningioma were treated according to symptomatology: 18 eyes were followed for minimal symptoms or total blindness, radiation was given for 6 eyes with progressive blindness, total resection was used in 10 eyes with visual loss and progressive enlargement, and surgery plus radiation was carried out for aggressive tumors (1).

Reference

1. Kennerdell JS et al: *Am J Ophthalmol* 106:450–457, 1988.

Results of Transsphenoidal Microsurgery for Growth Hormone-Secreting Pituitary Adenoma in a Series of 214 Patients
Ross DA, Wilson CB (Univ of California, San Francisco)
J Neurosurg 68:854–867, June 1988   18–16

Transsphenoidal microsurgery was carried out to remove a pituitary adenoma in 214 patients seen in a 14-year period with acromegaly. Nearly two thirds of tumors were grade II adenomas; there were relatively few true microadenomas less than 1 cm in size. The fasting growth hormone level exceeded 50 ng/ml in one third of patients. Only 28.5% of patients had been treated for acromegaly. One fifth of operations caused complications, but no deaths resulted.

A total of 174 patients were followed up for a mean of 76 months. The most recent growth hormone level was below 10 ng/ml in 93% of patients. Five patients (2.3%) were considered treatment failures. Nine patients had a second transsphenoidal exploration, and one required a third exploration; residual tumor was removed in seven cases. Anterior pituitary dysfunction was found in 5% of patients not given postoperative radiotherapy. Active acromegaly recurred in 4% of patients with growth hormone levels less than 5 ng/ml after initial operation.

Thirty surgical series of transsphenoidal microsurgery for growth hormone-secreting adenoma have been reported (table). The goals of this surgery are to eliminate mass effects of the tumor, as well as endocrine hyperactivity, while retaining existing anterior pituitary function, with minimal morbidity. Early surgery will improve the operative results. Acromegalics now have an excellent chance of obtaining a durable remission or cure by microsurgery, with adjuvant radiotherapy where indicated.

▶ This detailed report carried out over 18 years in 214 cases indicates the safety and efficacy of transsphenoidal microsurgery for acromegaly. Primary radiation therapy, however, does not seem to be as effective in control of this disorder. Postoperative radiation therapy will be occasionally required in cases with persistently elevated growth hormone levels. The role of somatostatin an-

Cumulative Results in 30 Surgical Series of Patients

| No. of Cases | Postop GH Levels (ng/ml) | | Deaths | New Hypopituitarism | Permanent Diabetes Insipidus | Complications |
	< 5	< 10				
1360	466/771	807/1094	12/1156	178/1014	22/847	66/982
	(60.4%)	(73.8%)	(1.04%)	(17.6%)	(2.6%)	(6.7%)

Note: Expressed as number of cases in each category/total cases reported, with percentages in parentheses. *GH*, growth hormone. Data derived from References. (Courtesy of Ross DA, Wilson CB: *J Neurosurg* 68:854–867, June 1988.)

alogues in the treatment of this disorder has not yet been defined but probably will be adjunctive.

Management of Large Pituitary Adenomas by Transsphenoidal Surgery
Black PM, Zervas NT, Candia G (Harvard Univ)
Surg Neurol 29:443–447, June 1988
18–17

Transsphenoidal surgery may be the best means of treating large as well as small pituitary adenomas. Experience with 113 patients having extrasellar extension was reviewed. These patients were among 255 consecutive subjects operated on for pituitary tumor between 1981 and 1984. In cases with extension, more than one fourth of the tumor mass was outside the sella. About one fifth of the extrasellar tumors were prolactinomas. Two thirds of patients with extrasellar extension had visual field defects.

There were no operative deaths in the entire series of 255 patients. Three patients with extrasellar extension had leaks of cerebrospinal fluid. Computed tomography was helpful in demonstrating the degree of tumor resection. Endocrine improvement was consistently observed, but fewer than half the patients were cured by current standards. Eight patients required hormonal replacement for the first time after transsphenoidal surgery. More than three fourths of patients had visual improvement after operation.

Transsphenoidal surgery is at least as effective as transfrontal operation in resecting large pituitary adenomas, with respect to both endocrine remission and visual improvement. Complications are substantially fewer after transsphenoidal operation.

▶ This important presentation demonstrates that transsphenoidal surgery is probably the treatment of choice even for extrasellar pituitary tumors as well as small adenomas. As carefully documented by the authors, the endocrine results and visual field improvements are at least as good as those recorded after transfrontal surgery, with a substantially lower morbidity and mortality. When one considers that postoperative radiation may be helpful in the further management of these tumors, with and without the adjunct of medical endocrinologic manipulation, the case for transsphenoidal surgery in these patients becomes even stronger.

Trigeminal Schwannoma: Surgical Series of 14 Cases With Review of the Literature
McCormick PC, Bello JA, Post KD (Columbia-Presbyterian Med Ctr, New York)
J Neurosurg 69:850–860, December 1988   18–18

Schwannomas arising from the intracranial part of the trigeminal nerve are rare. Data on 14 patients with histologically confirmed schwannomas at this site who were operated on during 1970–1986 were reviewed. No patient had a family history or physical evidence of neurofibromatosis. Eight tumors arose from the gasserian ganglion, and 5, from the trigeminal root. One lesion appeared to arise from the intracranial part of the maxillary nerve. The mean tumor diameter was 5 cm.

The surgical approach depended on the site and extent of tumor. All gross tumor was removed at initial operation in 6 patients, and most of it in 4 others. Abnormal trigeminal function was frequent and tended to be permanent, but some preoperative deficits improved. Two patients required cerebrospinal fluid shunt procedures. One patient died postoperatively, and 1 died of recurrent tumor after 4 years. All the other patients were clinically well after a mean follow-up of 4 years. Nine patients had some degree of trigeminal sensory loss when last examined.

No distinct syndrome is associated with trigeminal schwannoma. A subtemporal intradural approach is used in most cases. It may be dangerous to attempt removing all tumor when the inferomedial part is adherent to the posterolateral wall of the cavernous sinus.

▶ Much like acoustic neuroma, trigeminal schwannoma can often be excised with good results, according to this substantial study. In most of the cases total resection was possible; subtotal removal was achieved in cases in which the cavernous sinus was involved. Although it is technically possible to enter the cavernous sinus today for tumor removal, the risk of adding new cranial nerve deficits may not be justified. Because the tumors grow slowly, careful follow-up postoperatively is probably the best approach to avoid recurrence. In the case of recurrence, there may be a role for radiotherapy and radiosurgery, as demonstrated for acoustic neuroma.

Bordi and co-workers report that in 11 cases of trigeminal neuroma, total excision was possible in 4, with subtotal removal in the remainder and excellent outcome in 10 of 11 (1).

Reference

1. Bordi L et al: *Surg Neurol* 31:272–276, 1989.

Clinical Course and Surgical Prognosis of 33 Cases of Intracranial Epidermoid Tumors
Yamakawa K, Shitara N, Genka S, Manaka S, Takakura K (Univ of Tokyo Hosp)
Neurosurgery 24:568–573, April 1989   18–19

Epidermoid tumors are benign lesions of ectodermal origin that account for approximately 1% of all intracranial tumors. The most commonly involved sites are the cerebellopontine (CP) angle, the parapituitary in the middle fossa, and the chiasmal region near the skull base. Early detection and complete excision are the ideal treatment, but the tumor tends to grow by spreading and extending into surrounding areas. During a 25-year period, 45 patients were treated for epidermoid tumors, 33 of which were analyzed.

There were 15 (45.5%) tumors in the CP angle, 5 (15.1%) in the middle fossa, 5 (15.1%) in the cerebral hemisphere, 3 (9.1%) in the suprasellar region, 3 (9.1%) in the third ventricle, and 2 (6.1%) in the fourth ventricle. The tumor was removed totally or subtotally in 28 (85%) patients. The tumor was only partially removed in 5 patients, as the tumor capsule adhered to the surrounding structures, forcing the incomplete resection. The time from initial symptoms to operation averaged 11 months for tumors in the suprasellar region or third ventricle, but 7 years for tumors in other locations.

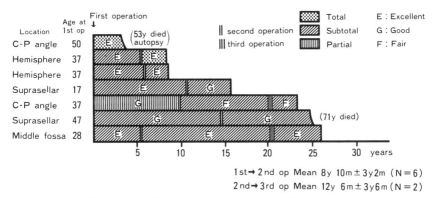

Fig 18–11.—Clinical course of 7 cases of recurrent intracranial epidermoid tumors. (Courtesy of Yamakawa K, Shitara N, Genka S, et al: *Neurosurgery* 24:568–573, April 1989.)

Of 29 patients who participated in a long-term follow-up survey, 7 (24.1%) had had recurrences after an average interval of 8 years 10 months for the first recurrence and 12 years 6 months for the second recurrence (Fig 18–11). All reoperations were successful. Most of the patients led independent and useful lives after operation, including those who had recurrences. Of the 29 patients, 3 (10.3%) had died at the late follow-up survey. The 20-year survival rate estimated by the Kaplan-Meier method was 92.8%.

▶ This report documents good results for surgery in cases of intracranial epidermoid tumor. In some cases total removal is possible, but the authors point out that adherence of the thin tumor membrane to delicate structures may necessitate partial removal. Because the tumor grows slowly, a patient may enjoy a long period without recurrence of symptoms that might indicate reoperation. With cautious application of judgment and precise technique, excellent surgical results are possible. It should be pointed out that the signal characteristics may be confused with other lesions, such as angiographically occult arteriovenous malformation or other gliomas.

Brief Notes on Surgical Management of Tumors

STEREOTACTIC SURGERY

The disadvantages of small sample size obtained through needle biopsy and CT-associated stereotaxis are overcome by a careful targeting and intraoperative frozen section examinations (Colbassani HJ et al: *J Neurol Neurosurg Psychiatry* 51:332–341, 1988).

Computer-assisted stereotactic resection provides maximum cytoreduction in high-grade glial tumors; it is most beneficial to patients with histologically circumscribed tumor such as pilocytic astrocytomas, metastases, and certain nonglial lesions (Kelly PJ: *Mayo Clin Proc* 63:1186–1198, 1988).

In 44 cases, computer-assisted stereotactic resection of metastatic lesions was carried out with no morbidity (Kelly PJ et al: *Neurosurgery* 22:7–17, 1988).

TRANSSPHENOIDAL SURGERY

Pituitary Adenoma.—Transsphenoidal surgery produces excellent results in microadenomas, curing about 70% to 80% of patients irrespective of whether the tumor produces ACTH, prolactin, or growth hormone. Macroadenomas secreting prolactin or growth hormone are also effectively treated, with only about 40% being cured. Invasive macroprolactinomas are not helped by surgery and are best treated with bromocriptine and radiotherapy. Radiotherapy should be used sparingly and has inevitable complications. Postoperative delayed visual deterioration is caused either by recurrent tumor or radiotherapy (Adams CBT: *Acta Neurochir (Wien)* 94:103–116, 1988).

Pituitary Adenoma.—DDAVP when given in 2-mcg doses every 12 hours over 3 days produces continuous antidiuresis in postoperative pituitary cases (Jedynak CP et al: *Presse Med* 17:723–726, 1988).

Pituitary Adenoma.—Routine glucocorticoid therapy is not needed in patients undergoing selective pituitary adenoma removal whose preoperative adrenal function is normal (Hout WM et al: *J Clin Endocrinol Metab* 66:1208, 1988).

Pituitary Adenoma.—Among 210 patients, late regrowth of pituitary adenoma had a median time to first failure of 3.8 years for surgery alone, 4.2 years for RT alone, and 10.2 years for surgery plus RT (Grigsby PW et al: *Cancer* 63:1308–1312, 1989).

Acromegaly.—Patients who undergo removal of pituitary adenoma for treatment of acromegaly have an excellent chance for cure, particularly if they have growth hormone levels less than 50 μg/L (Oyen WJG et al: *Acta Endocrinol (Copenh)* 117:491–496, 1988).

Acromegaly.—Among 15 acromegalics, adenectomy achieved endocrine cure in 3, and addition of radiation cured the other 12 (Guittard M et al: *Presse Med* 16:1217–1221, 1987).

Acromegaly.—Usually, improvement after operation for acromegaly is titrated by changes in growth hormone levels. Osawa, Kobayashi, Takemae, and Nakagawa, of Shinshu University, Nagana, Japan, evaluated improvement on clinical grounds (preoperative and postoperative symptoms), and correlated this with changes in the growth hormone response to thyrotropin-releasing hormone, and to somatomedin-C. Their conclusion was that somatomedin-C was more useful than growth hormone levels in predicting clinical improvement after surgery for acromegaly (*Neurol Med Chir [Tokyo]* 28:254–258, 1988).—Oscar Sugar, M.D.(Oscar Sugar, M.D., is Professor Emeritus and Former Head of the Department of Neurosurgery, University of Illinois College of Medicine at Chicago, and Clinical Professor of Neurosurgery, University of California at San Diego. Dr. Sugar was also Editor of the Neurosurgery section of the YEAR BOOK OF NEUROLOGY AND NEUROSURGERY from 1953 to 1985.)

Cushing's Disease.—In 64 patients treated with transsphenoidal surgery for Cushing's disease, 72% were well 6 years after surgery (Guilhaume B et al: *J Clin Endocrinol Metab* 66:1056, 1988).

Cushing's Disease.—Among 36 patients with Cushing's disease undergoing transsphenoidal surgery, 31 were initially cured without operative mortality or permanent neurologic sequelae (Bay JW, Sheeler LR: *Cleve Clin J Med* 55:357–364, 1988).

Cushing's Disease.—Transsphenoidal adenectomy cured 31 of 36 patients of Cushing's disease without operative mortality or permanent neurologic sequelae (Bay JW, Sheeler LR: *Cleve Clin J Med* 55:357–364, 1988).

TRANSLABYRINTHINE SURGERY FOR ACOUSTIC NEUROMA

Complications of translabyrinthine and suboccipital surgery for acoustic tumor removal were similar among 171 patients (Mangham CA: *Otolaryngol Head Neck Surg* 99:396, 403, 1988).

Translabyrinthe resection of acoustic neuromas is assisted by supine position, initial exposure of the facial nerve, and use of the ultrasonic aspirator (Sterkers JM, Desgeorges N: *Sem Hop Paris* 64:2341–2345, 1988).

SURGERY AND METASTASES

Among 652 patients with primary malignant melanoma, 55 patients had brain metastases (8.4%) (Mendez IM, Delmaestro RF: *Can J Neurol Sci* 15:119–123, 1988). Multiple lesions occur in 61% with a single metastasis in 39%. Six-month survival for patients with a single metastatic lesion was 58% if surgical excision was possible, and 25% of these patients survived greater than 2 years. Patients with a single metastasis appear to benefit from surgical removal of the lesion.

Synchronous onset of brain metastases from lung cancer does not necessarily contraindicate combined operations, which can provide long-term survival in selected cases (Torre M et al: *J Thorac Cardiovasc Surg* 95:994–997, 1988).

Experience with 19 cases undergoing resection of a primary lung tumor-associated brain metastasis yielded a 5-year survival of 45%, which is taken to justify continued application of this approach (Hankins JR et al: *Ann Thorac Surg* 46:24–28, 1988).

There is a high incidence of subtentorial lesions in patients with pelvic and gastrointestinal primary tumors (Delattre JY et al: *Arch Neurol* 45:741–744, 1988).

Adjunctive Therapy

Effective Preoperative Irradiation of Highly Vascular Cerebellopontine Angle Neurinomas
Ikeda K, Ito H, Kashihara K, Fujisawa H, Yamamoto S (Kanazawa Univ, Japan)
Neurosurgery 22:566–573, March 1988   18–20

Preoperative irradiation was used to lower the risk of intraoperative bleeding in three cases of hypervascular cerebellopontine angle neurinoma. Two patients had an acoustic neurinoma, and 1 had bilateral glossopharyngeal neurinomas. In two cases, massive tumor bleeding required partial removal at the initial operation. In one case, surgery was successfully carried out after preoperative radiotherapy. In the patients having repeat operation, the second procedure allowed complete tumor removal with little blood loss. Tumor vascularity was much reduced after the delivery of 30 Gy of radiation (Fig 18–12).

Hypervascular neurinomas with early venous drainage are being in-

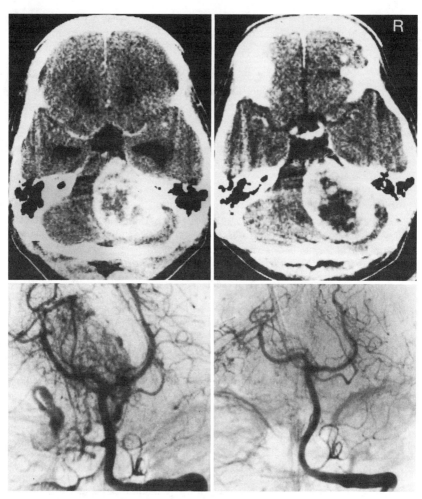

Fig 18–12.—Contrast-enhanced CT scan and vertebral angiogram before (**left**) and 1 month after irradiation (**right**). A central hypodense area is slightly enlarged and tumoral hypervascularity is markedly reduced, with disappearance of the early draining vein after irradiation with 3,000 rads. (Courtesy of Ikeda K, Ito H, Kashihara K, et al: *Neurosurgery* 22:566–573, March 1988.)

creasingly recognized. The present patients had large, hypervascular lesions with marked capsular and tumor stain and early draining veins. Radiotherapy is an alternative to embolizing feeding vessels in preparing these patients for tumor removal. Doses less than 3,000 rads have been effective when administered over 20 to 26 days. Radical surgery should be carried out 1–2 months after irradiation, when radiation effects on the vasculature are manifest.

▶ The authors report 3 cases of highly vascular posterior fossa neurinoma with effective reduction in vascularity by preoperation irradiation. I personally have had occasion to utilize this approach in 2 acoustic neuromas with remarkable vascularity and confirm the substantial utility of this approach. How are such cases to be recognized preoperatively? Ordinarily, angiography is not performed for cases of suspected cerebellopontine angle tumor. However, remarkable vascularity can also be detected on MRI; this could be the tip-off to such a case. It's been known for some time that cases with bilateral acoustic neurofibromatosis may have highly vascular lesions, and younger patients may have somewhat more vascular lesions (all of the patients in these reported cases were aged less than 30, and 1 of our patients was a 13-year-old girl). It's also worth remembering that radiotherapy may be an effective long-term therapy against enlargement of these lesions, as recently reported by the group from University of California, San Francisco

---

Central Nervous System Involvement in Malignant Melanoma
Retsas S, Gershuny AR (Westminster Hosp, London)
Cancer 61:1926–1934, May 1, 1988   18–21

After breast cancer and lung cancer, malignant melanoma (MM) is the third most common cause of metastases to the brain. Recent developments in the chemotherapy of this tumor have resulted in a somewhat improved survival among patients with cerebral metastases from MM. The case reports of 100 patients with brain tumors from MM metastatic to the central nervous system (CNS) were reviewed with regard to survival from the time of diagnosis of CNS involvement, response to treatment, characteristics of the primary lesion, and the course of the disease from initial diagnosis to the development of a brain tumor.

Of 451 patients who were treated during a 7-year study period for histologically confirmed malignant melanoma of all stages, 100 had clinical and radiologic evidence of cerebral metastases during the course of their illness. Of these 100 patients, who ranged in age from 26 to 77 years, 85 were investigated with computed axial tomography (CAT) and 15, with radioisotope scanning. Of the 85 patients who had a CAT scan, 25 had solitary brain lesions, and 54 had 2 or more brain lesions. The other 6 CAT scans were negative, but cerebral involvement was confirmed by other diagnostic techniques. Thirteen of the 15 radioisotope brain scans were positive for cerebral lesions corresponding to the clinical findings. The other 2 brain scans were negative, but extensive cerebral involvement was confirmed at autopsy in 1 of these patients.

After the diagnosis of CNS involvement, 76 patients underwent chemotherapy, of whom 10 (13%) experienced objective regression of their brain tumor. The median survival in these 10 patients was 11.5 months from the time of diagnosis of CNS involvement. In 11 other patients, cerebral lesions developed after an objective response of extracerebral metastases to earlier chemotherapy. The median survival in these 11 patients was 7 months from the time of diagnosis of CNS involvement. The other 24 patients did not have chemotherapy, as they had remained unresponsive to dexamethasone, and progressed rapidly from CNS involvement to death or had extensive extracerebral metastases resistant to earlier therapy. A total of 69 patients received cranial irradiation, combined in 62 with chemotherapy.

The median survival for all 100 patients was 2.5 months. However, 8 (8%) patients survived longer than 1 year from the time of diagnosis of cerebral metastases, 4 of whom survived longer than 2 years. One patient was still alive, disease-free, and in complete neurologic remission more than 82 months after the diagnosis of CNS involvement.

▶ The dismal results of this study indicate that radiation therapy and chemotherapy are ineffective for CNS malignant melanoma. In a recent review of 21 patients subjected to surgery at the University of Illinois for metastatic intracranial melanoma, Glick and co-workers noticed that all were alive at 3 months and 16 of 21 were alive at 1 year, with 5 surviving from 1 to 4.5 years.

Interstitial Brachytherapy for Metastatic Brain Tumors
Prados M, Leibel S, Barnett CM, Gutin P (Univ of California, San Francisco)
Cancer 63:657–660, Feb 15, 1989   18–22

Brain metastases develop in 20% to 50% of all patients with cancer. Up to 50% of these patients die from the metastases. Treatment for recurrent metastatic brain tumors after radiation therapy is difficult. Few patients benefit from further surgery, and systemic chemotherapy is generally unsuccessful. The results of treatment of such patients with temporary implantation of high-activity iodine 125 sources using stereotactic techniques were reported.

Results of Brain Tumor Brachytherapy

Patient	Prior Rx (brain)	MTD	Response	Survival
1	S/RT/C	8241	ST	23 wk (CNS/SYS)
2	RT	—	PR	59 wk (CNS/SYS)
3	RT	13,000	ST	24 wk (CNS/SYS)
4	RT	7125	PR	22 wk (SYS)
5	RT	—	PR	116 wk (CNS)
6	RT	5553	PR	239+ wk
7*	RT	3761	PR	86+ wk
8	S/RT	4664	ST	62+ wk
9	S/RT	4450	ST	64+ wk
10	RT	5250	PR	97+ wk
11*	S/RT	4760	ST	52+ wk
12*	RT	3443	ST	52+ wk
13	RT	4971, 4780	ST	54+ wk
14*	RT	12,500	ST	4 wk (SYS)

Abbreviations: S, surgery; *RT,* radiotherapy; *C,* chemotherapy; *MTD,* minimal tumor dose (rad); *PR,* partial response; *ST,* stable; *CNS,* central nervous system failure; *SYS,* systemic failure; +, remains alive.
*Brachytherapy done as "boost."
(Courtesy of Prados M, Leibel S, Barnett CM, et al: *Cancer* 63:657–660, Feb 15, 1989.)

Fourteen patients with progressive metastatic brain lesions have been treated since 1979. Four had had prior surgical resections, and 13 had undergone external whole-brain radiotherapy. Nine patients underwent brachytherapy at recurrence 4–16 months after conventional radiation therapy. The remaining 4 had implants as an adjuvant boost to the tumor area 2–4 weeks after external radiation. Six patients died. Two had stable brain lesions at 4 and 22 weeks, respectively; 3 had progressive systemic and central nervous system tumors at 23, 24, and 29 weeks, respectively; and 1 had progressive central nervous system disease 116 weeks after the implant. The remaining 8 patients, with a median follow-up of 63 weeks, were alive. Overall, the median survival was 80 weeks (table).

It is possible to palliate and sometimes significantly prolong survival with interstitial brachytherapy in patients with metastatic brain lesions. In this series, 10 of 14 patients survived a year or more.

▶ This preliminary study indicates that interstitial brachytherapy for progressive metastatic brain lesions was well tolerated and associated with a median survival of 80 weeks. Of course, these patients are very difficult to care for, and available treatment modalities appear to have little to offer. To establish that brachytherapy improves longevity or quality of life, careful follow-up studies, including assessment of quality of life, will be required in the future.

Systemic Gamma-Interferon Therapy for Recurrent Gliomas
Mahaley MS Jr, Bertsch L, Cush S, Gillespie GY (Univ of Alabama, Birmingham; Univ of North Carolina, Chapel Hill)
J Neurosurg 69:826–829, December 1988   18–23

Interferon-γ reportedly activates lymphocyte cytotoxicity against glioma cells in the presence of interleukin-2 and inhibits the growth of glioma cells in vitro. Recombinant interferon-γ was administered to 15 patients, 10 with glioblastoma, 2 with anaplastic astrocytoma, and 1 each with astrocytoma, oligodendroglioma, and ependymoma. All patients had a tumor volume less than 50 ml as detected with enhancing computed tomography (CT) and a Karnofsky rating of at least 70. Interferon was given intravenously in a dose of 2 mg/m^2 twice a week in 8-week courses.

Only 1 patient had CT evidence of a response; 3 other patients stabilized for 12 to 86 weeks. The median time to treatment failure in the 14 patients with documented progression was 7 weeks. The overall median survival was 24 weeks. One patient developed hypotension and was withdrawn from the study. Other toxicity was well tolerated except in 1 patient who died of acute renal failure of uncertain origin.

These results are disappointing, especially in view of the relatively early stage at which treatment was given. Future studies should utilize interferon-α or interferon-β unless interferon-γ is found to be effective when used with other interferons or with chemotherapy.

▶ This careful study from a very experienced team indicates that interferon-γ therapy for recurrent glioma is without value. One must be very careful in accepting claims of efficacy for unproved brain tumor therapies. The results, of course, do not bear on the possible efficacy of other interferons, including interferon-α and -β.

Intralesional Infusion of Lymphokine-Activated Killer (LAK) Cells and Recombinant Interleukin-2 (rIL-2) for the Treatment of Patients With Malignant Brain Tumor
Merchant RE, Merchant LH, Cook SHS, McVicar DW, Young HF (Virginia Commonwealth Univ)
Neurosurgery 23:725–732, December 1988   18–24

Anaplastic astrocytoma and glioblastoma multiforme comprise about 50% of all primary malignancies in the central nervous system (CNS). In the hope of improving patient survival, researchers are conducting many clinical trials using alternative forms of therapy involving combined modalities of radiation and chemotherapy as well as treatments with hyperthermia, radiation enhancing agents, blood-brain barrier modification, and immunotherapy. The application of intracerebral injections of human recombinant interleukin-2 (rIL-2) with autologous lymphocytes activated in vitro by rIL-2 for patients with recurrent and newly diagnosed tumors was reported.

Twenty patients with supratentorial, intracerebral lesions were treated with surgery and adoptive immunotherapy with lymphokine-activated killer (LAK) cells and rIL-2. Seventeen patients had glioblastoma; 2, high-grade oligodendroglioma; and 1, two metastatic sarcoma lesions. Lymphokine-activated killer cells were produced from blood mononuclear cells obtained by leukapheresis and cultured 3–5 days with 1,000 units of rIL-2/ml. Patients taking steroids or with a low Karnofsky functional status generated suboptimal LAK cell activity, on the average. Cultured mononuclear cells containing LAK cells were suspended in saline containing 10^6 units of rIL-2 and injected into tissue around the tumor cavity during craniotomy. For 3 postoperative days, patients were given 10^6 units of rIL-2 into the tumor cavity through an Ommaya reservoir. All patients had some degree of headache, fever, or lethargy that cleared within a few days of the last rIL-2 injection. Computed tomographic scans taken just after treatment depicted areas of low density, suggesting a greater-than-normal extent of edema around the operative site. The tumors of 7 patients recurred, with an average disease-free interval of 25 weeks. Eight patients have been alive and tumor free for 6 months or more after treatment.

The immunotherapeutic regimen described is safe, with toxicity most closely associated with increased cerebral edema that probably develops as a result of locally high, extracellular concentrations of rIL-2 or cytokines secreted by the infused cells. Immunotherapy with LAK cells and rIL-2 probably has its greatest potential in patients not dependent on steroids to control cerebral edema and whose tumors are in an area where near-complete resection of the mass can be done.

▶ This very careful study from a well-established and experienced neuro-oncology group indicates that intracerebral injection of rIL-2 with autologous lymphocytes was well tolerated by patients with recurrent or freshly diagnosed brain tumors. The frequency of recurrence and interval of tumor-free survival are encouraging but do not demonstrate any clear benefit. Some evidence of extended peritumoral edema was noticed in these cases. The experience of the Richmond group was encouraging and warrants further investigation of this treatment adjunct. Utilization of this method should be confined to experimental protocols at this time.

Whiteside and associates report that with 48-hour activation by rIL-2 adherence to plastic, it was not possible to enrich inactivated NK cells from the blood of patients with CNS tumors (1).

Reference

1. Whiteside TL et al: *Cancer Res* 48:1669–1675, 1988.

Adoptive Immunotherapy for Recurrent Glioblastoma Multiforme Using Lymphokine Activated Killer Cells and Recombinant Interleukin-2
Merchant RE, Grant AJ, Berchant LH, Young HF (Virginia Commonwealth Univ)
Cancer 62:665–671, Aug 15, 1988   18–25

Intracerebral injections of autologous lymphocytes and human recombinant interleukin-2 (rIL-2) were used to treat 13 patients with recurrent glioblastoma. Mononuclear cells from these patients were exposed to rIL-2 in vitro to allow differentiation of some lymphocytes into lymphokine-activated killer (LAK) cells.

Of the 13 patients, 9 received LAK cells and rIL-2 by injection into the brain tissue around the tumor cavity during craniotomy. These patients received rIL-2 boosters into the tumor cavity for the next 3 days. After 1 to 2 weeks, the LAK/rIL-2 injection was repeated into the tumor cavity. The remaining 4 patients received both LAK treatments by intracavity injection. The ability of the patients to make LAK cells was not influenced by age, sex, Karnofsky score, treatment history, anticonvulsant dosage, or steroid dosage. The therapy was well tolerated. All patients experienced headache, fever, and malaise on treatment days. This therapy did not appear to significantly influence patient survival.

This study of adoptive immunotherapy in 13 recurrent glioblastoma patients found that it was safe. However, the effectiveness of this treatment was not demonstrated. The authors suggest that phase II trials be conducted in patients with newly diagnosed or recurrent glioma.

▶ In this careful study of 13 cases in a recognized tumor center, adoptive immunotherapy was found to be safe. The stage is set for phase-II trials in patients with newly diagnosed or recurrent glioma.

Delivery of Melanoma-Associated Immunoglobulin Monoclonal Antibody and Fab Fragments to Normal Brain Utilizing Osmotic Blood-Brain Barrier Disruption

Neuwelt EA, Barnett PA, Hellström I, Hellström KE, Beaumier P, McCormick CI, Weigel RM (Oregon Health Sciences Univ, Portland; Oncogen, Seattle; NeoRx, Seattle; VA Hosp, Portland)
Cancer Res 48:4725–4729, Sept 1, 1988   18–26

Specific monoclonal antibodies offer a new approach to the diagnosis and treatment of brain tumors. Because disruption of the blood-brain barrier increases antibody delivery, iodinated monoclonal antibodies were administered to melanoma-associated antigens after osmotic barrier opening in normal rats. The barrier was opened with 25% mannitol solution, delivered by intracarotid injection.

Monoclonal antibody delivery increased significantly after opening of the blood-brain barrier. The Fab concentration in disrupted brain was higher than that of immunoglobulin G (IgG), and it was cleared more rapidly. Plasma clearance also was more rapid for Fab than for IgG. Antibody recovered from disrupted brain retained immunologic reactivity.

This approach may prove especially useful for relatively impermeable tumors or tumor-infiltrated normal brain. Specifics of antibody dosing are being studied in nude rats having human tumors implanted intracerebrally.

▶ This interesting paper combines monoclonal antibodies and blood-brain barrier opening technology for delivery of antibody to melanoma-associated antigens. Initial results in laboratory animals are promising, and it may be that this strategy will be effective in the clinical setting. Also of note is a pilot study of ^{131}I monoclonal antibodies for leptomeningeal tumors, which showed minimal acute toxicity and objective response to treatment in 4 of 5 patients (1).

Reference

1. Lashford LS et al: *Cancer* 61:857–868, 1988.

Preoperative Treatment of Acromegaly With Long-Acting Somatostatin Analog SMS 201-995: Shrinkage of Invasive Pituitary Macroadenomas and Improved Surgical Remission Rate

Barkan AL, Lloyd RV, Chandler WF, Hatfield MK, Gebarski SS, Kelch RP, Beitins IZ (University and VA Hosps; Univ of Michigan, Ann Arbor)
J Clin Endocrinol Metab 67:1040–1048, November 1988   18–27

The effects of the long-acting somatostatin analogue SMS 201-995 were studied in 10 previously untreated patients with acromegaly with invasive pituitary macroadenomas more than 10 mm in diameter. Most patients received a dose of 100–250 µg every 6 or 8 hours for 3 to 30 weeks before the adenoma was resected transsphenoidally or subfrontally. The last injection was given on the morning of surgery.

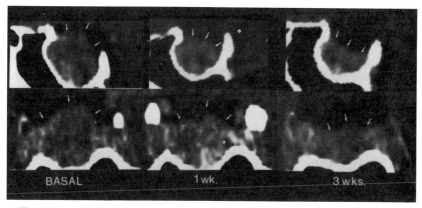

Fig 18–13.—Reformatted sagittal (**upper panel**) and coronal (**lower panel**) views of CT imaging in patient before and during SMS 201-995 treatment. (Courtesy of Barkin AL, Lloyd RV, Chandler WF, et al: *J Clin Endocrinol Metab* 67:1040–1048, November 1988.)

Growth hormone levels became normal in 8 of the 10 patients preoperatively. Tumors decreased in size by 20% to 54% during analogue treatment (Fig 18–13). Suprasellar expansion was eliminated in 5 patients, and cavernous sinus invasion lessened in 3 patients. Pituitary function remained normal postoperatively in all patients, and growth hormone dynamics became normal in 8 patients. The tumors exhibited decreased total cell areas, perivascular fibrosis, and dense granularity.

Preoperative treatment with SMS 201-995 can improve the surgical outcome in patients with invasive growth hormone–producing macroadenomas of the pituitary gland. Treated patients have had a high remission rate, contrasting with the usual poor surgical outcome in patients with macroadenoma.

▶ Long-acting somatostatin analogue (SMS 201-995) produces normalization of growth hormone levels and decrease in tumor size, with elimination of suprasellar and cavernous sinus invasion in some. This important communication indicates that medical therapy is highly likely to have a role in the treatment of acromegaly, whether as adjunct or primary treatment to be determined by future studies.

Brief Notes on Adjunctive Tumor Therapy

RADIATION

Prophylactic cranial irradiation appears to be effective in greatly reducing the incidence of brain relapse in patients with limited non-small cell lung cancer (Griffin BR et al: *Cancer* 62:36–39, 1988).

In 196 patients treated with whole brain irradiation for metastatic tumor, neurologic status improved in 37% and mean survival was 6.6 months with 11% alive at 1 year (Chassard JL et al: *Rev Neurol [Paris]* 144:489–493, 1988).

Brain metastasis in renal carcinoma carries a poor prognosis and is usually unresponsive to conventional radiation therapy. In selective cases, alternative treatment with surgery or neutron therapy should be considered (Maor MH et al: *Cancer* 62:1912–1917, 1988).

Irradiation of the whole brain at 40–45 Gy over 4.5 weeks for cerebral metastases led in 196 cases to a mean survival of 6.6 months with 11% survival at 1 year (Chassard JL et al: *Rev Neurol [Paris]* 144:8–9, 49–493, 1988).

BRACHYTHERAPY

High activity iodine 125 permanent implantation has been advocated for recurrent skull base tumors (Kumar PP et al: *Cancer* 61:1518–1527, 1988).

Interstitial iodine 192 implantation has been utilized for malignant brain tumors with a simple and accurate CT-guided dosimetry and planning technique (Wu A et al: *Br J Radiol* 62:154–157, 1989).

A contrast enhancing computed tomographic ring may occur after brachytherapy for glioblastoma multiforme without recurrent tumor (Kumar PP et al: *Cancer* 61:1759–1765, 1988).

CHEMOTHERAPY

Supraoptic arterial infusion of BCNU in high-grade glioma is safe and may be helpful to the patient (Fontaine S et al: *J Can Assoc Radiol* 39:178–181, 1988).

Nimuftine and ramustine can induce DNA lability in rat glioma cells (Mineura K et al: *J Neurol Neurosurg Psychiatry* 51:1391–1394, 1988).

Melphalan cytotoxicity is enhanced after glutathione depletion in a human medulloblastoma transplanted to athymic mice (Skapek SX et al: *Cancer Res* 48:2764–2767, 1988).

Etoposide may cause acute neurologic dysfunction after high-dose therapy for malignant glioma (Leff RS et al: *Cancer* 62:32–35, 1988).

In 11 patients treated with steroids, reduced size in brain tumor mass and reduction of enhancement intensity occurred in most of the cases (Cairncross JG et al: *Neurology* 38:724–726, 1988).

Chemotherapy has been recommended in cases of bilateral acoustic neuromas in an effort to save the remaining hearing (Jahrstoerfer RA, Benjamin RS: *Otolaryngol Head Neck Surg* 98:273–282, 1988).

19 Vascular

Introduction

In the area of **ischemia,** the most dramatic changes have to do with the decrease in the number of carotid endarterectomies performed in the United States (Abstract 19–1). The dramatic 22% decline in 1986 is undoubtedly related to the intense scrutiny of this procedure that has arisen in recent times, surely fueled by the negative results of the extracranial-intracranial bypass study. Rational indications for endarterectomy await the conclusion of carefully done, well-controlled trials of carotid endarterectomy in the prevention of stroke. Until then, endar-terectomy should be offered to symptomatic patients with proven stenosis. For 53 such patients aged more than 70 at the University of Iowa, carotid endarterectomy led to excellent surgical results and no perioperative mortality (Abstract 19–2).

In a related area, the Mayo Clinic group report radiation-associated atheromatous disease of the cervical carotid artery (Abstract 19–3). The results of surgery in this series were good, but for many surgeons the difficult and worse results in this group of patients may well warrant a medical treatment program. Lee and Davis report long-term studies after carotid endarterectomy (Abstract 19–4). Among 211 patients who underwent 256 carotid endarterectomies over a 22-year period, there were 10 ipsilateral strokes, many fewer than predicted actuarially. The findings confirm that carotid endarterectomy protects against late ipsilateral stroke. However, coronary artery disease with myocardial infarction is a major cause of premature death in these patients.

There was intense activity regarding cerebral **aneurysms** in 1989. Magnetic resonance imaging for acute subarachnoid hemorrhage is very helpful, particularly in problem cases (Abstract 19–5). Magnetic resonance imaging discloses the extent of bleeding but often provides more information of the site and source of hemorrhage as compared with computed tomography. Intra-arterial digital subtraction angiography has been used for definitive diagnosis of intracranial aneurysms (Abstract 19–6). Even aneurysms down to the diameter of 1–2 mm can be detected. In certain cases, in which the aneurysm is visualized vaguely or not at all, cut-film technique will still have a role.

Early surgery has come to the fore: as reported by Adams and colleagues at the University of Iowa, results in patients undergoing aneurysm surgery within 7 days of bleeding are now rather satisfactory (Abstract 19–7). Of 150 patients, 107 had a favorable outcome, 17 had disabilities, and 26 have died. It may be that nimodipine, 21 aminosteroids, and volume expansion can improve these numbers yet further. Professor Suzuki and colleagues (Abstract 19–8) have recommended a bifrontal interhemispheric approach for wide exposure of carotid-ophthalmic aneurysms. Solomon and Stein (Abstract 19–9) have described surgical approaches to aneurysms of the vertebral and basilar arteries. They advocate a subtemporal or pterional approach to distal basilar lesions, a combined supratentorial and infratentorial approach to trunk lesions, and a suboccipital approach to distal vertebral aneurysms.

Aneurysms of the basilar artery have been successfully treated with circulatory arrest and barbiturate protection (Abstract 19–10). An aneurysmal microendarterectomy has been performed in the treatment of giant middle cerebral artery aneurysms (Abstract 19–11). In a multicenter, double-blind placebo-controlled trial of nimodipine treatment in patients with poor grade aneurysm, there is convincing evidence that nimodipine improves the outcome (Abstract 19–12). This substantial study adds confirmatory weight to the evidence in favor of nimodipine, which is now recommended for all patients with aneurysmal subarachnoid hemorrhage. Dr. Weir and his group have demonstrated the safety and efficacy of intrathecal thrombolytic therapy in a primate model of cerebral vasospasm (Abstract 19–13). Whether intrathecal tPA will be helpful for patients with subarachnoid hemorrhage remains to be seen.

In the management of intracranial *arteriovenous malformations* (AVMs), MR imaging is extremely valuable for demonstration of the extent of AVM nidus, relationships to feeding and draining vessels, and associated parenchymal abnormalities (Abstract 19–14). Stable xenon CT evaluation of cerebral blood flow appears to be useful in evaluating blood flow near an arteriovenous malformation (Abstract 19–15). Höllerhage reports 53 patients operated on for AVM with 29 excellent results, 20 good results, and 4 moderate disabilities (Abstract 19–16). He adds weight to the opinion that AVM should be excised whether or not there has been a hemorrhage unless the AVM is in the speech region or brain stem. Micro AVMs are reported by Willinsky and co-workers (Abstract 19–17). They found among 152 malformations 13 that were less than 1 cm in size but still visualized on angiography.

The Henry Ford Hospital group reported successful removal of 6 AVMs of the basal ganglia with 4 excellent and 2 good results (only 1 worse). These remarkable results show what can be done and suggest that surgical excision of even some very difficult lesions may be recommended. On the other hand, complications can occur with AVM surgery: the Mayo Clinic reports 3 catastrophic bleeding problems, possibly related to perfusion breakthrough, complicating surgery for vein of Galen malformation (Abstract 19–19). In this era, when surgery, embolization, and radiosurgery may be used for arteriovenous malformation, we must consider carefully the various risks and benefits for a patient with AVM before recommending a treatment program.

Ischemia

Dramatic Changes in the Performance of Endarterectomy for Diseases of the Extracranial Arteries of the Head

Pokras R, Dyken ML (Ctrs for Disease Control, Hyattsville, Md; Indiana Univ, Indianapolis)
Stroke 19:1289–1290, October 1988   19–1

Concerns have been raised about the lack of well-defined indications for endarterectomy and the unusually high complications rates associated with this procedure in some institutions and communities. Trends in the performance of carotid endarterectomy were investigated.

Updated estimates from the National Hospital Discharge Survey (NHDS) for the United States were analyzed. The estimated number of carotid endarterectomies increased substantially from 1971 through 1982, from 15,000 to 82,000. In-hospital mortality for patients undergoing this procedure in this period was about 3%.

The estimated number of these procedures continued to rise for 3 years after 1982 to 95,000 in 1983, 103,000 in 1984, and 107,000 in 1985. However, a dramatic 22% decline was noted in 1986. The combined mortality for those years was 2.6% (Fig 19–1). The 22% decrease for 1986 may have a favorable effect on stroke mortality and morbidity.

▶ These data certainly indicate a dramatic fall in the performance of endarterectomy for diseases of the extracranial arteries of the head. Certainly it is gratifying that the morbidity of these operations is decreased by the decreasing frequency of surgery. On the other hand, it is unknown what benefits will also

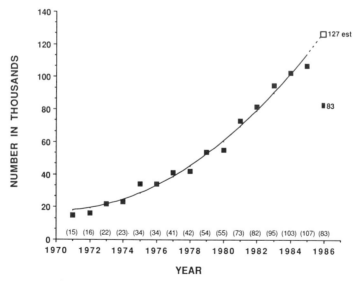

Fig 19–1.—Number of carotid endarterectomies estimated from NHDS for 1971–1986. Quadratic regression function describing points for 15 years. $Y = (year - 1970)^2 \times B + A$, where Y is predicted number of carotid endarterectomies; year is year of estimate; A and B are regression coefficients; A = 17.684; B = 0.428. (Courtesy of Pokras R, Dyken ML: *Stroke* 19:1289–1290, October 1988.)

be lost. In other words, let's not throw out the baby with the bath water. In order to avail to patients the benefits of carotid surgery, we must know the precise indications of this surgery. Such indications can only be established in a scientific and valid fashion by prospective, randomized, controlled studies.

Several carotid endarterectomy trials are ongoing. The Asymptomatic Carotid Artery Stenosis Study got under way in early 1988, with 17 participating studies. So far, 115 patients have been randomized prospectively to surgical therapy or medical therapy. Patients with hemodynamically significant carotid atherosclerosis, which is asymptomatic, are randomized to surgery with postoperative aspirin therapy or medical treatment with aspirin therapy. The end point is transient ischemic attack (TIA) or cerebrovascular accident (CVA). In a consensus statement, the organizers of this trial have suggested that baseline evaluation of carotid stenosis is appropriate to determine the pathoanatomy of the carotid bifurcation in persons considered to be at high risk for extracranial carotid arterial disease, including those with carotid bruit, those with a family history of coronary and cerebrovascular disease, those who are candidates for coronary or peripheral vascular reconstructive surgery, and those who have evidence of a carotid artery event. Recommended studies are ophthalmoplethysmography; Doppler, B-mode, or duplex Doppler examination; and digital subtraction angiography of carotid arteries in the neck. Subsequent management will depend on the findings disclosed by such atraumatic evaluation.

The North American Symptomatic Carotid Endarterectomy Trial is now under way. The objectives will be achieved by the randomized allocation of 3,000 eligible patients to one of two treatment arms: best medical management or best medical management plus carotid endarterectomy. Patients will be observed for an average of 5 years. Eligibility includes an episode of amaurosis fugax, TIA, retinal infarction, or minor nondisabling stroke in the territory of the internal carotid artery within 120 days of randomization. In these patients cerebral angiography must reveal an accessible ipsilateral carotid stenosis between 30% and 99%. Patients are excluded who do not meet entry criteria, are unable to give informed consent, have serious intercurrent disease, or are older than 80 years. Forty-one centers are participating. An extensive data management center and statistical group are integral to this study. To date, more than 500 patients have been entered into the study. There is good balance between the medical and surgical arms of the study.The Veterans Administration Cooperative Studies Program No. 309 is evaluating the role of carotid endarterectomy in preventing CVA from symptomatic carotid stenosis. Men seen at the hospital within 30 days after symptoms of TIA, retinal ischemia, or recent small completed CVAs are examined through rigorous neurologic medical and cardiologic screening processes. When the symptoms relate to a hemodynamically significant carotid stenosis (greater than 70% reduction of lumen), randomization is made to treatment with endarterectomy plus aspirin or aspirin alone. Patients are prestratified according to symptoms. Accrual over 4 years is expected to accumulate 600 patients. Treatment failure is a cerebral infarction or crescendo TIA.

Carotid Endarterectomy in Symptomatic Elderly Patients

Loftus CM, Biller J, Godersky JC, Adams HP, Yamada T, Edwards PS (Univ of Iowa)

Neurosurgery 22:676–680, April 1988   19–2

An attempt was made to confirm that advanced age alone does not increase the risk of carotid artery surgery in symptomatic patients. Of 203 carotid endarterectomies done between 1978 and 1986, 53 were in patients aged more than 70 years. These patients had a mean age of 74 years. A majority were seen with transient ischemic attacks. Medical risk factors were frequently present. The EEG was monitored continuously during surgery.

Forty-three percent of the older patients had 75% or greater carotid stenosis on angiography. Eight patients had contralateral carotid occlusion. The mean cross-clamp time was 48.5 minutes. Six patients required shunt insertion. One patient had a postoperative myocardial infarct, and 1 had a stroke; there were no perioperative deaths. Minor self-limited complications occurred in 15% of patients. No new neurologic events were identified in 45 patients followed up at a mean of 12.7 months.

Excellent surgical results were obtained in these older patients, and there was no perioperative mortality. Carotid endarterectomy may be done in symptomatic older patients with a risk-benefit ratio equal to that of younger patients.

▶ The group at the University of Iowa reports excellent results after carotid endarterectomy in symptomatic elderly patients. Among 53 cases, there was less than a 4% incidence of neurologic and cardiac complications. Of interest in this report was a poor correlation between noninvasive studies and definitive angiography. Centers with similar morbidity and mortality statistics may pursue an aggressive approach as recommended, but where such fine results have not been documented, a more conservative, medically oriented program may be more appropriate. In the final analysis, the results of the North American Symptomatic Carotid Endarterectomy Trial will provide relevant scientific information on the appropriate utilization of carotid endarterectomy in symptomatic patients.

Radiation-Associated Atheromatous Disease of the Cervical Carotid Artery: Report of Seven Cases and Review of the Literature

Atkinson JLD, Sundt TM Jr, Dale AJD, Cascino TL, Nichols DA (Mayo Clinic, Rochester, Minn)

Neurosurgery 24:171–178, February 1989   19–3

Because prolonged survival after radiation and combination adjuvant therapy for malignancy is becoming more prevalent, more patients have long-term side effects from radiotherapy. Radiation-induced atheromatous disease affecting large vessels in a variety of locations has been reported.

Seven patients had radiation-induced carotid atheromatous disease after treatment for cervical proximity malignancies. They underwent 9 carotid endarterectomies and were followed for an average of 49 months. Of the 7, 1 patient who had primary closure at the arteriotomy site and was not treated with a vein patch graft needed postoperative anticoagulation after sustaining 2 transient hemispheric events. Also, 2 patients had transient cranial nerve palsies involving the hypoglossal and vagus nerves. Although there may be increased risk to the surrounding neural structures, the neurovascular results were judged to be favorable and possibly comparable to those of endarterectomy procedures in nonirradiated patients.

It was recommended that any patient surviving 5 years after radiotherapy be followed with accurate noninvasive procedures for carotid occlusive disease. Attempts should be made to decrease known risk factors, such as hypertension and serum cholesterol. If surgery is needed, these patients should be approached as if radiation changes were not a major factor for reconstructive arterial surgery.

▶ Unfortunately, the results of surgery on radiation-induced atheromas in other hands have not been as good as the results of the Mayo Clinic group. Cases summarized in the report show that 19% of these had new neurologic deficits, with postoperative thrombosis in an additional 12%. These complications rates would negate any benefit from the procedure unless it could be shown that radiation angiopathy is a particularly malignant cause of stroke. Because of these technical challenges, it may be well for many surgeons to defer carotid endarterectomy on these patients until further data are available.

Stroke, Myocardial Infarction, and Survival During Long-Term Follow-Up After Carotid Endarterectomy
Lee KS, Davis CH Jr (Wake Forest Univ Med Ctr, Winston-Salem, NC)
Surg Neurol 31:113–119, February 1989   19–4

Only 1 previous prospective, randomized, multicenter trial found that carotid endarterectomy in the treatment of extracranial cerebrovascular disease is superior to nonsurgical treatment. All other evidence that carotid endarterectomy protects against stroke has been obtained from retrospective follow-up studies. A review was made of the epidemiologic data concerning 211 patients aged 36–80 who underwent 256 carotid endarterectomies during a 22-year period. The data were analyzed by the actuarial method to determine the incidence of stroke, myocardial infarction, and survival among these patients.

Indications for carotid endarterectomy included transient cerebral ischemia in 91 (36%) patients, stroke in 72 (28%), asymptomatic stenosis of greater than 80% in 55 (21%), and amaurosis fugax in 38 (15%). The main atherosclerotic risk factors were hypertension in 134 (64%) patients and smoking in 87 (41%). There were 6 (2.8%) perioperative deaths, and 8 patients had a stroke within the first 30-day postoperative period. The median follow-up period in the surviving 205 patients was 7

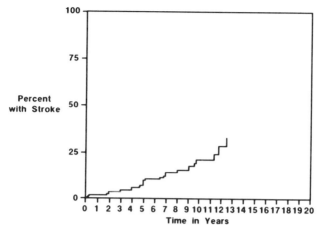

Fig 19–2.—Cumulative incidence of late stroke. (Courtesy of Lee KS, Davis CH Jr: *Surg Neurol* 31:113–119, February 1989.)

years, ranging from 1 month to 23.2 years; 14 (7%) patients were unavailable for follow-up.

Of the remaining 191 patients, 44 (22%) died within 5 years of endarterectomy, 62 (30%) died more than 5 years after endarterectomy, and 85 (41%) were alive at last follow-up. The actuarial 5-year survival rate was 77%; the 10-year survival rate was 49%; the mean annual death rate was 4%. Comparison with the age-matched general population showed that the study population had significantly lower survival rates. Of 27 (13%) patients who sustained a stroke during follow-up, 10 (4.9%) had an ipsilateral stroke, 12 (5.9%) had a contralateral stroke, and 5 (2.2%) had a posterior circulation stroke; 9 (4.4%) strokes were fatal. Actuarial freedom of stroke was 91% at 5 years and 80% at 10 years (Fig 19–2). The annual ipsilateral stroke rate after endarterectomy was 0.41%, which was comparable to that of the general population. During follow-up, 69 (34%) patients sustained a myocardial infarction, 52 of which were fatal. Infarction accounted for 49% of all late deaths.

Carotid endarterectomy protects against late ipsilateral stroke. However, coronary artery disease with myocardial infarction is a major cause of premature death in these patients.

▶ This nice study from Bowman Gray College of Medicine demonstrates with actuarial data that carotid endarterectomy does in fact largely reduce the risk of ipsilateral ischemic stroke. It also shows that myocardial infarction is a major cause of premature death in these patients.

Brief Notes on Ischemia

Carotid Endarterectomy: Techniques

In a randomized study, routine saphenous vein patch closure did not produce superior results despite increased operative time and higher incidence of early recurrence (Clagett CP et al: *J Vasc Surg* 9:213–223, 1989).

For exposure of the internal carotid artery near the skull base, the sternomastoid muscle is dissected from the mastoid, the posterior belly of the digastric is divided, the facial nerve may be dissected, and the tail of the parotid resected for additional exposure (Shaha A et al: *J Vasc Surg* 8:618–622, 1988).

Hemodynamic studies during carotid endarterectomy showed that distal internal carotid artery (ICA) pressure fell 8 mm Hg in only 3 of 11 patients with severe pressure reduction across the ICA stenosis (Sillesen H: *J Vasc Surg* 2:309–313, 1988).

A study in a neurosurgical training program noted that the use of an intraluminal shunt during carotid endarterectomy significantly reduced the risk of intraoperative neurologic deficit without increasing other complications (Gumerloch MK, Neuwelt EA: *Stroke* 19:1485–1490, 1988).

CAROTID ENDARTERECTOMY: RESULTS

In 106 carotid endarterectomies performed under local anesthesia, strokes occurred in 2%, and there was no mortality (Zuccarello M et al: *Neurosurgery* 23:445–450, 1988).

Among 2,000 carotid endarterectomies performed under local anesthesia, operative ischemia accounted for 0.5% of neurologic deficits, whereas cerebral embolization and intercerebral hemorrhage each accounted for 0.5% with a total of 2.5% cerebral deficits (Imparato AN: *World J Surg* 12:756–762, 1988).

In Medicare patients in Kentucky undergoing carotid endarterectomy in 1983 and 1984, 85% had symptoms of carotid disease and postoperative stroke rate was 3.7% with a mortality of 2% (Richardson JD, Main KA: *J Vasc Surg* 9:65–73, 1989).

In a community-based teaching hospital, 148 carotid endarterectomies were performed from 1984 to 1989 with 2.7% strokes and no deaths (Friedmann P et al: *Stroke* 19:1323–1327, 1988).

CAROTID ENDARTERECTOMY: SPECIAL CONCERNS

Fourteen patients underwent reoperation for symptomatic recurrent carotid stenosis after previous carotid endarterectomy (Kazmers A et al: *Am J Surg* 156:346–352, 1988). Most patients had carotid patch angioplasty with repeated endarterectomy, and 1 patient had a replacement vein graft. Outcome was good in all cases. Reluctance to reoperate is unwarranted because of the good results obtainable.

Twenty-seven carotid endarterectomies were performed within 30 days of cerebral infarction. All did well save for 2 of 3 patients with preoperative progressive neurologic deficit, 1 of whom died. Patients with recent stroke and normal CT results are at low risk for carotid endarterectomy, those with stroke and CT evidence of infarct are at medium risk, and those with progressive infarct are at high risk (Little JR et al: *Neurosurgery* 24:334–338, 1989).

Twenty-two patients underwent 27 external carotid artery revascularizations without perioperative strokes or death and no strokes during a 46-month mean follow-up (Friedman SG et al: *Arch Surg* 123:497–499, 1988).

Extracranial carotid artery disease may lead to chronic ocular ischemia and neovascular glaucoma (Wagner WH et al: *J Vasc Surg* 8:551–557, 1988).

OTHER SURGERY FOR ISCHEMIA

Emergency embolectomy for acute middle cerebral artery embolus can lead to recovery of function if flow is reestablished within 5–7 hours of the onset of symptoms (Opalak ME et al: *Microsurgery* 9:188–193, 1988).

For distal anterior cerebral ischemia, an interposition graft of left superficial temporal artery was placed between the right superficial temporal artery and a branch of the anterior cerebral artery, with postoperative angiographic patency (Iwata Y et al: *Microsurgery* 9:14–17, 1988).

Successful management of sagittal sinus thrombosis was carried out with ventricular drainage and pentobarbital coma (Hanley DF et al: *Stroke* 19:903–909, 1988).

CAROTID ARTERY: ARTERIOSCLERSOSIS

Serial B-mode ultrasonography suggests that the rate of progression of carotid atherosclerosis may be slow in people who quit smoking compared with those who don't (Tell GS et al: *JAMA* 261:1178–1180, 1989).

Multicenter evaluation of ultrasonography, arteriography, and pathology leads to the conclusion that development of a morphological standard for carotid stenosis is hindered by a number of problems (Schenk EA et al: *Stroke* 19:289–296, 1988).

Weinberger and co-workers (*J Am Coll Cardiol* 12:1515–1521, 1988) report correlation of development of symptomatology with growth of atherosclerotic plaque in the carotid artery bifurcation demonstrated on sequential imaging by real-time D-mode ultrasonography.

Quantitative ultrasound pulsation studies in the human carotid artery have detected loss of wall flexibility associated with arteriosclerotic lesion formation (Barth JD et al: *Arteriosclerosis* 8:778–781, 1988).

Macrophages in intimal thickening of rat carotid arteries have been identified by cytochemical localization of purine nucleoside phosphorylase (Verheyen AK et al: *Arteriosclerosis* 8:759–767, 1988).

Biomechanical studies show that the common carotid artery in women has a stiffer arterial wall (VanMerode T et al: *Ultrasound Med Biol* 14:571–574, 1988).

CAROTID ARTERY: INTRAPLAQUE HEMORRHAGE

On duplex ultrasonography, heterogeneous plaque appearance suggesting intraplaque hemorrhage correlates with ipsilateral cerebral symptoms (Leahy AL et al: *J Vasc Surg* 8:558–562, 1988).

On CT study of the cervical carotid artery, a lucent defect is an image of intraplaque hemorrhage or necrosis (Culebras A et al: *Stroke* 19:723–727, 1988).

In evaluation of 62 carotid artery bifurcation plaques, intraplaque hemorrhage was not correlated with symptoms (Bassiouny HS et al: *J Vasc Surg* 9:202–212, 1989).

Magnetic resonance imaging of a dissected internal carotid artery demonstrated a hyperintense lesion expanding the wall (the hematoma) with narrowing of the lumen (Hommel N et al: *Rev Neurol [Paris]* 144:8–9, 512–513, 1988).

CAROTID ARTERY: ANOMALOUS BRANCHES

Distal cervical internal carotid artery (ICA) branches may maintain patency of distal ICA after proximal cervical ICA occlusion, thus making possible carotid endarterectomy (Littooy FN et al: *J Vasc Surg* 8:634–637, 1988).

The occipital artery may arise from the distal cervical internal carotid artery (Benson MT, Hamer JD: *J Vasc Surg* 8:643–645, 1988).

CAROTID OCCLUSION

Among 40 patients with unilateral carotid occlusion, no strokes occurred in 19 patients whose vessels had already occluded and the stroke rate was 3.8% for those whose vessels occluded during follow-up (Bornstein NM, Norris JW: *Neurology* 39:6–8, 1989).

In a survey of 1,836 angiograms, the incidence of silent ICA occlusion in the population aged more than 60 years was estimated at less than 1% (Pierce GE et al: *J Vasc Surg* 8:74–80, 1988).

Seventy-four patients with bilateral ICA occlusion were treated conservatively over a mean of 42 months with 13% strokes per patient-year and 8% death per year (Wode JPH et al: *Brain* 110:667–682, 1987).

Among 17 patients with common carotid artery occlusion, 10 (59%) suffered stroke, 7 of which were ipsilateral to the occlusion (Levine SR, Welch KMA: *Neurology* 39:178–186, 1989).

Tissue plasminogen activator (tPA) has gained prominence in the treatment of acute coronary occlusion. Studies have demonstrated efficacy in the ultra acute phase of myocardial ischemia, although heparinization has been required to prevent rethrombosis. Successful application of this thrombolytic agent has prompted studies of tPA in acute cerebrovascular accident (CVA). A number of laboratory investigations have indicated that the agent is effective in the lysis of thrombus in the intracranial setting, but intracranial hemorrhage is a feared complication. Currently, there are several ongoing studies of this agent in the treatment of acute CVA. In one study, directed by Del Zoppo, tPA is used only in the acute setting, less than 8 hours from symptom onset. Following initial clinical assessment, computed tomography (CT) scan and angiography, each patient with a documented cerebral arterial occlusion appropriate to the clinical syndrome may receive a preassigned intravenous dose of tPA over 60 minutes. Angiography and CT are repeated after infusion to document recanalization in the absence of hemorrhage. This study thus far has not provided evidence to suggest that tPA is safe or beneficial in this particular setting. Another study by Brott and colleagues has utilized an infusion beginning within 90 minutes of symptom onset but without angiographic study. This dose escalation study has been applied in 21 patients; 9 had rapid neurologic improvement during the 60-minute tPA infusion or within 90 minutes after the end of infusion. Three of these patients deteriorated after cessation of tPA. On the 24-hour CT scan, 2 of the 21 patients had small areas of hemorrhagic change within a larger area of infarction. Hemorrhagic conversion was clinically silent. Twelve of the 21 patients showed no early improvement. Two died, both from cerebral edema and herniation. Further data will be required to establish efficacy and safety of tPA in the setting of acute cerebral thrombosis.

OTHER STROKE TOPICS

The Scandinavian Stroke Study Group (*Stroke* 18:691–699, 1987) performed a multicenter trial of hemodilution in acute ischemic stroke with no overall beneficial effects detected.

Hemiparesis with few brain stem signs may herald basilar artery occlusion (Fisher CM: *Arch Neurol* 45:1301–1303, 1988).

Very low dose aspirin failed to reduce risk of TIAs stroke, heart attack, and vascular death (Boysen G et al: *Stroke* 19:1211–1215, 1988).

Aneurysms

Magnetic Resonance Imaging of Acute Subarachnoid Hemorrhage
Jenkins A, Hadley DM, Teasdale GM, Condon B, Macpherson P, Patterson J
(Southern Gen Hosp, Glasgow, Scotland)
J Neurosurg 68:731–736, May 1988   19–5

Magnetic resonance (MR) imaging is being used more often as the initial investigation for a wide range of central nervous system disorders but only in patients with nonacute lesions. The usefulness of MR in spontaneous subarachnoid hemorrhage may be limited, as there is doubt about its ability to display acute intracranial hemorrhage. Moreover, the strong magnetic field created during MR imaging may be hazardous to patients with metallic implants.

To investigate the safety and usefulness of MR imaging before and after surgery, 30 patients aged 15–69 years who had MR imaging between 8 hours and 5 days after onset of SAH symptoms were evaluated. Twenty-seven patients also had 4-vessel catheter angiography. All 30 patients underwent computed tomography (CT) within 48 hours after MR imaging and within 3 days after the ictus. Ten patients had MR imaging after aneurysm clipping; 4 also underwent postoperative CT within 24 hours after MR.

Comparison of Preoperative CT and MRI Findings in 30 Patients
With Clinical Evidence of SAH

Feature	No. of Cases	
	CT	MRI
Subarachnoid blood	24	25
Intracerebral blood	10	12
Intraventricular blood	11	10
Shift/space-occupying effect	9	8
Hydrocephalus	11	8
Ischemia	0	0
Localization of bleeding	11	16
Visualization of aneurysm	0	14

CT, computed tomography; *MRI*, magnetic resonance imaging; *SAH*, subarachnoid hemorrhage.
(Courtesy of Jenkins A, Hadley DM, Teasdale GM, et al: *J Neurosurg* 68:731–736, May 1988.)

Angiography showed an aneurysm in 25 patients; 12 had multiple aneurysms. None refused to undergo MR studies, and none deteriorated while undergoing MR imaging. Findings on MR imaging were similar to those of CT in the detection of intracranial bleeding in the subarachnoid space and ventricles, and in identification of intracerebral clots. However, MR detected subarachnoid blood more often and provided more information about the site and source of the hemorrhage than did CT (table). Postoperative MR imaging showed changes corresponding with those seen on CT. Both MR imaging and CT studies detected hydrocephalus and space-occupying effect.

Magnetic resonance imaging appears safe for investigating patients with a suspected subarachnoid hemorrhage. For the present, CT will most likely remain the first-line imaging strategy in cases of subarachnoid hemorrhage because it is quicker, more accessible, and may be cheaper.

▶ Magnetic resonance imaging provides more information than CT regarding the site and source of subarachnoid hemorrhage. In some instances MR can also demonstrate cerebral angiomas and aneurysms. In questionable cases MR is a useful addition, but for now, CT is cheaper and quicker and will remain the initial study of choice in these patients for the present.

In a related report, Satoh and Kadoya found that MRI is useful in imaging subarachnoid hemorrhage (1). Among 30 patients evaluated with MR and CT, 4 of 4 appearing normal on CT showed high-intensity subarachnoid hemorrhage on T2-weighted MRI. Thirteen of 24 aneurysms larger than 5 mm were detected on T2 images. In 1 case of multiple aneurysms the hemorrhagic lesion was indicated by blood shown on MR but not CT.

Reference

1. Satoh S, Kadoya S: *Neuroradiology* 30:361–366, 1988.

Intraarterial Digital Subtraction Angiography for Definitive Diagnosis of Intracranial Aneurysms

Touho H, Karasawa J, Tazawa T, Nakagawara J, Yamada K, Kobayashi K, Asai M, Kagawa M, Yasue H (Osaka Neurological Inst, Osaka, Japan)
AJNR 9:1157–1161 November–December 1988   19–6

Angiography is the primary radiologic diagnostic procedure for diseases affecting blood vessels. Intravenous digital subtraction angiography is now widely used for detecting cervicocerebrovascular lesions. Recent advances have extended to diagnostic and therapeutic intra-arterial digital subtraction angiography (IA-DSA). A review was made of 1 series of patients with intracranial aneurysms studied with IA-DSA.

No conventional angiography was used in the 101 patients examined. High-quality images were consistent with IA-DSA, facilitating accurate, definite diagnosis of intracranial aneurysm. Magnification radiography and stereography using IA-DSA were performed for a more precise diagnosis. This enabled detection of 5 small aneurysms, with diameters of 1–2 mm. The procedure was judged to be as safe and reliable as conventional angiography.

In this series, IA-DSA was found to facilitate the accurate and definitive diagnosis of intracranial aneurysms. Important advantages of this technique include decreased procedural time and contrast agent burden, factors that will ensure broader application for definitive diagnosis of intracranial aneurysms as experience with the technique grows.

▶ Certainly intra-arterial digital subtraction angiography is helpful in the analysis of many cases of intracranial aneurysm. On the other hand, the resolution for this technique is still surpassed by cut-film angiography in many institutions. When there are questions, cut-film angiography may be preferable.

Intracranial Operation Within Seven Days of Aneurysmal Subarachnoid Hemorrhage: Results in 150 Patients
Adams HP Jr, Kassell NF, Kongable GA, Torner JC (Univ of Iowa)
Arch Neurol 45:1065–1069, October 1988   19–7

The combined mortality and morbidity among patients with aneurysmal subarachnoid hemorrhage (SAH) who reach a major medical center alive approaches 45% 6 months after SAH has occurred. In the past, operation on patients with SAH has been delayed until 7–14 days after the event because of poor results with early operation. Although delayed surgery allows the patient to recover from the effects of the initial SAH before undergoing operation, postponing surgery leaves the patient at risk for rebleeding. To date, the outcomes of interim early medical treatment and delayed intracranial operation have been disappointing. With the advances in neuroanesthesia, perioperative care, and operative techniques, early operation within 1 week of SAH may now be more practical. The outcome of early intracranial operation in patients with SAH was studied.

One hundred fifty patients with SAH, 92 women and 58 men, were operated on within 7 calendar days of SAH. Patients in all clinical grades, except those who were moribund, and patients with either anterior or posterior circulation aneurysms were treated.

At follow-up evaluation 1 month to 7 years after operation, 107 patients (71.3%) had favorable outcomes, 17 (11.3%) had major disabilities, and 26 (17.3%) had died. Symptomatic vasospasm was the most commonly diagnosed complication of SAH, occurring in 63 (42%) patients. Rebleeding occurred in 39 (26%) patients. The adjusted overall rates of good recovery were 69% in those operated on during days 0–3 and 52% in those operated on during days 4–7. Neurologic condition on admission had a major influence on outcome, regardless of the time of operation.

These results were similar to those of other reports of series of early operations on SAH.

▶ This important report describes 150 patients operated on within 7 days of SAH by the same surgeon in a single center. The outcome was favorable for 71%, with 11% having major disabilities and 17% dying. Despite early operation, rebleeding occurred in 26%. Vasospasm was present in 42%. Thus, these 2 important complications of cerebral aneurysm are not eliminated by the early surgical effort. Early surgery should not be excluded because of depressed level of consciousness, deep location of aneurysm, size of aneurysm, or age of the patient. In my opinion, the report offers moderate encouragement for a policy of early aneurysm surgery, but the neurosurgeon and his center must be prepared to deal with these patients on an emergency basis and to accept the higher rate of surgical complications super-added from those patients conventionally treated with medical therapy alone.

Bifrontal Interhemispheric Approach for Carotid-Ophthalmic Aneurysms
Mizoi K, Suzuki J, Kinjo T, Yoshimoto T (Tohoku Univ, Sendai, Japan)
Acta Neurochir (Wien) 90:84–90, 1988   19–8

Direct operation on a carotid-ophthalmic aneurysm is difficult because of the aneurysm's location. Unilateral frontotemporal craniotomy is most often used to repair carotid-ophthalmic aneurysms. A bifrontal interhemispheric approach, reported to facilitate operation, was evaluated when 18 women and 11 men aged 31–67 years underwent operation for a carotid-ophthalmic aneurysm in a 20-year period. A bifrontal interhemispheric approach was used in 28 of the 29 patients.

Technique.—Before dissecting the aneurysm, the common carotid artery (CCA) and the external carotid artery (ECA) were temporarily occluded with tape in the neck. Wide dissection of the sylvian fissures and the interhemispheric fissure was performed through a bifrontal craniotomy. When necessary, the anterior clinoid process and the roof of the optic canal were removed. The neck of the aneurysm could then be viewed from various angles, thus facilitating treatment of the aneurysm.

Twenty (69%) of the 29 patients had excellent results with no postoperative neurologic deficits. Seven (24%) patients had postoperative loss of vision on the side of the aneurysm. However, they were rated as having good results, as they had no other neurologic deficits and were able to lead normal lives. There were 2 (7%) deaths. In 1 patient with a giant aneurysm, stenosis of the internal carotid artery developed during ligation of the neck. The other patient who had multiple aneurysms had re-rupture of an untreatable aneurysm that had been wrapped only.

None of the patients experienced postoperative complications because of temporary occlusion of the CCA and the ECA. Treatment of the aneurysm consisted of clipping alone in 17 patients with 18 aneurysms, ligation and clipping in 5, ligation alone in 2, and muscle wrapping alone in 5.

The interhemispheric approach used in surgery for carotid-ophthalmic aneurysms provides a much larger operative field and exposes the aneurysm much better than do other surgical approaches.

▶ This interesting report from Professor Suzuki's group documents results in 29 patients treated with an interhemispheric approach for carotid-ophthalmic aneurysms. As the authors suggest, a very wide exposure is possible in this fashion. The authors used temporary clipping with mannitol protection in most cases. They reported death in 2 and visual disturbance or blindness in 7 (almost a quarter). Results appear similar to those reported by Dolenc, who used a combined epidural and subdural approach (1), and Yasargil, who used a pterional approach (2). It is clear that, whatever the approach, removal of the anterior clinoid process and unroofing of the optic canal are useful maneuvers in obtaining proximal control of the internal carotid artery and exposing the neck of the aneurysm.

From the data, it is not clear that the interhemispheric approach produces superior results as compared with the other approaches. In addition, particularly for giant aneurysms in this area and most especially in the older patient, consideration should be given to the possible utilization of balloon occlusion of the internal carotid artery with or without extracranial-intracranial bypass, as indicated by CBF studies.

References

1. Dolenc: *J Neurosurg* 62:667, 1985.
2. Yasargil: *Surg Neurol* 8:155, 1977.

Surgical Approaches to Aneurysms of the Vertebral and Basilar Arteries
Solomon RA, Stein BM (Columbia Presbyterian Med Ctr, New York)
Neurosurgery 23:203–208, August 1988   19–9

Aneurysms of the vertebral-basilar system were inoperable until the development of microsurgery and improved instrumentation. Surgical treatment, however, remains difficult. The authors report operative techniques and outcomes in 44 patients with these aneurysms.

Thirty-four of the patients experienced a sudden subarachnoid hemorrhage and 10 had unruptured aneurysms. The operative method was chosen according to the location of the aneurysm (Fig 19–3). A frontotemporal pterional craniotomy was performed on 30 patients with an aneurysm adjacent to the basilar apex (Fig 19–4). A unilateral suboccipital craniectomy was the method of choice for 8 patients with aneurysm of the vertebral artery or adjacent to the vertebral basilar junction. For midbasilar aneurysms (5 patients), combined supratentorial and infratentorial approaches were employed.

Aneurysms were clipped in 37 patients and wrapped in 3 patients. Four large fusiform aneurysms were treated by occlusion of the basilar or

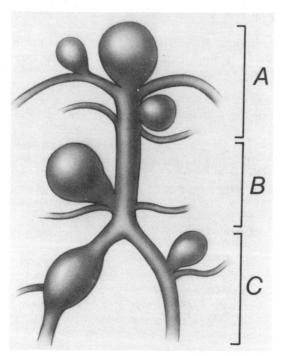

Fig 19–3.—Schematic diagram of the various aneurysm locations on the vertebral-basilar arteries. *A*, aneurysms that can be approached from the pterional subtemporal approach. *B*, aneurysms that are best approached by the combined supratentorial and infratentorial approaches. *C*, aneurysms best approached via the suboccipital route. (Courtesy of Solomon RA, Stein BM: *Neurosurgery* 23:203–208, August 1988.)

vertebral artery. As a result of operation, 1 patient died, 4 patients had significant, long-lasting morbidity, and 32 patients returned to normal activities.

Computed tomography and magnetic resonance imaging proved in-

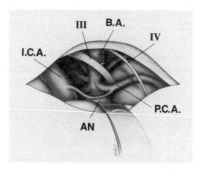

Fig 19–4.—Drawing of the operative exposure of the basilar apex aneurysms as seen from the pterional subtemporal approach. *I.C.A.*, internal carotid artery; *B.A.*, basilar artery; *P.C.A.*, posterior cerebral artery; *A.N.*, basilar apex aneurysm. The *Roman numerals* signify the location of the corresponding cranial nerves. (Courtesy of Solomon RA, Stein BM: *Neurosurgery* 23:203–208, August 1988.)

valuable in determining the exact location of the aneurysm and its relationship to the tentorium and brain stem. Brain relaxation and intraoperative hypotension are both necessary for a successful surgical outcome, as are specially trained neurosurgeons and facilities for neurosurgical intensive care.

▶ Solomon and Stein present a logical division of approaches to vertebrobasilar aneurysms: subtemporal for the upper basilar lesions, combined supratentorial-subtentorial for trunk lesions, and suboccipital for the vertebral and vertebrobasilar junction lesions. Impressively good results support the application of this program. It is worth knowing that serious complications occurred in 20% of the cases, even in the hands of this highly experienced team. Therefore, these lesions require the attention of an experienced neurosurgical operator and institution.

In a series of some 50 cases we have used a similar approach and concur in the application of this breakdown. Resection of a small portion of the inferomesial temporal lobe is sometimes helpful in the pterional-subtemporal approach rather than excessive retraction of the temporal lobe. For basilar superior cerebellar aneurysms, the pterional approach is superior because the line of sight gives one a perpendicular approach to the neck of the aneurysm while avoiding the third nerve. Although the basilar trunk lesions can be reached through a strictly lateral approach, I agree that the tentorial section offers a wider field of view and in the long run is probably safer.

Aneurysms of the Basilar Artery Treated With Circulatory Arrest, Hypothermia, and Barbiturate Cerebral Protection
Spetzler RF, Hadley MN, Rigamonti D, Carter LP, Raudzens PA, Shedd SA, Wilkinson E (Barrow Neurological Inst, Phoenix)
J Neurosurg 68:868–879, June 1988   19–10

Giant and large intracranial basilar artery aneurysms remain a difficult challenge for the neurosurgeon. Even in the hands of the most competent surgeons, the associated incidence of perioperative morbidity and mortality is significant. Several investigators have reported improved results with complete circulatory arrest in the treatment of complex intracranial vascular lesions.

Seven patients aged 41–77 years underwent intracranial procedures under complete cardiac arrest, deep hypothermia, and prearrest barbiturate cerebral protection. Six had giant basilar artery aneurysms, and 1 had a large basilar artery aneurysm. In 1 patient a giant basilar artery aneurysm was discovered incidentally during the diagnostic work-up after mild head trauma had occurred. Of the other 6 patients, 2 were in grade I of subarachnoid hemorrhage (SAH), 1 was in grade II, 2 were in grade III, and 1 was in grade IV before operation.

All 7 patients survived surgery and the techniques of circulatory arrest and cardiopulmonary bypass. In each patient circulatory arrest allowed detailed dissection of the aneurysm with modest manipulation and direct

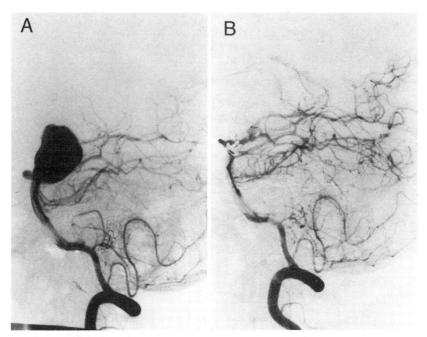

Fig 19–5.—A, preoperative angiogram, lateral view, depicting a giant basilar artery aneurysm. B, postoperative angiogram, lateral view, revealing complete elimination of the aneurysm without compromise of associated vessels. (Courtesy of Spetzler RF, Hadley MN, Rigamonti D, et al: *J Neurosurg* 68:868–879, June 1988.)

clipping of the aneurysm base. However, 1 patient with a preoperative grade III SAH who initially responded well after operation sustained a large brain stem infarction and died 8 weeks later of severe pneumonitis. Another patient who initially did well after operation died 7 months later of myocardial infarction. Of the 5 survivors, 1 had ipsilateral third-nerve palsy and contralateral hemiparesis postoperatively that improved steadily. The other 4 patients had excellent outcomes without neurologic sequelae, including the patient with the unruptured aneurysm (Fig 19–5). No association was found between a patient's preoperative SAH grade and postoperative course.

These patients illustrate that the inherent risk associated with the surgical treatment of giant basilar artery aneurysms can be reduced with the use of extracorporeal circulation, cardiac arrest, deep hypothermia, and barbiturate cerebral protection.

▶ The authors report excellent results in 4, good in 1, and fair in 1, with an early postoperative death. These are very encouraging results for this extremely difficult type of case. In particular, there is no evidence of postoperative intracerebral hemorrhage, the problem that convinced Drake this method was not feasible. This is evidently a result of newer developments in cardiopulmonary bypass and strict adherence to the technical details described. Even with these good results, of course, some significant operative morbidity and mortality remain.

Thus it is appropriate to consider alternative modes of therapy. Hunterian ligation, often utilizing balloon catheter technology and involving one or both vertebral arteries or the basilar artery (depending on the location of the aneurysm), can be used for giant aneurysms in the vertebral basilar circulation. We have used such techniques for the obliteration of 4 giant aneurysms without morbidity. The technique was effective in obliterating 3 of the 4 aneurysms completely. In his much larger series, Drake has reported reasonably good results, but with some morbidity and treatment failures. The establishment of the superiority of any treatment methodology will await further data on the results.

Endaneurysmal Microendarterectomy in the Treatment of Giant Cerebral Aneurysm: Technical Note
Hylton PD, Reichman OH (Loyola Univ, Maywood, Ill)
Neurosurgery 23:674–679, November 1988   19–11

Surgical treatment of the giant cerebral aneurysm is complicated by the laminated intramural thrombus that often is present, as well as calcified atheroma at its neck. Endaneurysmal microendarterectomy, preserving or reconstructing the parent artery, is a feasible approach to these lesions. Two patients with giant aneurysms were managed by temporary trapping of the aneurysm, intramural thrombectomy, and end-aneurysmal microendarterectomy. Both did well after the operation.

The use of delicate atraumatic vascular clips will minimize the risk of injuring the vascular endothelium. Intramural thrombectomy (Fig 19–6) is required to accurately delineate the calcified atheroma. Precise dissection under high magnification and good illumination is the key to successful microendarterectomy. Application of a clip or clips to the aneurysm neck is the best means of obliterating the orifice. If there is any doubt about the patency of the parent vessel or its branches, immediate angiography is indicated.

This approach presently is used for carotid bifurcation, middle cerebral artery, and paraclinoid giant aneurysms where calcified atheroma is present at the base of the aneurysm. The aneurysm can be totally obliterated while preserving the native cerebral vessels.

▶ This excellent paper shows that after careful complete dissection some giant aneurysms may be opened for precise removal of mural thrombus and atheroma to permit accurate clipping of the neck. Temporary clipping with cerebral protection is needed in these cases. In our experience with temporary clipping, mannitol, hypertension, and intermittent opening of the clips permit cross-clamping of up to an hour for internal carotid artery and middle cerebral artery lesions. Although direct repair of this sort can be done, it carries a substantial

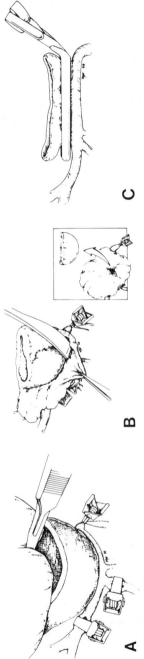

Fig 19–6.—Principal operative steps required for endaneurysmal microendarterectomy with parent vessel preservation. **A,** temporary trapping with resection of the aneurysm dome above the cuplike calcified atheroma followed by intramural thrombectomy for precise visualization of the atheroma. **B,** endarterectomy of the calcified atheroma. **C,** parent vessel reconstruction by clip application to the now supple aneurysm neck. (Courtesy of Hylton PD, Reichman OH: *Neurosurgery* 23:674–679, November 1988.)

risk. In selected patients, alternative treatment with an indirect technique utilizing proximal parent vessel occlusion (with or without bypass) may carry a lower risk.

Nimodipine Treatment in Poor-Grade Aneurysm Patients: Results of a Multicenter Double-Blind Placebo-Controlled Trial

Petruk KC, West M, Mohr G, Weir BKA, Benoit BG, Gentili F, Disney LB, Khan MI, Grace M, Holness RO, Karwon MS, Ford RM, Cameron GS, Tucker WS, Purves GB, Miller JDR, Hunter KM, Richard MT, Durity FA, Chan R, Clein LJ, Maroun FB, Godon A (Univ of Alberta)
J Neurosurg 68:505–517, April 1988   19–12

Delayed neurologic deterioration caused by vasospasm is a major cause of a poor outcome in survivors of initial subarachnoid hemorrhage. These patients have a large volume of subarachnoid blood and provide a good test of nimodipine for preventing delayed ischemic deficits secondary to vasospasm. Seventeen centers in Canada enrolled 154 patients in a placebo-controlled double-blind trial of nimodipine. Adult patients with aneurysm rupture during the previous 4 days, who were grade 3 or worse, received 90 mg of nimodipine or placebo at 4-hour intervals.

A good outcome was present 3 months after bleeding in 29% of nimodipine-treated patients and 10% of placebo recipients. Delayed ischemic deficits caused by vasospasm were significantly less frequent in the nimodipine group (Fig 19–7). Both grade 3 and grade 4 patients did better when given nimodipine, but grade 5 patients did not.

Repeated angiography showed no significant difference in moderate or

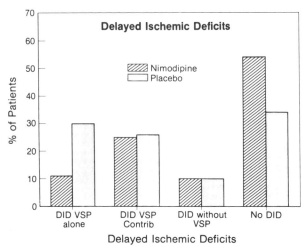

Fig 19–7.—Incidence of permanent delayed ischemic deficits *(DID)* and their etiology in the nimodipine and placebo groups. *VSP*, vasospasm. (Courtesy of Petruk KC, West M, Mohr G, et al: *J Neurosurg* 68:505–517, April 1988.)

severe diffuse spasm in the nimodipine and placebo groups. Rebleeding occurred in 24% of nimodipine-treated patients and 21% of the placebo group. Antifibrinolytic therapy did not influence the outcome.

Nimodipine improves the outcome in poor-grade patients with subarachnoid hemorrhage. Prevention of large-vessel spasm is not the explanation. The treatment is quite safe.

▶ This substantial controlled double-blind trial adds confirmatory weight to the evidence in favor of nimodipine for the prevention of delayed ischemic deficit after subarachnoid hemorrhage. Although the exact mechanism remains unclear, there is a statistically significant improved outcome for poor-grade aneurysm patients with nimodipine treatment.

Safety and Efficacy of Intrathecal Thrombolytic Therapy in a Primate Model of Cerebral Vasospasm

Findlay JM, Weir BKA, Gordon P, Grace M, Baughman R (Univ of Alberta, Edmonton; Genentech Inc, South San Francisco)
Neurosurgery 24:491–498, April 1989   19–13

A recent controlled trial with a primate model of subarachnoid hemorrhage showed that human recombinant tissue plasminogen activator (rt-PA), administered intrathecally at a dose of 1.5 mg over 24 hours, can effectively lyse a unilateral subarachnoid hematoma and prevent vasospasm without initiating system fibrinolysis or causing brain damage. The following studies were a continuation of this work.

To test the safety of high doses of rt-PA, 6 cynomolgus monkeys received 10 mg of rt-PA through an Ommaya reservoir 24 and 36 hours after undergoing craniectomy and dissection of the basal cisterns. All 6 monkeys remained clinically normal throughout the observation period. Plasma thrombin times were unchanged by the administration of rt-PA. At autopsy, the brain and meninges of all 6 were normal, and there were no signs of systemic fibrinolysis.

In a second study, a randomized, placebo-controlled trial was used to assess the safety and efficacy of a single, unilateral, intraoperative rt-PA injection administered in a more diffuse, bilateral subarachnoid hemorrhage. The 16 monkeys underwent frontotemporal craniectomy and induction of a subarachnoid hemorrhage on both the left and right sides of the brain. Before closure on the right side, 0.5 mg of rt-PA suspension plus 1.25 mg of slow-release rt-PA gel was injected into the subarachnoid space in 8 monkeys. An equal volume of placebo was injected in the other 8 monkeys.

Significant vasospasm developed in all 8 control animals in all the major right- and left-sided anterior cerebral vessels, whereas vasospasm did not occur in any of the rt-PA–treated monkeys. At autopsy, all placebo-treated animals had gross subarachnoid clots, but only 1 of the 8 treated animals had a small fragment of a subarachnoid clot (Fig 19–8).

It appears that unilateral administration of rt-PA in the form of a sus-

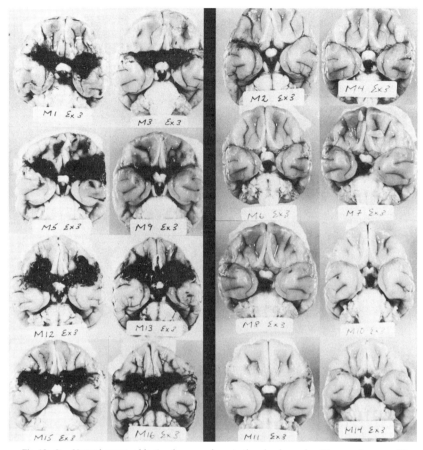

Fig 19–8.—Ventral aspect of brains from monkeys in the placebo and rt-PA-treated groups. Note the remaining subarachnoid blood present bilaterally in the brains from the placebo group. (Courtesy of Findlay JM, Weir BKA, Gordon P, et al: *Neurosurgery* 24:491–498, April 1989.)

pension plus a slow-release gel can effectively lyse a diffuse bilateral subarachnoid clot and prevent vasospasm on both sides of the anterior cerebral circulation in primates.

▶ In a primate model of cerebral vasospasm, the authors have documented the efficacy of t-PA in resorbing clot from the subarachnoid space and decreasing vasospasm on angiography. This report brings us closer to the point of clinical trials.

Brief Notes on Aneurysms

DIAGNOSTIC STUDIES

Computed tomographic and CSF findings in 100 patients with ruptured aneurysms were reviewed (MacDonald A, Mendelow AD: *J Neurol Neurosurg Psychiatry* 51:342–344, 1988). There was no blood visible on CT scans of 20 patients. Of these, 7 had blood in the CSF but no xanthochromia. It is concluded that bloodstained CSF is important in the diagnosis of subarachnoid hemorrhage. A normal CT scan in the absence of xanthochromia does not exclude a ruptured aneurysm.

Intra-arterial digital subtraction angiography (DSA) detects aneurysms down to 1.0 mm and is considered as reliable and safe as standard angiography (Tonko H et al: *AJNR* 9:1157–1161, 1988).

In 25 patients with SAH and a normal initial angiogram, aneurysms were noted in 5 of 20 when angiography was repeated. Subsequent review of the initial angiogram disclosed the aneurysm in 4 of 5 cases. Review by a second neuroradiologist may avoid the second angiogram (Shuaib A et al: *Can J Neurol Sci* 15:413–416, 1988).

Cross-compression during DSA gave adequate visualization of the circle of Willis in 93%, of which 3.7% had no or inadequate collateral to the carotid artery (Fermand M et al: *Presse Med* 17:910–913, 1988).

A study of complications in cerebral angiograms performed with Isopaque and Omnipaque disclosed no important difference between the 2 contrast media (Skalpe IO: *Neuroradiology* 30:69–72, 1988).

Spinal cord arteriograms of 96 patients were associated with 8.2% local complications, 3.7 systemic-nonneurologic, and 2.2% neurologic complications with full recovery within 1 week. There were no lasting complications (Forbes G et al: *Radiology* 169:479–484, 1988).

Selective transbrachial carotid and vertebral DSA can be performed safely in an outpatient setting (Barnett FJ et al: *Radiology* 170:535–539, 1989.)

Early Surgery

Among 56 patients operated on within 7 days after SAH and treated with prophylactic hypervolemic hypertension, 41 returned to their prior occupations, 4 were independent without deficit, 4 were independent with deficit, 3 were dependent on care, and 4 died (Solomon RA et al: *Neurosurgery* 23:699–704, 1988.)

Among 47 consecutive patients with ruptured intracranial aneurysms, prophylactic volume expansion therapy and early aneurysm surgery led to excellent results in 41 without delayed ischemic damage (Solomon RA et al: *Arch Neurol* 45:325–332, 1988).

Good results are reported after early operation for saccular aneurysm with nimodipine treatment in a small neurosurgical unit (Hillman J et al: *Acta Neurochir [Wien]* 94:28–31, 1988).

Extensive cerebrospinal fluid drainage may lead to hydrocephalus after early operation for ruptured aneurysms (Ogura K et al: *Surg Neurol* 30:441–444, 1988).

Experience with 53 patients suggests an advantage for clipping the aneurysm and evacuating a significant hematoma at the same surgical procedure (Seifert V et al: *Theor Surg* 3:83–88, 1988).

Additional Surgical and Therapeutic Approaches

Induced hypertension in patients with symptomatic vasospasm is recommended for anesthesia for cerebral aneurysm surgery (Buckland MR et al: *Anesthesiology* 69:116–119, 1988).

Superficial temporal aneurysms are generally traumatic and best treated by ligation or excision under local anesthetic (Peick AL et al: *J Vasc Surg* 8:606–610, 1988).

A review of the literature indicates that patients with brain stem hematomas fare quite well after surgical therapy (Mangiardi JR, Epstein FJ: *J Neurol Neurosurg Psychiatry* 51:966–976, 1988).

Autoregulation remains intact at 32C and 27C after surface-induced hypothermia (London MJ et al: *J Surg Res* 45:491–495, 1988).

Super giant cerebral aneurysms (larger than 6 cm) may be treated by clipping and resection or bypass and parent artery occlusion with good results (Sakaguchi M et al: *Surg Neurol* 31:300–309, 1989).

In *Giant Intracranial Aneurysms, Therapeutic Approaches* (Springer-Verlag, Berlin, 1988), Yves Keravel and Marc Sindou provide an overview of current French management of giant aneurysms. The book is based on a monograph published by the French-speaking Neurosurgical Society in *Neurochirurgie* in 1984, with 309 cases contributed by French neurosurgeons. Drs. Keravel and Sindou have added 85 personal cases and updated the literature through 1985. The detailed reporting of results and excellent bibliography are the greatest strengths of the book; the delay in its appearance is the principal drawback.

The biology of giant aneurysms is summarized clearly with coverage of pathology, hemodynamics, and experimental models. The section on neuroradiology includes useful material on angiography and especially on computed tomography, but only early magnetic resonance images were available for publication.

Direct neck clipping is well presented. Available clips are discussed, along with their metallurgical and mechanical properties. Methods of clip application are presented clearly, including creative applications of multiple clips (including fenestrated and angled versions), always with the goal of neck occlusion and maintenance of patent normal arteries. A fine exposition is given by Dolenc's important method for exposure of the proximal internal carotid artery and mobilization of the optic nerve for clipping of carotid ophthalmic aneurysms. Dolenc's method of attack on intracavernous aneurysms is also well presented. In summarizing literature on clipping of giant carotid aneurysms, the authors note good results in carotid-ophthalmic (65%) and carotid-posterior communicating lesions (70%), but high mortality (77%) in bifurcation lesions. For middle cerebral aneurysms, 58% good results with 22% mortality were achieved; results for anterior communicating and selected vertebrobasilar lesions were similar.

Wrapping, transmural wiring à la Mullan, and extracorporeal circulation are reviewed without much new being added.

Hunterian ligature of parent arteries is reviewed in some detail. On the basis of published literature and personal experience, it was concluded that internal carotid occlusion is more effective than common carotid occlusion for internal carotid artery giant aneurysms. Gradual occlusion is believed to be safer than abrupt occlusion. Drake's data on intentional vertebrobasilar occlusion is reviewed, and the section concludes with description of an ingenious implantable vascular occluder with a Doppler probe to assure cessation of flow. The authors briefly summarize data regarding revascularization for giant aneurysms; its value in prevention of ischemia is difficult to evaluate objectively. Tests for tolerance of therapeutic occlusion are reviewed, but data and conclusions are limited. A more extensive treatment of known cerebral blood flow thresholds for ischemia is available elsewhere (e.g., Wood's volume on cerebral blood flow).

Balloon catheters are discussed, with presentation of 21 of DeBrun's cases. It is concluded that Hunterian ligature is preferable to intra-aneurysmal thrombosis. This was written before the recent spectacular successes of Schcheglov and Hieshima with intra-aneurysmal balloon occlusions.

The book concludes with a well-organized and exhaustive bibliography (through 1985).

Giant Intracranial Aneurysms belongs on the shelf of every neurosurgeon (or interventionist) with a serious interest in treating these lesions. The volume thus takes its place alongside the important monographs on aneurysms by Suzuki, Yasargil, and Weir.

NIMODIPINE

Thromboxane B_2 levels in serum during nimodipine treatment for aneurysmal subarachnoid hemorrhage do not support the idea that nimodipine exerts an effect on platelet function (Vinge E et al: *Stroke* 19:644–647, 1988). The recently concluded British Aneurysm Nimodipine Trial showed a beneficial effect upon morbidity and mortality after SAH.

In a study of 116 consecutive patients, early aneurysm surgery and intravenous nimodipine effectively prevented symptomatic vasospasm (Gilsbach JN, Harders AG: *Acta Neurochir [Wien]* 96:1–7, 1989).

A controlled trial of nimodipine in 213 patients demonstrated fewer total deaths and fewer deaths due to ischemia (Ohman J, Heiskanen O: *J Neurosurg* 69:683–686, 1988).

The recent support for the use of nimodipine for the prevention of delayed ischemic deficit after subarachnoid hemorrhage (*KEY Neurol Neurosurg* 3[4]:39, 1988) adds to the need to know what causes ischemia when blood is spilled. Watanabe and his coworkers in Tokyo (*Neurol Med Chir [Tokyo]* 28:645–649, 1988) studied changes in lipid peroxidases (measured as thiobarbituric acid reactive substances, TRS) and their scavenging enzyme, glutathione peroxidase, in the blood and cerebrospinal fluid of patients with subarachnoid hemorrhage compared with normal subjects. Cerebrospinal fluid (CSF) is almost devoid of TRS and glutathione peroxidase. Glutathione peroxidase appears in the CSF after subarachnoid hemorrhage, presumably from that which is in the blood. It diminishes in 2 to 4 days, whereas TRS increases, presumably as a result of blood clotting within the subarachnoid space. Thereafter the glutathione peroxidase again increases. The lipid peroxides present in CSF and serum of patients with subarachnoid hemorrhage may be responsible for development of delayed vasospasm, and serum glutathione peroxidase might play an important role in controlling it.—Oscar Sugar, M.D. [Professor Emeritus and Former Head of the Department of Neurosurgery, University of Illinois College of Medicine at Chicago and Clinical Professor of Neurosurgery, University of California at San Diego; Editor of the Neurosurgery section of the YEAR BOOK OF NEUROLOGY AND NEUROSURGERY from 1953 to 1985.]

INTRA-ANEURYSMAL BALLOON OCCLUSION

Intra-aneurysmal balloon occlusion of a giant carotid ophthalmic aneurysm led to visual improvement (Higashida RT et al: *Surg Neurol* 30:382–386, 1988).

Hema polymerizes in 40–60 minutes at body temperature to provide long-lasting inflation of detachable intracranial vascular balloons (Goto K et al: *Radiology* 169:787–790, 1988).

Neuroleptanesthesia is a preferred technique for anesthesia during closed embolization of cerebral arteriovenous malformations to permit immediate neurologic assessment (Omahony BJ, Bolsin SNC: *Anesth Intens Care* 16:318–323, 1988).

In December of 1988, Dr. Victor Schcheglov addressed the Radiological Society of North America on the subject of "endoaneurysmal balloon obliteration." He reported on 617 cases. In this group treated by Professor Schcheglov at the Kiev Neurological Institute over the past 12 years, there was obliteration of the aneurysm alone in 91% and obliteration of the aneurysm and the parent vessel in 9%. Among the cases treated were 301 internal carotid aneurysms, 207 anterior communicating aneurysms, 64 middle cerebral aneurysms, 17 vertebrobasilar lesions, and 28 multiple lesions.

Schcheglov selected a group of 409 cases that, according to his estimate, could have been done microsurgically with similar results. Of these cases, 376 were treated with aneurysmal occlusion alone and 33 had occlusion of the parent artery as well. There were 22 deaths, or 5% of the total. With regard to the preoperative status, 338 were in good condition, and mortality was 1.8%. Among the 71 poor grade patients, mortality was 22%. It should be noted that, among this total population of cases, only 17 were treated within the first 5 days after subarachnoid hemorrhage; all others were treated 5 days to 5 months after hemorrhage.

The description of the technique indicates that a standard detachable balloon has been used in many cases. In addition, a double balloon is described with 2 small chambers, 1 distal to the other. In some cases a thrombin glue tip is utilized for fixing the balloon in a specific zone of the aneurysm. In some cases, a balloon within a balloon has been used to help with the problem of dead space.

A special group of patients with giant aneurysms was described. Of 69 cases, 54 were treated with aneurysmal occlusion alone, with an additional 5 undergoing parent-vessel occlusion. Up to 4 balloons were used for the occlusion effort. In 17 vertebrobasilar giant aneurysms, 15 cases could be occluded with preservation of the parent vessel and 2 had occlusion of the parent vessel as well. Among this particular group, there was 1 death and 2 complications (both strokes).

Overall, the results are impressive and encouraging. It is remarkable that balloon catheter occlusion of lesions in these various locations can be achieved by a highly experienced surgeon. On the other hand, it should be noted that these patients were by and large operated on during a chronic phase when standard microsurgical dissection can eliminate these lesions with excellent results. In fact, one may question whether the results of microsurgery might be superior in a number of these instances. Nonetheless an advancing role for balloon occlusion of aneurysms seems likely. Certainly further experience will be needed before the role of this form of therapy can be established. Selected lesions, those especially difficult for the surgeon, will probably be especially amenable to the balloon treatment. It remains to be seen what the balloon technique can do for aneurysms in the acute phase when we know that the results of surgery are unfortunately marred by complications (see Abstract 19–7). It appears important that neurosurgeons and interventionists work together in this promising new field to obtain maximal benefit for our patients.

OTHER REPORTS ON HEMORRHAGE

Autopsy of a patient with Marfan's syndrome showed 2 early aneurysms with mural thinning and fragmentation of elastica, changes typical of aneurysms in non-Marfan's patients (Stebbens WE et al: *Surg Neurol* 31:200–202, 1989).

Among 19 cases of pericallosal aneurysm, none were fusiform lesions, 7 were multiple, and 16 were operated on with 15 good or excellent results and no mortality (Sindou M et al: *Surg Neurol* 30:434–440, 1988.)

Arteriovenous Malformations

MR Imaging in the Management of Supratentorial Intracranial AVMs
Smith HJ, Strother CM, Kikuchi Y, Duff T, Ramirez L, Merless A, Toutant S
(Univ Hosp and Clinics; Saint Marys Hosp; Dean Med Ctr, Madison, Wis)
AJNR 9:225–235, March–April 1988   19–14

Magnetic resonance (MR) imaging and computed tomography (CT) have nearly equal sensitivity for detecting angiographically evident intracranial arteriovenous malformations (AVMs). However, planning an operation that will eliminate the risk of intracranial hemorrhage requires much detailed information. A retrospective study attempted to determine which imagine technique would be most useful in defining the size, characteristics, and location of the AVM nidus, its arterial supply and venous drainage, and the precise anatomical location of all these structures. The imaging studies were also evaluated for their ability to depict changes occurring after embolization. The MR images, CT scans, and angiograms were independently reviewed.

Of 9 males and 6 females aged 16–68 years, with angiographically confirmed intracranial supratentorial AVMs, 5 had chronic headaches and 7 had seizures. Three patients had recently had an intracranial hemorrhage. Two others had a history of intracranial hemorrhage in the distant past. One patient had a symptomatic spinal AVM but no symptoms related to his intracranial AVM.

Magnetic resonance imaging was superior to both CT and angiography in showing the exact anatomical relationships of the nidus, the feeding arteries, and the draining veins. Although angiography showed a larger number of feeding arteries and draining veins than either MR or CT, the precise relationships of these vessels to other structures were better visualized with MR imaging and CT. Because of its multiplanar capabilities,

MR imaging was still superior to CT in this regard. Magnetic resonance was also superior in demonstrating the extent of AVM nidus obliteration after embolization and was more sensitive than CT in visualizing associated parenchymal abnormalities and subacute hemorrhage. Magnetic resonance is generally more sensitive than CT in detecting subacute and old hemorrhage. In this study, however, MR imaging had a low sensitivity for detecting remote hemorrhages within an AVM nidus, probably because of the flow-related artifacts and low sensitivity for distinguishing calcifications from rapid flow or hemosiderin or both.

Magnetic resonance is superior to both CT and angiography in the diagnosis of AVM, but angiography provides the detailed vascular and hemodynamic information needed for planning optimal surgical or endovascular intervention.

▶ This important communication documents the value of MRI in the management of supratentorial AVMs. The authors demonstrate that MR is extremely valuable in demonstrating the exact relationships of nidus, feeding arteries, and draining veins. These studies can also demonstrate the relationship of the nidus to critical parenchymal structures. In many aspects in the analysis of the AVM, the MRI is actually superior to the cerebral angiogram. As Fabrikant has discussed, MRI may disclose obliteration of the arteriovenous malformation, as zones of signal void begin to show higher signal. For the detection of residual arteriovenous malformation, however, angiography remains the gold standard at this time.

A very important subject in the management of arteriovenous malformation is the question of preoperative evaluation of risk. Often it is this estimate that determines whether surgical, embolic, or radiosurgical therapy will be recommended. Spetzler and Martin have developed a practical and useful grading system for this purpose. (1) However, in their proposal, MRI was not included. In a series of 40 patients, many with surgical correlation, we have found MRI of substantial additional value in the preoperative evaluation of risk and in development of surgical strategies. A modification of Spetzler and Martin's classification probably will be usefully enhanced by the addition of MRI criteria. These criteria will surely involve the proximity of nidus to crucial structures such as the internal capsule, "dense" or "loose" packing of the lesion, engorgement of peripherally located vascular channels, adjacent edema, presence of adjacent fresh hematoma as an aid to dissection, and the like.

Reference

1. Spetzler, Martin: *J Neurosurg* 65:476–483, 1986.

Cerebral Blood Flow Evaluation of Arteriovenous Malformations With Stable Xenon CT
Marks MP, O'Donahue J, Fabricant JI, Frankel KA, Phillips MH, DeLaPaz RI, Enzmann DR (Stanford Univ; Univ of California, Berkeley)
AJNR 9:1169–1175, November–December 1988   19–15

Arteriovenous malformations (AVMs) are functionally low-resistance shunts bypassing the normal capillary vascu ar bed in brain parenchyma. Although the serious hemorrhagic complica ions of AVMs are well known, the physiologic and clinical consequences of hemodynamic disturbances resulting from a high-flow shunt are not we understood. The most likely regions of decreased flow with AVMs were studied to quantify and more accurately localize them.

To determine cerebral blood flow, 20 patients with AVMs were assessed with angiography, conventional computed tomography (CT), and stable xenon CT. Contralateral and ipsilateral areas of interest were assessed from cerebral blood flow maps and correlated with angiography. A significant reduction in cerebral blood flow was seen in the ipsilateral cortical gray matter adjacent to the AVM relative to the corresponding contralateral cortex. Larger AVMs were associated with a more marked reduction with a mean difference of 12.22 ml/100 gm/minute. Other areas of interest were studied on the basis of angiographic findings that suggested areas of decreased flow. These areas were compared with analogous contralateral areas and also showed a significant decline in cerebral blood flow. This decline was greater with larger AVMs, with a mean difference of 11.38 ml/100 gm/minute.

The results of flow studies were analyzed by using rigidly defined anatomical regions of interest and coordinating them with angiographic results obtained at the same time in each of 20 patients. The regions most likely to have reduced flow from an AVM were pinpointed.

▶ This report shows a nice resolution of cerebral blood flow by the stable xenon CT technique sufficient to characterize areas near AVMs. Application of this approach may be helpful in the management of patients with AVMs undergoing treatment, including embolization and surgery. It may be that preoperative clues regarding risk of perfusion breakthrough may be discovered in analysis of such CBF data.

Neurosurgical Treatment of Cerebral Arteriovenous Malformations
Höllerhage H-G (Med Univ, Hannover, West Germany)
Neurochirurgia 31:139–143, 1988   19–16

Cerebral arteriovenous malformations (AVMs) are considered benign lesions that can be treated conservatively. However, patients who have these lesions are at risk for spontaneous hemorrhage and subsequent neurologic complications. Previous studies have shown that, without surgical intervention, only one third of all patients will be completely asymptomatic 20 years after the initial diagnosis and that 10% of the patients will have died. Experience with surgical and conservative treatment of intracranial AVMs is reported.

During the 4-year study period, 61 patients were treated for AVMs, including 28 with acute hemorrhage and 33 with seizures, neurologic deficits, or intractable headaches. Fifty-five of the 61 patients underwent op-

Surgical Results

Neurologic Status at Follow–Up	I	II	III	IV	V	( )
With hemorrhage	10	10	4	–	–	24
Without hemorrhage	19	10	–	–	–	29
Total	29	20	4	–	–	53

(Courtesy of Höllerhage H-G: *Neurochirurgia* 31:139–143, 1988.)

eration, 4 patients refused operation, and 2 had AVMs not amenable to surgical treatment. Of 55 patients followed up for 6–67 months, 53 had been operated on. No patient died.

At follow-up examination, 29 of the 53 patients operated on had excellent results, 20 had good results, and 4 had moderate disability. All 4 patients with moderate postoperative neurologic deficits had had hemorrhage before surgery (table). Nine of the 18 patients who before operation had sporadic epileptic seizures were completely free of epileptic seizures after surgery, even without antiepileptic drug therapy. Two of 9 patients with overt preoperative epilepsy also became free of seizures without the use of antiepileptic drug therapy after operation. Of the 6 patients not operated on, only 2 were completely asymptomatic, 1 was slightly disabled, and 3 were severely disabled at follow-up.

Patients with intracranial AVMs should be advised to undergo operation, whether or not they have had an intracranial hemorrhage, unless the AVM is located in the speech region or in the brain stem.

▶ These good results from Germany (29 good or excellent results in 53 cases) bolster the case for surgical excision of intracranial arteriovenous malformations. It is interesting that 9 of 18 patients with preoperative seizures were seizure free postoperatively, which corresponds to Heros's recent experience. As noted by the author, careful preoperative evaluation risk is important in case selection. The classification method of Spetzler and Martin, modified by the addition of MRI criteria, is helpful in this respect. Such experiences give strong support to the concept of excision of most arteriovenous malformations, which can be removed with low risk. There remain very large and deep lesions, and those in eloquent zones, where other modalities such as embolotherapy or radiosurgery may be a lower risk treatment. Careful follow-up studies, together with the use of standardized reporting methodology, will likely help sharpen the indications for the various treatment methodologies.

Cerebral Micro Arteriovenous Malformations (mAVMs): Review of 13 Cases

Willinsky R, Lasjaunias P, Comoy J, Pruvost P (Hôpital Bicêtre, Bicêtre, France)
Acta Neurochir (Wien) 91:37–41, 1988   19–17

A series of 152 cerebral vascular malformations included 13 that were less than 1 cm in size, with a small nidus or fistula and a single feeding artery and draining vein of normal size. All 13 patients had intracerebral hematoma when first seen. The average age was 31 years. Eleven of the small arteriovenous malformations (AVMs) were demonstrated angiographically. The malformations, all peripheral, were surgically removable without perioperative morbidity. Ten lesions were cortical and supratentorial, 2 were infratentorial, and 1 was at the brain surface on the optic tract. None of the lesions were demonstrated with CT or MRI.

These lesions are occult with respect to studies such as CT and MRI because the feeding artery and draining vein are of normal size. Micro AVMs are suspected of causing many intracerebral hematomas in young, previously healthy persons. The congenital or "acquired" nature of an arteriovenous shunt cannot be delineated by angiography. With a small AVM, the small bridging arteries that anchor the cortical veins are a mechanical obstacle, disposing to increased upstream pressure and rupture. It is not clear whether small AVMs become large ones. Nevertheless any micro AVM should be treated.

▶ AVMs are likely to be invisible to CT or MR demonstration. They are clearly delineated by angiographic study and thus are easily distinguished from cavernous angioma, a histologically distinct variety of intracranial vascular abnormality. Surgical excision is recommended in the majority of these lesions because of the safety and efficacy of the treatment.

Microsurgical Removal of Arteriovenous Malformations of the Basal Ganglia
Malik GM, Umansky F, Patel S, Ausman JI (Henry Ford Hosp, Detroit)
Neurosurgery 23:209–217, August 1988   19–18

To evaluate the surgical treatment of intracranial arteriovenous malformations (AVMs) involving the basal ganglia and internal capsule, data on 6 of 140 patients who had surgery for AVMs in an 11-year period were reviewed. Of these 2 males and 4 females aged 14–53, 5 had intracranial bleeding and 1 had recurrent subarachnoid hemorrhage. The AVMs in all 6 patients were fed primarily by the perforating branches of the middle cerebral artery and secondarily by perforating vessels arising from the anterior cerebral artery. In all 6 patients the efferent vessels led to the deep venous system. The arterial supply and venous drainage of the AVMs were identified with cerebral angiographic studies. Only 1 patient had a 2-stage operation.

All 6 patients survived surgery. Four were able to return to their previous activities. Two patients with hemiparesis and dysphasia before operation had persistent symptoms after operation, with worsening in 1. However, both were much improved at follow-up and are now living independently. Complete excision of deep-seated AVMs in the basal ganglia remains the treatment of choice.

▶ The authors present excellent results in 6 cases of microsurgical removal of arteriovenous malformations of the basal ganglia. It is worth noting that 5 of the 6 had hemorrhages and 1, a progressive neurologic deficit. Careful preoperative planning using angiographic, CT, and MRI data is critical. In each instance, approach through normal tissue is required, the precise cortisectomy being determined by the location of the lesion and the associated hematoma. Few would argue against operation in patients with hemorrhage; however, the role of prophylactic surgery in asymptomatic patients remains undefined. The alternative of focal stereotactic radiation may be considered in patients without bleeding, especially in lesions smaller than 3 cm, which reportedly have high rates of obliteration (as high as 90% obliteration in 2 years, according to Steiner).

Normal Perfusion Pressure Breakthrough Complicating Surgery for the Vein of Galen Malformation: Report of Three Cases
Morgan MK, Johnston IH, Sundt TM Jr (Mayo Clinic, Rochester, Minn; Royal Alexandra Hosp for Children, Sydney, Australia)
Neurosurgery 24:406–410, March 1989   19–19

Mortality among untreated neonates with a vein of Galen malformation is as high as 95%, but surgical treatment of this lesion is still associated with an 80% mortality among neonates and a 44.5% mortality among all children aged less than 1 year. The degree of systemic circulatory disturbance, intraoperative blood loss, and myocardial ischemia have previously been identified as contributing factors in the unfavorable outcomes. However, the normal perfusion pressure breakthrough syndrome may also have a significant role in the development of catastrophic postoperative complications. The case reports of 3 infants with malignant brain swelling after surgery for vein of Galen malformations are presented.

The infants, whose ages ranged from 10 days to 12 weeks, had large arteriovenous (AV) shunts sufficient to create at least some degree of cardiac failure and possibly some loss of cerebral parenchyma. In all 3 patients, the AV shunts were completely obliterated and the outflow channel was occluded. Generalized brain swelling rapidly developed in each infant after operation, and 1 patient also had a cerebral hemorrhage remote from the initial malformation, occurring within a short time of the final obliteration of the AV fistula.

All 3 patients had a rapid and malignant clinical course and died soon after. Because other causes for their sudden decline could be excluded, the sudden brain swelling was believed to be caused by cerebral hyperperfusion resulting from the surgical closure of the high-flow fistulas. The large increase in perfusion pressure appeared to have overwhelmed the autoregulatory mechanisms in these patients.

Breakthrough edema and hemorrhage have previously been associated with the treatment of cerebral AV malformations but not with the treatment of vein of Galen malformations.

▶ This paper emphasizes the difficulties involved in surgery for neonates with vein of Galen malformation. The mortality from the untreated condition is extremely high, but even in the microsurgical era, the risk of total obliteration of the malformation is still quite high. In these cases obliteration of the vein of Galen itself may well have been a factor in the catastrophic outcomes. It may be that partial obliteration of the shunt, adequate to permit cardiac recovery, should be the initial goal of therapy. Encouraging results have been reported with both transarterial obliteration (Berenstein) or transtorcular occlusion (1). The best treatment for these menacing lesions has yet to be established.

Reference

1. Mickle JP, Quisling RG: *J Neurosurg* 65:731–735, 1986.

Brief Notes on AVMs

DIAGNOSTIC TECHNIQUES

Vascular intracranial lesions are rapidly demonstrated by GRASS imaging as high intensity, sometimes in relation to neoplasm, also assisting in the detection of vascular thrombosis, occult vascular malformations, and hemorrhagic complications of vascular lesions (Atlas SW et al: *Radiology* 169:455–461, 1988).

Cerebral venous angiomas show up on MRI as flow void with a stellate configuration but without mass effect, scar, or hemorrhage (Toro VE et al: *J Comput Assist Tomogr* 12:935–940, 1988).

Coronal spin-echo MR imaging can demonstrate dural arteriovenous malformations of the orbit (Hirabuki N et al: *Neuroradiology* 30:390–394, 1988).

Radio-xenon tomography has been validated by experimental studies that suggest this may be a convenient method of assessing perfusion in vascular territories in the brain (Rezai K et al: *J Nucl Med* 29:348–355, 1988).

Stable xenon CT permits clinical and pathologic correlation of ischemia in baboons (Yonas H et al: *Stroke* 19:228–238, 1988).

Eight patients tolerated temporary balloon occlusion of intracranial aneurysm (ICA) with little change in xenon CT cerebral blood flow; all tolerated resection of a portion of ICA and skull base tumor without deficit (Sekhar L et al: *Laryngoscope* 98:960–966, 1988).

Xenon single photon emission computed tomography (SPECT) is a sensitive noninvasive method of diagnosis of cerebrovascular disease and may help identify patients with hemodynamic ischemia with possible benefit from EC-IC bypass surgery (Leinsinger G et al: *Nucl Med* 27:127–134, 1988).

Reversible cerebral ischemia can be present before infarction as shown by positron emission tomography (PET), but this technique is not as widely available as single-photon tomograms. A. H. Maurer of Temple University points out that even the "gold standard" for confirming or excluding cerebrovascular disease, i.e., selective carotid angiography, fails to assess functional hemodynamic significance of a lesion or reserve capacity of cerebral perfusion. Early xenon studies have shown the presence of perfusion abnormalities in early stroke and in patients with transient ischemic attacks (TIAs). Newer agents useful in SPECT include amines labelled with ^{123}I, especially [123]I-*N*-isopropyl-*P*-iodoamphetamine (IMP). With this, SPECT can show large perfusion defects well before CT evidence of infarction. Recently, IMP has shown ischemia in TIAs; in early images there is decreased IMP uptake, which redistributes ("fills in") 2 to 3 hours after injection. Correction of such perfusion abnormalities before and after revascularization procedures have been shown with SPECT. A new compound using ^{99m}Tc hexamethylpropylenamine oxine has also shown retention in the brain proportionate to regional cerebral blood flow. Both compounds show essentially the same brain retention for 60 minutes, with luxury perfusion being manifested with the Tc compound but not with IMP; the latter shows a redistribution pattern not seen with Tc.

It seems possible to use these techniques, with various imaging agents, not only for more accurate diagnosis of extent of cerebrovascular disease, but for directing therapy to those patients most likely to benefit.

This material is included in vol 1, no. 2 of *Advances in Functioning NeuroImaging,* a quarterly published by Macmillan Healthcare Information (Florham Park, NJ 07932), sponsored ultimately by Hoffmann-LaRoche, Inc.—Oscar Sugar, M.D. [Professor Emeritus and Former Head of the Department of Neurosurgery, University of Illinois College of Medicine at Chicago and Clinical Professor of Neurosurgery, University of California at San Diego; Editor of the Neurosurgery section of the YEAR BOOK OF NEUROLOGY AND NEUROSURGERY from 1953 to 1985.]

A new publication, *Advances in Functional NeuroImaging,* has been sent to doctors by a subsidiary of Hoffmann-LaRoche, Inc. It is designed to bring into the open new diagnostic approaches in medicine. Although the first number is devoted to imaging in psychiatry, the type of case involved is such that neurology and neurosurgery must also be considered because symptoms such as progressive dementia are of interest to all 3 disciplines.

N-isopropyl iodoamphetamine (IMP) has been used by van Heertum and O'Connell (pp. 4–11) for SPECT in psychiatric illness. A number of schizophrenic patients have shown evidence of diminished IMP uptake in the frontal lobes that is more pronounced than any changes of frontal lobe atrophy in CT scans. In addition, some increased uptake of IMP has been noted in the head of the caudate nucleus. Unipolar depressed patients tend to show decreased IMP uptake in the cerebral cortex; an increase in uptake of IMP in the temporal lobe is seen in some manic and schizophrenic patients. The scanning is done with relative ease and without emotional trauma. Repeated scanning to assay effect of therapeutic measures is easily done.

Tikofsky of the University of Wisconsin has used SPECT studies in assaying differential hemispheric responses of normal persons and chronic aphasics; the two groups respond differently to stimulation. The pattern of chronically phasic patients who continue to recover language is different from that of chronically aphasic patients who do not improve or who regress. The Boston Naming Test was used as a stimulating procedure; this requires subjects to name a series of

60 pictures of a number of different subjects. Stimulation with IMP-SPECT assays may be useful in detection of learning disorders.—Oscar Sugar, M.D.

Using HIPDM-SPECT in patients with medically intractable complex partial seizures may be helpful in identifying epileptic foci for surgery (Lee BI et al: *Arch Neurol* 45:397–402, 1988).

Technetium 99m HMPAO may be helpful in the study of regional cerebral blood flow in stroke patients (Smith FW et al: *Br J Radiol* 61:358–361, 1988).

TREATMENT

Twenty-five patients with cerebral AVM were managed conservatively for a mean of 10.6 years after diagnosis. Nineteen had unaffected occupational status, 3 had moderate to severe deficits, and 5 had moderate to severe intellectual deficits. No hemorrhages occurred in follow-up. Conservative treatment may be as effective as surgery (Andersen EB et al: *J Neurol Neurosurg Psychiatry* 51:1208–1212, 1988).

Mapping and corticography have been used for the excision of arteriovenous malformations in sensorimotor and language-related neocortex (Burchiel KJ et al: *Neurosurgery* 24:322–327, 1989).

In his beautiful volume *Microneurosurgery, Volume 3B: Arteriovenous Malformations,* Professor M. G. Yasargil shows what can be done surgically with arteriovenous malformations. In a series of more than 400 operated cases, he illustrates the technical details used to excise even the largest and deepest arteriovenous malformations with exceptionally good clinical results. Time and again one is stunned to find that he has removed a large deep lesion (for example, in the insula) in a few hours' time with no neurologic deficit nor even the need for blood transfusion. Only a very few master neurosurgeons will be able to approach these results; the most difficult lesion should be reserved for such surgeons, but all neurosurgeons may be helped by emulation of the Yasargilian example in more accessible lesions.

The volume is beautifully presented. The organization is typically Teutonic, with a breakdown of lesions logically by parenchymal zone and vascular territory. Anatomy is given in detail and is wonderfully illustrated, often in color. Pathoanatomy is particularly brilliantly portrayed in the section on vein of Galen abnormalities. Surgical methodology, including positioning, approach, and microsurgical technique, is extensively presented and illustrated. Still, the genius of this master can only be surmised by the reader from the results that are extensively documented in preoperative and postoperative angiograms and statistical tabulations. (One can get closer to this special, virtually unique capacity through the medium of 3-dimensional video presentation; details are in the book's introduction).

An interesting portion of the book is devoted to patients who did not have surgery. It is clearly documented that a substantial proportion of these cases went on to operate in certain cases of thalamic and brain stem AVMs. Some of these cases have been referred to radiosurgery. A generally poor opinion of this approach is offered, though all 5 of the cases undergoing gamma radiosurgery in Stockholm enjoyed total obliteration. It is also of note that Professor Yasargil does not use lasers for AVM surgery, nor has embolization been used as a helpful adjunct.

This is a monumental contribution and should be in the library of every neurosurgeon as well as of others interested in the management of AVM. Future experience will indicate how microneurosurgery, especially in the hands of other neurosurgeons, compares with alternative therapy, including embolotherapy and radiosurgery.

Nine of 21 patients with venous angioma had hemorrhage when first seen, and 2 of these had recurrent hemorrhage. All 9 were resected with limited morbidity and no mortality (Malik GM et al: *Surg Neurol* 30:350–358, 1988).

Deep Arteriovenous Malformations.—In the semi-annual all-English issue of *Neurologia Medico-Chirurgica (Tokyo)* for January 1988, deep arteriovenous malformations continue to be discussed at length. Surgical indications and approaches to malformations in the basal ganglia are discussed by Matsushima and colleagues of the Kyushu University (pp. 49–56) on the basis of 18 cases. (The series excluded malformations restricted to the thalamus.) Based on locations, feeders, and drainers, four groups were established:

lateral: nidus in putamen and insula, fed by lateral lenticulostriate arteries or branches of the middle cerebral cortical arteries or both

medial: nidus mainly in caudate head, one portion facing anterior horn of lateral ventricle, and feeders mainly from medial lenticulostriate arteries; drainage mainly internal cerebral vein via caudate vein

mixed: nidus relatively large and involving not only basal ganglia, but also thalamus or internal capsule or both; lenticulostriate, insular, cortical, choroidal, and perforating arteries give feeders, and drainage is via superficial cortical (including sylvian veins) and deep cerebral (including internal cerebral veins)

anteroinferior: fed from recurrent artery of Heubner or lenticulostriate artery, lying mainly in anterior perforated substance, anteroinferior to anterior limb of internal capsule and putamen; drainage to via basal vein and deep middle cerebral vein.

Small nidus refers to one less than 2.5 cm on angiogram, medium-sized is from 2.5 to 5 cm, and large is more than 5.0 cm. Seven patients underwent surgery to remove the malformation: 6 malformations were totally removed, and one had its feeding artery occluded. Total removal was attempted only for lateral (4) or medial (2) cases. In 11 cases, surgery either was not attempted or was directed at hydrocephalus or some other palliative procedure. These, and one large malformation on which operation was not attempted (era before use of operating microscope), were followed; in 8 with reports, 4 died of rebleeding at intervals of from 2 to 16 years. The authors consider medial and lateral malformations in the basal ganglia candidates for total removal; small malformations elsewhere in the depths may be candidates if the nidus is accessible via a hematoma cavity and do not involve major arteries.

From the Akita University School of Medicine, Kikuchi and co-workers (pp. 66–69) report successful removal of a midline arteriovenous malformation on the floor of the third ventricle. It was fed by right medial posterior choroidal, posterior thalamoperforating, and thalamogeniculate arteries, and drained into the vein of Galen. Through a 2.5-cm incision in the anterior corpus callosum the malformation was visualized by coming through the right foramen of Monro. The size is not given, but the CT scan with enhancement shows the lesion near the bottom of the ventricle, at about 1 cm in size. Postoperative hydrocephalus was successfully treated by ventriculoperitoneal shunt. There was no neurologic or psychologic sequela of the small incision in the corpus callosum in constrast to those made in other places and involving more crossing fibers.— Oscar Sugar, M.D.

Preoperative embolization was helpful in excision of 3 deep AVMs, but in a fourth case an inaccessible portion of the lesion in the basal ganglia bled fatally 3 days after surgery (Adelt D et al: *J Neurol* 235:355–358, 1988).

In a series of 50 patients with arteriovenous malformation, cerebrovascular vasospasm after subarachnoid hemorrhage was relatively common but caused no important symptoms (Von Holst H et al: *Acta Neurochir [Wien]* 94:129–132, 1988).

Brief Notes on Laboratory Vascular Studies

Ischemia Models

Reversible occlusion of the middle cerebral artery (MCA) without craniectomy may be performed in rats with 4-0 Nylon suture inserted through the internal carotid artery into the MCA (Longa EZ et al: *Stroke* 20:84–91, 1989).

A tethered ball may be introduced via the carotid artery to produce temporary MCA occlusion without craniectomy in rabbits (Molnar L et al: *Stroke* 19:1262–1266, 1988).

Transvascular placement of middle cerebral artery copper wire can lead to local thrombosis as a model of cerebral thrombosis in dogs (Hirschberg M, Hofferberth B: *Stroke* 19:741–746, 1988).

Proximal basilar artery occlusion in the primate circulation produced most flow changes most distal to the occlusion (Bentivoglio P et al: *Acta Neurochir [Wien]* 95:61–71, 1988).

Ischemia Therapies

In a controlled rabbit study, tPA was effective in dissolving MCA emboli and reestablishing flow (Chehrazi BB et al: *Neurosurgery* 24:355–360, 1989).

Tissue type plasminogen activator dissolved MCA emboli in 7 of 8 rabbits (Phillips DA et al: *AJNR* 9:899–902, 1988).

Nagao and co-workers (*J Trauma* 28:1650–1655, 1988) report in experimental animals beneficial effects of intravenous lidocaine on cortical ischemia and electrophysiology after experimental injury.

In an experimental study in dogs, there was no correlation between cerebral blood flow and neurologic recovery after total reversible cerebral ischemia (LaManna JC et al: *Exp Neurol* 101:234–247, 1988).

Endorphin mechanisms are responsible for beneficial effect of opioid antagonists on cerebral function during cerebral ischemia in rats (Skarpagdinsson J, Thoren P: *Acta Physiol Scand* 132:281–288, 1988).

Aminophylline reduces postischemic edema and brain damage in cats (Seida N et al: *Stroke* 19:1275–1282, 1988).

Revascularization

Larger inflow vessel diameter and higher graft flow improve patency in venous bypass grafts of 3–5 mm (Periera BM et al: *Neurosurgery* 31:195–199, 1989).

Kanaujia (*J Hand Surg* 13B:44–49, 1988) reports a microvascular anastomosis of femoral epigastric arteries in rats with 2 sutures and cuff yielding 98% patency.

ANEURYSMS

In experimental saccular aneurysms in dogs, intra-aneurysmal pressure measurements are similar to intracarotid measurements but are remarkably altered when the carotid is stenosed by 50% (Sekhar LN et al: *Stroke* 19:352–356, 1988).

A laser-sealed arterotomy produces aneurysms of the rat aortic bifurcation similar to those occurring in humans (Quigley MR et al: *Surg Neurol* 30:445–451, 1988).

SUBARACHNOID HEMORRHAGE

The 21-aminosteroid U74006F greatly reduced basilar artery narrowing induced by subarachnoid hemorrhage in rabbits (Vollmer DG et al: *Surg Neurol* 31:190–194, 1989).

Cerebral arteries after ischemia show impairment of dilatation with preserved vasoconstriction, which may contribute to impaired reperfusion (Mayhan WG et al: *Am J Physiol* 255:H879–H884, 1988).

In cat studies, subarachnoid blood placed upon the adventitial surface of intact cerebral arteries activates platelet aggregation within those vessels (Honma Y et al: *Neurosurgery* 24:487–490, 1989).

Selective endothelial injury of arteries abolishes dilatation caused by the ionophore A-23187 (Rosenblum WI, Nelson GH: *Stroke* 19:1379–1382, 1988).

Plasma catecholamines and their metabolites are increased after SAH, and their monitoring may be clinically useful (Minegishi A et al: *Arch Neurol* 44:423–428, 1987).

20 Spine

Introduction

A number of advances occurred in the area of *spinal degeneration* management. A follow-up report on 164 cases of anterior *cervical* diskectomy without fusion indicated no mortality and a single myelopathic worsening without other neurologic deficits (Abstract 20–1). In essence, the communication tends to confirm the attitude of Robertson that fusion is not required for these cases. Cervical laminoplasty to enlarge the spinal canal has been recommended for ossification of the posterior longitudinal ligament and cervical spondylosis with myelopathy (Abstract 20–2 and 20–3). The initial results are encouraging, but further data will be needed to establish this new form of treatment.

For *thoracic* herniated disk, a transthoracic approach was used from T-4 down to T-12 with good results (Abstract 20–4).

In the area of *lumbar* spine, Abdullah and colleagues (Abstract 20–5) report experience with extreme lateral disk herniation in 138 cases. The diagnosis is suspected with thigh pain, and lateral bending may reproduce the pain. Computed tomography is used to make the diagnosis, and often a portion of the facet may be removed for excellent results. A survey of complications in lumbar disk surgery indicates that overall frequency of complications might be as high as 13.75%, but important complications were quite uncommon (Abstract 20–6). Among 100 patients receiving percutaneous lumbar diskectomies, 87 were believed to have a successful outcome, but validation of the method will require control trials by neuroscientific clinicians (Abstract 20–7). For evaluation of the postoperative lumbar spine, gadolinium-enhanced MRI is helpful for the discrimination of postoperative epidural scar and retained disk (Abstracts 20–8 and 20–9).

Spinal *tumors* were highlighted in 1988. Magnetic resonance imaging (MRI) accurately clarifies the anatomy of intraspinal tumors, often providing histologic diagnosis (Abstract 20–10). Extramedullary hematopoiesis in thalassemia may cause spinal cord compression (Abstract 20–11). The diagnosis is made on hematologic grounds, and MRI can demonstrate the cause of spinal cord compression. Low-dose radiotherapy offers satisfactory decompression. For primary and metastatic vertebral tumors in the thoracic and lumbar spine, one-stage posterolateral decompression and stabilization are effective and relatively safe treatment (Abstract 20–12).

The management of *syringomyelia* received attention. Tator and Bercino (Abstract 20–13) report 29 good or excellent results in 40 cases with syringosubarachnoid shunting. On the other hand, Batzdorf (Abstract 20–14) reports goods results in 5 cases treated with suboccipital craniectomy and duroplasty. These cases all had Chiari malformations, and the precise indications for these 2 different approaches to syringomyelia have yet to be established.

Cervical

Clinical Long-Term Results of Anterior Discectomy Without Fusion for Treatment of Cervical Radiculopathy and Myelopathy: A Follow-Up of 164 Cases
Bertalanffy H, Eggert H-R (Univ of Freiburg im Breisgau, West Germany)
Acta Neurochir (Wien) 90:127–135, 1988   20–1

Cervical degenerative disk disease can cause nerve root compression, spinal cord compression, or both. Nerve root compression may lead to symptoms of radiculopathy, whereas spinal cord compression may cause symptoms of myelopathy. Anterior cervical decompression, with or without interbody fusion, is increasingly gaining acceptance. The preoperative and operative findings in 251 patients with degenerative cervical disk disease who underwent anterior cervical diskectomy without interbody fusion were reviewed. Long-term clinical follow-up data were available for 164 reexamined patients.

Of the 251 surgical patients, 146 (58%) had symptoms of lateral cervical disk syndrome and 105 (42%) had symptoms of medial cervical disk syndrome when first seen. Thirty-six (14%) patients had a history of prior cervical injury, 4 (1.6%) of whom had had a previous cervical disk operation. Associated lumbar discopathy was present in 106 (42%) patients, 13 (5%) of whom had already undergone lumbar disk surgery. Symptoms lasted from 5 days to 25 years.

Of 164 patients who were reexamined after a mean postoperative period of 3.3 years, 109 had been operated on because of radiculopathy and 55, because of myelopathy. Seventy-two of the 164 patients had soft disk lesions, and 92 had hard disk lesions. Patients with soft disk lesions and radiculopathy had significantly better long-term outcome than those with hard disk lesions and myelopathy. There was no significant association between clinical outcome and sex, preoperative occupation, preoperative trauma, or associated lumbar discopathy. Factors that did influence outcome were type of disk lesion, age at the time of operation, duration of symptoms, number of involved levels, and pattern of symptoms at onset. In all, 82% of the radiculopathy patients and 55% of the myelopathy patients had good to excellent long-term results. These findings are in agreement with other published data.

▶ Bertalanffy and Eggert report excellent results from anterior diskectomy without fusion. There was no mortality and a single myelopathic worsening without other neurologic long-lasting deficits. It is clear both from the self-estimation and from objective evaluation that patients with soft disk and radiculopathy fared better than those with hard disk or myelopathy. In the case of myelopathy, progression of the disease was arrested in 93% of the cases; 80% of patients improved, and 55% achieved a desirable end-result. These results overall compare favorably with results obtained with the anterior diskectomy without fusion or with laminectomy. In essence, the communication tends to confirm the attitude of Robertson (1) that fusion is not required in any of these cases.

Reference

1. Robertson: *Clin Neurosurg* 20:259–261, 1973.

Cervical Laminoplasty to Enlarge the Spinal Canal in Multilevel Ossification of the Posterior Longitudinal Ligament With Myelopathy
Tomita K, Nomura S, Umeda S, Baba H (Kanazawa Univ, Kanazawa, Japan)
Arch Orthop Trauma Surg 107:148–153, April 1988   20–2

Ossification of the posterior longitudinal ligament (OPLL) is a major cause of severe cervical myeloradiculopathy among the Japanese. The ideal treatment is resection of ossified tissue in the spinal cord anteriorly if the OPLL is limited to 3 vertebral bodies. However, in advanced myelopathy, with multiple levels of OPLL, it is difficult to resect ossified tissue without damaging the spinal cord. Results with posterior decompression are reported with laminoplasty used to enlarge the spinal canal and bone grafting to support the opened laminae. The resected spinous processes were used as bone grafts (Fig 20–1).

This expansive laminoplasty was performed in 20 men and 3 women aged 37–74 with severe myeloradiculopathy involving more than 3 levels of OPLL of the cervical spine. All patients were evaluated before and after surgery using a Japanese scoring system to grade the cervical myelopathy. Results were compared with those in 14 patients who had extensive laminectomy without bone grafting and in 17 who had undergone anterior decompression.

After an average of 31.5 months, neurologic recovery was observed in 81.2% of patients who had expansive laminoplasty, in 72.4% of those who underwent laminectomy, and in 63.6% of those who had anterior decompression. Postoperative computed tomography scans showed neither contact nor compression of the lamina or bone graft with the spinal cord in any of the patients. None experienced postoperative instability, malalignment, subluxation, or swan neck deformity, and none have had a recurrence of myeloradiculopathy.

▶ Cervical laminoplasty to enlarge the spinal canal is an interesting idea, but futher data will be required to confirm this concept and make it available for general use. Pathophysiology of cervical myelopathy caused by ossification of the posterior longitudinal ligament probably involves direct compression by the opacified structures together with the congenitally narrow spinal canal and superadded spondylosis (1).

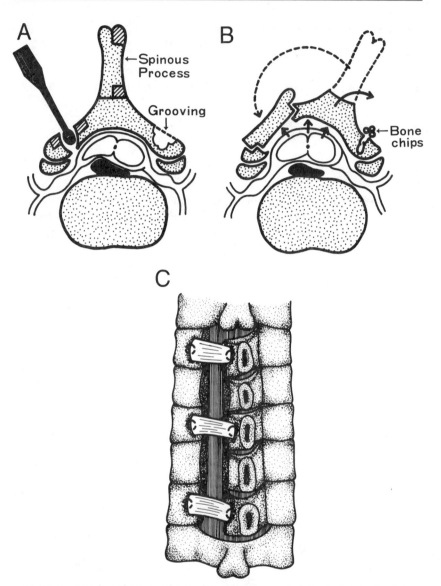

Fig 20–1.—Procedure of expansive laminoplasty. **A,** grooves are drilled on both sides of each lamina, 1 side just to the internal cortex and the other side through. The *hatched areas* show the trimming design of the bone graft. **B,** laminae are then reflected back in a way analogous to opening a door, and the trimmed spinous processes are inserted between the spaces. Bone chips fill the hinge groove. **C,** bone grafts to support the reflected laminae should be applied every 2 or 3 laminae. (Courtesy of Tomita K, Nomura S, Umeda S, et al: *Arch Orthop Trauma Surg* 107:148–153, April 1988.)

Reference

  1. Yu YL et al: *Brain* 111:769–783, 1988.

Comparison of the Results of Laminectomy and Open-Door Laminoplasty for Cervical Spondylotic Myeloradiculopathy and Ossification of the Posterior Longitudinal Ligament
Nakano N, Nakano T, Nakano K (Nakano Orthopaedic Hosp; Hokkaido Univ, Sapporo, Japan)
Spine 13:792–794, 1988   20–3

Laminectomy usually gives good results in treating cervical spondylotic myeloradiculopathy and ossification of the posterior longitudinal ligament, but complications can occur. Laminoplasty has been used as an alternative in Japan since 1978. The 2 procedures and their long-term results are compared.

In 14 patients treated with laminectomy, the outcomes showed an average improvement score of 81.1%. Laminoplasty offered an improvement percentage of 81.4. Operative time was similar for both procedures, although blood loss was greater during laminoplasty. Time before ambulation averaged 3 days after surgery for laminoplasty and 2 weeks for laminectomy. In 3 cases presented, numbness in fingers had progressed to inability to walk. Both surgical procedures offered patients good long-term results.

In the Nakano laminoplasty, a hole is made in each spinous process.

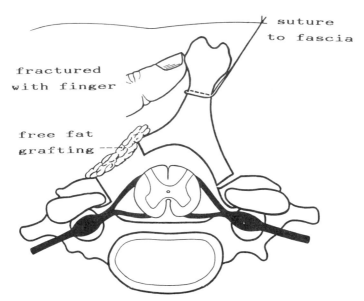

Fig. 20–2.—Surgical technique of Nakano laminoplasty. (Courtesy of Nakano N, Nakano T, Nakano K: *Spine* 13:792–794, 1988.)

Using an air drill, the surgeon performs a 6-mm resection of the left lamina. A hinge is made near the facet joint, and a fracture is induced. The spinous processes are sutured to the right side of the fascia, then free fatty tissue is grafted over the open-door laminoplasty created when the lamina is raised (Fig 20–2). Bone grafting is not required to obtain stability. Even a small enlargement of the spinal canal brings about improvement, probably a result of improved circulation in the spinal cord and nerve roots.

▶ Open door laminoplasty is an interesting technique for cervical decompressions that could be effective without threatening destabilization. Further results will be needed to clarify the usefulness and safety of the method.

Brief Notes on the Cervical Spine

IMAGING TECHNIQUES

For cervical spine MR imaging, the best sequence appears to be one with a very short repetition time, short echo-time, and small flip angles within a narrow range (Enzmann DR, Rubin JB: *Radiology* 166:467–472, 1988).

The most important clinical parameters of rheumatoid arthritis of the cervical spine (including atlantodental interval, dens erosion, osteophytes of the upper spine, and subluxation) are well seen in MR evaluation (Bundschuh C et al: *AJR* 151:181–187, 1988).

FUSION

In 18 patients with rheumatoid arthritis affecting the cervical spine, fusion of an unstable rheumatoid cervical spine relieved pain and prevented progression of existing neural lesions without undue risk to the patient (Santavirta S et al: *J Bone Joint Surg [Am]* 70A:658–667, 1988).

In a study of 26 rheumatoid arthritic patients, results suggest that fusion without decompression leads to remission (Heywood AWB et al: *J Bone Joint Surg [Br]* 70B:702–707, 1988).

Atlantoaxial instability may be corrected with lowered risk by utilization of a Steinmann pin drilled through the base of C2 spinous process (Apran H, Harf R: *Orthopedics* 11:1687–1693, 1988).

For subaxial injuries, subluxation and facet dislocations are most reliably treated with posterior 1-level fusion; Halo jacket immobilization has few indications (Stauffer ES: *Clin Orthop* 239:30–39, 1989).

Halo brace can be used for early mobilization and early discharge in patients with no neurologic deterioration (Parry H et al: *Paraplegia* 26:226–232, 1988).

Chronic atlantoaxial dislocation may lead to a spontaneous bony fusion with progressive spastic quadriparesis (Heselson NG, Maruf G: *Clin Radiol* 39:555–557, 1988).

INSTRUMENTATION

The internal spinal fixation device of Dick consists of transpedicular screws attached by hinged coupling clamps to ipsilateral square-rounded threaded spanning rods. Application of these devices bilaterally provides remarkable solidarity for immediate fusion (Thalgrett JS et al: *Orthopedics* 11:1465–1468, 1988).

According to L. B. Bone and co-workers (*J Orthop Trauma* 2:195–201, 1988) the broad dynamic compression produced by the Armstrong NRC plate appears, on the basis of in vitro studies, to fulfill most nearly the ideal attributes of an anterior spinal implant for the treatment of burst fractures of the thoracic and lumbar spines.

Segmental spinal instrumentation has been described for passage of wire through the base of the spinous process without the neurologic risks of sublaminar instrumentation (Douglas DF, Keene JS: *Orthopedics* 11:1403–1410, 1988).

A T-plate screwed to occiput and screwed and wired to C-2 produced fusion in 12 of 14 cases (Heywood AWB et al: *J Bone Joint Surg [Br]* 70B:708–711, 1988).

Thoracic

Anterior Excision of Herniated Thoracic Discs
Bohlman HH, Zdeblick TA (Case Western Reserve Univ)
J Bone Joint Surg [Am] 70-A:1038–1047, August 1988   20–4

Herniation of the thoracic disk is relatively uncommon. Laminectomy of a herniated thoracic disk by the posterior midline approach involves manipulation of the spinal cord. Decompression by this route has historically yielded poor postoperative results. A transthoracic anterior or anterolateral approach via a costotransversectomy has significantly increased the number of successful decompressions. The case reports of 10 men and 9 women aged 25–73 years who underwent excision of 22 herniated thoracic disks between 1972 and 1984 were reviewed.

Preoperative symptoms included back pain, pain and weakness in the lower extremities, spastic gait, bowel or bladder dysfunction, and numbness. The diagnosis of a herniated thoracic disk was confirmed with spinal radiography and myelography. Eleven patients underwent decompression via a costotransversectomy; the others were operated on with a transthoracic approach. Three patients in each group had an arthrodesis. Continuous intraoperative monitoring of the spinal cord with cortical evoked potentials was used in all patients.

Thoracotomy was performed at the level of the rib, which corresponded with the level of herniation. After the midlateral portion of the herniated disk was removed, a high-speed bur was used to create a trough in the vertebral bodies on either side of the disk space while leaving the posterior aspect of the cortex and the protruding disk intact. A diamond-tipped bur was used to thin the posterior aspect of the cortex (Fig 20–3).

After an average of 48.8 months, 10 of the 19 patients reported complete pain relief, 8 had partial pain relief, and 1 reported no change. Functional outcome was rated excellent or good in 16 patients, fair in 1 patient, and poor in 2 patients. The latter 2 patients experienced tran-

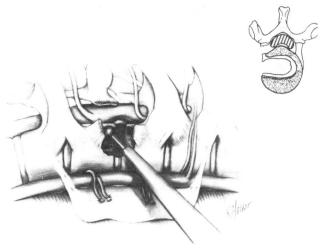

Fig 20–3.—A high-speed bur is used to create a trough in the vertebral bodies on either side of the disk space. The posterior part of the cortex of the bodies is thinned using a diamond-tipped burr. (Courtesy of Bohlman HH, Zdeblick TA: *J Bone Joint Surg [Am]* 70-A:1038–1047, August 1988.)

sient postoperative paraparesis, but both had a hard herniated upper thoracic disk of long standing with atrophy of the spinal cord.

Although surgical decompression of a herniated thoracic disk still carries a risk of spinal cord injury, the anterior or anterolateral approach to thoracotomy has greatly lowered this risk.

▶ The authors demonstrate the possibility of good results via transthoracic excision of herniated thoracic disks from T4 to T12. The operating microscope probably makes the surgery more precise. Intraoperative monitoring is probably useful in minimizing complications, and motor evoked potentials in the future will likely be best of all.

Brief Notes on the Thoracic Spine

In 4 surgically proven cases, thoracic disk herniation was differentiated from spinal metastasis with magnetic resonance imaging (Goldberg AL et al: *Skeletal Radiol* 17:423–426, 1988).

Among 680 myelograms only 3 cases of multilevel thoracic disk herniations were found (Alvarez O et al: *J Comput Assist Tomogr* 12:649–652, 1988).

Surgical treatment, despite its difficulty and complications, may be the best alternative in some cases of adult scoliosis (*Clin Orthop* 229:70–86, 1988).

Spinal epidural hematoma in hemophilia was successfully treated with serial factor VIII transfusions (Narawong D et al: *Pediatr Neurol* 4:169–171, 1988).

Lumbar

Surgical Management of Extreme Lateral Lumbar Disc Herniations: Review of 138 Cases

Abdullah AF, Wolber PGH, Warfield JR, Gunadi IK (Washington County Hosp, Hagerstown, Md)
Neurosurgery 22:648–653, April 1988   20–5

Lumbar disk herniations compressing the nerve root that exists at the same level are termed *extreme lateral herniations* and comprise about 10% of all lumbar herniations. The great majority of extreme lateral herniations in 138 patients occurred at the L3-L4 and L4-L5 interspaces. The Lasègue sign was negative in 65% of cases. It is important to distinguish between conjoined nerve roots (Fig 20–4) and extreme lateral herniation on computed tomographic study.

An extruded fragment was found in 82 cases, and a circumscribed protrusion, in 56 others. Double disk herniation on the same side at the same level occurred in 15% of patients. Pain was totally relieved 3 months after operation in 113 cases. Twenty patients had good relief and resolution of the neurologic deficit. Five patients delayed their return to work but had no objective abnormality or physical incapacity. In 1 patient, a pseudomeningocele developed from a persistent lumbar puncture hole at the level of surgery. Of 93% of patients after 10 years or longer, only 1 patient had surgery at the same level for recurrent symptoms.

Radical diskectomy is done in these cases, with thorough curettage of the interspace. Adequate foraminotomy will prevent later encroachment on the neural elements from narrowing of the interspace.

▶ The main point of this presentation is to emphasize that this clinical condition should not be overlooked. For the L2 root, pain is in the medial thigh; for L3, it is in the knee; and for L4, in the anterolateral thigh. Lateral bending toward the side of the lesion often reproduces the pain. The excellent diagnostic possibilities of computed tomography obviate the need for diskography. Access to the lesion typically involves removal of a portion of the medial facet. For surgical management, good results can be expected in this group of patients.

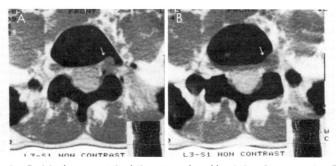

Fig 20–4.—Conjoined nerve root simulating extreme lateral herniation: **A,** upper section; **B,** section immediately below. Decompression affords good relief, but the surgeon should be knowledgeable beforehand about the presence of this anomaly. (Courtesy of Abdullah AF, Wolber PGH, Warfield JR, et al: *Neurosurgery* 22:648–653, April 1988.)

Intra- and Postoperative Complications in Lumbar Disc Surgery

Stolke D, Sollmann W-P, Seifert V (Med School, Hannover, West Germany)
Spine 14:56–59, January 1989   20–6

Complications occurring during and after lumbar disk surgery are discussed in only a few retrospective studies. Because of an increasing number of malpractice suits for failed low-back surgery, intraoperative and postoperative complications in lumbar disk surgery were studied prospectively.

Analyzed were 412 primary operations and 69 reoperations for herniated lumbar disk. Each of the surgeons had experience with more than 100 surgical procedures on lumbar disks. Perforations of the dura, generally without nerve root damage, occurred in 1.8% of microdiskectomies and in 5.3% of macrotechniques. The dura was perforated in 17.4% of patients undergoing reoperations. Bleeding from the venous plexus or spongiosa was notable when repeated electrocoagulation and a longer tamponade with gelfoam or the application of bonewax was needed.

Such bleeding occurred in 3.2% of microdiskectomies, 4.2% of macrodiskectomies, and 8.7% of reoperations. Problems in identifying the correct interspace occurred in 2.8%, 4.3%, and 2.9% of microtechniques, macrotechniques, and reoperations, respectively. Nerve root damage, caused by rongeurs, was noted in 2 patients having primary operations and in 1 having reoperation. Postoperative complications included delayed wound healing in 2.4% of microdiskectomies and 3.7% of macrodiskectomies. Interspace infection developed in 0.5% and 1.4% of macroprocedures and microprocedures, respectively. A preoperatively documented paresis worsened in 2 patients undergoing macrodiskectomies and 1 patient undergoing reoperation. Of the patients having primary procedures, 2 had persisting sciatica after surgery. Additional surgery was necessary for 15.

The incidence of intraoperative complications in lumbar disk surgery was found to range from 7.8% in microdiskectomies and 13.7% in macrodiskectomies to 27.5% in reoperations. Postoperative complications occurred in 1.4% of reoperations, 3.9% of microdiskectomies, and 4.2% of macrodiskectomies. The risk of complications correlated with patient age and operating time.

▶ Complications of lumbar disk surgery are described in this extensive survey of experienced disk surgeons. Some of the complications are clearly of more significance than others. Although ooze from the venous plexus may be considered an intraoperative complication, it is clearly not as important as a wound infection or pulmonary embolus. The frequency of important complications is very low in usual cases. The 15 reoperations were performed for such problems as abscess, secondary wound closure, and repair of leakage of cerebrospinal fluid, with 1 death from pulmonary embolism.

Percutaneous Lumbar Discectomy: Review of 100 Patients and Current Practice

Kambin P, Schaffer JL (Univ of Pennsylvania, Philadelphia)
Clin Orthop 238:24–34, January 1989   20–7

Lumbar disk herniation is a major national health problem, with an estimated 80% of the population suffering low back pain at some time in their lives. The percutaneous posterolateral approach to the lumbar intervertebral disk is an alternative to conventional treatment for lumbar disk protrusion and its associated radiculopathy.

One hundred patients with 102 herniations of the nucleus pulposus at L2-L3, L3-L4, L4-L5, and L5-S1 and unremitting radicular pain were treated with percutaneous lumbar diskectomy. Ninety-three patients were available for follow-up evaluation. The 7 not available for this review had all been followed up for at least 1 year, at which time they were judged to have an excellent result. Fifty-nine patients were followed up for 2–6 years. Evaluations of outcomes were based on modified MacNab criteria and patient interview, questionnaire, and examination. Eighty-seven percent of the patients were judged to have a successful outcome; they were pain free and had returned to preinjury activities. Thirteen percent of the outcomes were considered failures and repeat procedures were done in these cases. There were no major complications, including superficial or deep infections, diskitis, or neurovascular compromise (table).

Percutaneous lumbar diskectomy is a valuable method for the treatment of herniated disks. In this series, the results were successful in 87% of the cases and unsuccessful in 13%. Meticulous patient selection for the procedure is the key to success.

▶ This communication acclaims remarkable results for percutaneous lumbar diskectomy: 87% of patients were believed to have a successful outcome without significant morbidity and no mortality. This is an interesting approach, but to gain wide acceptance, confirmation by other investigators will be required and validation by clinicians specifically trained in the evaluation of the nervous system will be important. Moreover, alternative therapy should be con-

Results of Percutaneous Lumbar Diskectomy

Surgical Level	Successes	Failures	Available for Follow-up	Unavailable for Follow-up	Total
L3–L4	9 (90%)	1 (10%)	10	2	12
L4–L5	69 (90%)	8 (10%)	77	5	82
L5–S1	3 (50%)	3 (50%)	6	—	6
Total	81 (87%)	12 (13%)	93	7	100

Surgical Results

(Courtesy of Kambin P, Schaffer JL: *Clin Orthop* 238:24–34, January 1989.)

sidered, such as microdiskectomy or percutaneous nucleotome treatment. Controlled trials provide the best validation of any proposed therapy.

Gadolinium-DTPA-Enhanced MR Imaging of the Postoperative Lumbar Spine: Time Course and Mechanism of Enhancement
Ross JS, Delamarter R, Hueftle MG, Masaryk TJ, Aikawa M, Carter J, VanDyke C, Modic MT (Case Western Reserve Univ)
AJR 152:825–834, April 1989   20–8

Magnetic resonance (MR) imaging is an effective means of distinguishing between epidural fibrosis, or scar, and recurrent disk herniation when gadolinium-DTPA (Gd-DTPA) is used in a way analogous to the use of iodinated contrast material. Just after intravenous injection of Gd-DTPA, epidural scar is enhanced, whereas disk material is not. The optimal timing for MR imaging after injection in patients after surgery and the reason for such intense scar enhancement have not been established. The time course and mechanism of epidural fibrosis enhancement after Gd-DTPA were examined.

A 3-part study included humans and dogs with epidural scar after spine injury. First, the dynamic in vivo contrast-enhancing properties of epidural scar were evaluated with sequential fast spin-echo sequences af-

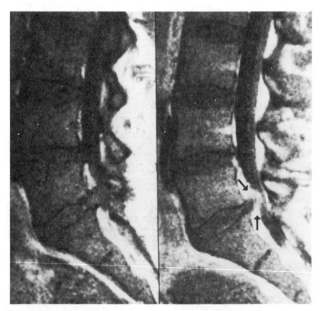

Fig 20–5.—Gd-DTPA enhancement in human scar and muscle. Scar enhancement *(top curve)* follows a course similar to that in dogs, with a peak around 6 minutes and subsequent slower decline. Muscle follows a similar pattern, but with less overall intensity. Curves are averages from signal-intensity values of 3 patients with enhancing epidural scar. (Courtesy of Ross JS, Delamarter R, Hueftle MG, et al: *AJR* 152:825–834, April 1989.)

ter contrast injection. In dogs, epidural scar was enhanced rapidly. Peak enhancement occurred 6 minutes after injection, with a slower decline toward baseline to 45% after 44 minutes. In humans, epidural fibrosis followed a similar pattern, with maximal enhancement at 73% after 5 minutes. Paraspinal muscle had a lower peak enhancement in humans and dogs, at 36% and 22%, respectively (Fig 20–5). Vascular injection in 2 dogs with india ink then demonstrated multiple small vessels throughout the epidural scar. Light and electron microscopy was done on epidural scar obtained at reoperation in humans and dogs. Light microscopy revealed multiple small capillaries scattered throughout a background of collagen, and electron microscopy showed a wide variation in the junctions between endothelial cells, ranging from tight to loose. Areas of endothelial discontinuity were also seen.

These findings suggest that Gd-DTPA is diffused rapidly into the extravascular space in epidural scar, with a slower net movement toward the intravascular compartment as the agent is filtered renally. The agent probably transgresses the endothelium through leaky intercellular junctions and regions of endothelial discontinuity.

▶ This study demonstrates clearly the mechanism of gadolinium enhancement of postoperative epidural scar. Such basic studies clearly illuminate the basic biology of our diagnostic techniques and may, in fact, suggest wider use in various other clinical settings.

Lumbar Spine: Postoperative MR Imaging With Gd-DTPA
Hueftle MG, Modic MT, Ross JS, Masaryk TJ, Carter JR, Wilber RG, Bohlman HH, Steinberg PM, Delamarter RB (Case Western Reserve Univ)
Radiology 167:817–824, June 1988   20–9

Patients with the failed back surgery syndrome (FBSS) have intractable pain and varying degrees of functional incapacitation. The FBSS is commonly caused by epidural fibrosis or herniated disk; differentiating between these causes is essential because reoperation on scar unaccompanied by disk material usually has a poor surgical outcome.

Researchers studied 30 patients with FBSS to evaluate the effectiveness of magnetic resonance (MR) imaging with gadolinium-diethylene-triaminepenta-acetic acid/dimeglumine in differentiating scar from recurrent disk herniation. Precontrast and postcontrast MR images were evaluated without knowledge of other findings.

In 17 patients, surgical and pathologic findings correlated with MR at 19 disk levels. Precontrast studies had a sensitivity of 100%, a specificity of 71%, and accuracy of 89%. Epidural fibrosis showed heterogeneous enhancement on the early T_1-weighted spin-echo images obtained within 10 minutes of contrast administration. Herniated disk was not significantly enhanced on the early studies but did show enhancement on delayed images in 9 of 12 patients. Enhancement patterns were the most useful criteria.

Precontrast and early postcontrast T_1-weighted spin-echo studies can accurately differentiate between epidural fibrosis and herniated disk in patients with FBSS. Patients treated either conservatively or with surgery after MR examination should be followed for further study.

▶ In the postoperative lumbar spine, epidural fibrosis is bright on T_1, and herniated disk showed enhancement on delayed images in 9 of 12 cases. This ability to distinguish between herniated disk and fibrosis is of obvious assistance to the spinal surgeon.

Brief Notes on the Lumbar Spine

LAMINECTOMY

Among 40 patients treated surgically for lumbar canal stenosis by laminectomy without diskectomy, 85% of cases experienced a reduction of clinical symptoms (Spanu G et al: *Acta Neurochir [Wien]* 94:144–149, 1988).

Widening the lumbar vertebral canal seems an effective alternative to laminectomy for lumbar stenosis (Senegas J et al: *Fr J Orthop Surg* 2:93–99, 1988).

Epidural morphine just before closing a lumbar laminectomy reduces postoperative pain (Presper JH, Denion J: *Spine* 13:1688, 1988).

An annotated bibliography on spinal stenosis is provided by Haglund and coworkers (*Pain* 35:1–37, 1988).

PERCUTANEOUS DISK SURGERY

Ten-year follow-up was carried out on 50 patients with percutaneous removal of L4-L5 herniated disk under local anesthesia, and 43 patients (86%) had relief of sciatica and sensory deficit (Hoppenfeld S: *Clin Orthop* 238:92–97, 1989).

Percutaneous nucleotome resection of lumbar disk results in a 70% success ratio (Maroon JC et al: *Clin Orthop* 238:64–71, 1989; the nucleotome is a suction device, similar to a "Roto-Rooter.")

Six athletes underwent percutaneous automated diskectomy and returned to their sports within 6 months (Maroon JC et al: *Physician Sports Med* 16:61–64, 1988).

Seventy-nine of 109 patients (72.5%) had success after percutaneous nucleotomy for herniated lumbar disks (Schreiber A et al: *Clin Orthop* 238:35–42, 1989).

Percutaneous disk surgery in 48 patients offered results comparable with those of open surgery and the advantages of reduced trauma (Shepperd JAN et al: *Clin Orthop* 238:43–47, 1989).

A curved cannula may be utilized for automated percutaneous diskectomy at L5-S1 (Onik G et al: *Clin Orthop* 238:71–76, 1989).

SURGICAL COMPLICATIONS

Diskitis occurred in 12 of 1,796 cases of lumbar diskectomy (Peruzzi P et al: *Neurochirurgie* 34:394–400, 1988). Nine of these were staphylococcus, suggesting intraoperative contamination. Needle aspiration and bone scan were of greatest diagnostic utility.

Soft tissue biopsies of postlaminectomy arachnoiditis in 14 cases of 26 demonstrated fibrillary foreign material consistent with surgical patties (*J Bone Joint Surg [Br]* 70B:659–662, 1988).

Epidural fat-grafting may cause a cauda equina syndrome (Pousick et al: *J Bone Joint Surg [Am]* 70A:1256–1258, 1988).

In biopsies of 26 patients with symptomatic radiculopathy after prior laminectomy, dense fibrous connective tissue was found in and about the nerve roots and fibrillary foreign material was seen in 55% (Hoyland JA et al: *J Bone Joint Surg [Br]* 70B:659–662, 1988).

Four cases of cauda equina syndrome are reported after fusion in situ and decompressive laminectomy for severe spondylolisthesis (Maurice HJ, Morley TR: *Spine* 14:214–216, 1989).

Ohrya and associates (*Paraplegia* 26:350–354, 1988) report acute intermittent mesenteric insufficiency after use of spinal Harrington rods.

MR Imaging

Magnetic resonance imaging effectively distinguishes fibrosis and recurrent disk herniation in the lumbar spine (Bundschuh et al: *AJR* 150:923–932, 1988).

Magnetic resonance imaging can image degenerative disk disease, both in standard spin sequences, with gadolinium enhancement and with spectroscopy (Modic MT et al: *Radiology* 168:177–186, 1988).

Szyprit and co-workers (*J Bone Joint Surg [Br]* 70B:717–722, 1988) examined 30 patients with MRI and myelography in search of lumbar disk protrusion. Surgical verification indicates that MRI was slightly better than myelography in the diagnosis of lumbar disk protrusion.

Magnetic resonance imaging can detect traumatic spinal arachnoid cyst (Mirich DR et al: *J Comput Assist Tomogr* 12:862–865, 1988).

Chymopapain

The Chief of the Division of Orthopedics at the Medical College of Pennsylvania (Philadelphia) has written the annual chapter on "What's New in Surgery for Orthopedics" for the *Bulletin of the American College of Surgeons* (73:24–28, January 1988). He reports that injections of chymopapain into the lumbar disks were made in 57,000 patients in 1983 and in fewer than 8,000 patients in 1986. Although the enzyme did relieve symptoms for the long term in 75% of patients, its use was associated with muscle spasm and back pain for up to 6 weeks in most of the patients who received it. Furthermore, there has been a low but frightening incidence of serious adverse reactions and complications. At the clinical conference of the ACS in 1987, there appeared to be a preference for surgery instead of enzyme injection for patients who have failed to respond to conservative therapy. Some of this, he contends, is also due to the advances in surgical techniques—the use of magnification and "even percutaneous devices"—so there is less muscle stripping and less facet disruption at the time of surgery; thus, postoperative morbidity should decline.—Oscar Sugar, M.D. [Professor Emeritus and Former Head of the Department of Neurosurgery, University of Illinois College of Medicine at Chicago and Clinical Professor of Neurosurgery, University of California at San Diego; Editor of the Neurosurgery section of the Year Book of Neurology and Neurosurgery from 1953 to 1985.]

Computed tomography after chemonucleolysis failure in 8 cases demonstrated persistent nerve root compromise (Burkus JK et al: *Orthopedics* 11:1677–1682, 1988).

According to Grammer and associates (*Clin Orthop* 234:12–15, 1988), chymopapain anaphylaxis may be prevented by screening with cutaneous chymopapain testing.

In an experimental model, chymopapain caused degenerative changes in dorsal nerve roots and fibrosis in the adjacent arachnoid without arachnoid fibrosis (Haughton VM et al: *Radiology* 169:475–478, 1988).

EXPERIMENTAL STUDIES

Cadaver studies suggest that tears in the anulus fibrosis are common with bulging disks (Yu S et al: *Radiology* 169:761–763, 1988).

In human cadaver experiments with motion, inward and outward bulging of the disk wall causes stresses within the disk leading to disruption of the adjacent anulus (Seroussi RE et al: *J Orthop Res* 7:122–131, 1989).

In human cadaver studies of the lumbar spine, during flexion-extension the ligamentum flavum did not appear to be a significant factor regarding dimensions of the spinal canal (Schoenstroem N et al: *J Orthop Res* 7:115–121, 1989).

Articular cartilage and intervertebral disk proteoglycans differ in structure (Buckwalter JA et al: *J Orthop Res* 7:146–151, 1989).

β-endorphin is diminished in the cerebrospinal fluid of monkeys with arachnoiditis (Lipman BT, Haughton VM: *Invest Radiol* 23:190–192, 1988).

Drummond and Moore (*Anesthesiology* 70:64–70, 1989) report that elevated blood dextrose causes worse neurologic outcome after temporary spinal cord ischemia in the rabbit.

Bower and co-workers (*J Vasc Surg* 9:135–144, 1988) report that drainage of cerebrospinal fluid in dogs during thoracic aortic occlusion maintains spinal cord perfusion above critical levels, diminishes reperfusion hyperemia, and improves neurologic outcome.

Tumors

MR Imaging of Intraspinal Tumors: Capability in Histological Differentiation and Compartmentalization of Extramedullary Tumors

Takemoto K, Matsumura Y, Hashimoto H, Inoue Y, Fukuda T, Shakudo M, Nemoto Y, Onoyama Y, Yasui T, Hakuba A, Nishimura S, Ban S (Osaka City Univ, Osaka; Baba Mem Hosp, Osaka; Kobe Municipal Central Hosp, Kobe, Japan)
Neuroradiology 30:303–309, August 1988   20–10

Magnetic resonance imaging (MRI) was evaluated for its ability to distinguish intraspinal tumors. These tumors are classified according to location as intramedullary, intradural extramedullary (consisting primarily of meningiomas and nerve sheath tumors), and extradural (often a metastasis). In this series, MRI scans of 29 patients were reviewed retrospectively.

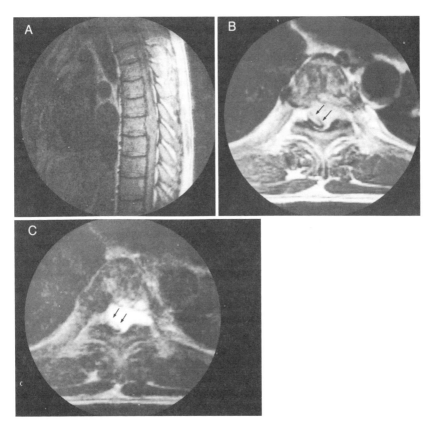

Fig 20–6.—A 38-year-old man with an extradural cavernous hemangioma. **A,** saggital SE (TR, 600 msec; TE, 40 msec); **B,** axial SE (TR, 800 msec; TE, 40 msec); **C,** axial SE (TR, 2,000 msec; TE, 120 msec). Spinal cord appears to be enlarged because of partial volume effect on the sagittal image at T9 level (**A**). On axial short SE (**B**) and long SE (**C**) images, a curvilinear low intensity band *(arrows)* is well seen between the tumor and the markedly compressed cord. The tumor is hypointense on the T $_1$-weighted image (**B**) and hyperintense on the T$_2$-weighted image (**C**). *SE* = spin echo; *TR* = repetition time; *TE* = echo time. (Courtesy of Takemoto K, Matsumura Y, Hashimoto H, et al: *Neuroradiology* 30:303–309, August 1988.)

Nine of the patients had intramedullary tumors, 14 had intradural extramedullary tumors, and 6 had extradural tumors. MRI correctly classified the 9 intramedullary tumors. One of the 20 extramedullary tumors was misjudged as intramedullary on both sagittal and axial images. With axial images the others were correctly identified as extramedullary. A low intensity band was seen between the tumor and spinal cord in all 6 extradural tumors (Fig 20–6).

Magnetic resonance imaging is judged to be quite specific in classifying intraspinal mass lesions. When sagittal images are inconclusive, coronal or axial images may be more specific. In this study, 5 of 6 extradural lesions exhibited the "extradural sign," a well-defined low intensity band.

Magnetic resonance imaging was also found to be reliable in distinguishing meningiomas from schwannomas.

▶ This careful study demonstrates that MRI accurately classifies the anatomy of intraspinal tumors, often providing histologic diagnosis. Occasional misses suggest that in some instances myelography will still be needed.

Spinal Cord Compression Due to Extramedullary Hematopoiesis in Thalassemia: Long-Term Follow-Up After Radiotherapy

Jackson DV Jr, Randall ME, Richards F II (Wake Forest Univ)
Surg Neurol 29:389–392, May 1988   20–11

Mass lesions of extramedullary hematopoiesis may compress the spinal cords of patients with thalassemia or other hematologic disorders. A rapid, durable response was obtained by low-dose radiotherapy alone in a thalassemic patient with this complication, with no side effects.

Man, 24, with a diagnosis of β-thalassemia major since age 4, was first seen with slowly progressive bilateral leg weakness and numbness and urinary hesitancy. The spleen was palpated 8 cm below the left costal margin. The lower limbs were moderately spastic and weak. Pinprick sensation was reduced to T11 or T12 bilaterally, and position and vibratory senses were reduced in the legs. Paraspinous masses were present in the thorax, and a bone scan showed wide-

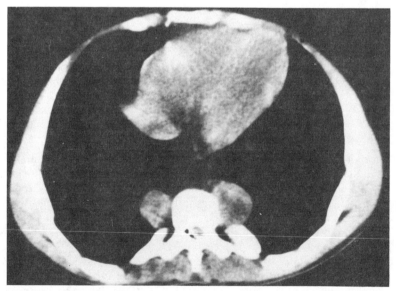

Fig 20–7.—Computed tomography scan through region of T10 demonstrating paraspinal soft tissue masses, representing sites of extramedullary hematopoiesis. (Courtesy of Jackson DV Jr, Randall ME, Richards F II: *Surg Neurol* 29:389–392, May 1988.)

spread activity representing marrow expansion. A total block was present at the T10 level and another at T4, corresponding to the area of the paravertebral masses (Fig 20–7). Generalized enlargement of the marrow cavities was noted. Indium scanning showed increased uptake in the masses. Radiotherapy directed at the lesions compressing the cord was followed by improved leg strength and resolution of symptoms. Neurologic function was normal both subjectively and objectively after delivery of 2,000 rads in 3 weeks.

Low-dose irradiation was an effective treatment of cord compression caused by extramedullary hematopoiesis in this thalassemic patient.

▶ Extramedullary hematopoiesis in thalassemia may cause spinal cord compression. The diagnosis is made on hematologic grounds with bone scan demonstration of marrow expansion. The cause of the spinal cord compression can be demonstrated with MRI. With the diagnosis secure, low-dose radiotherapy appears to offer satisfactory decompression and good long-term results, without the need for surgery.

One-Stage Posterolateral Decompression and Stabilization for Primary and Metastatic Vertebral Tumors in the Thoracic and Lumbar Spine
Shaw B, Mansfield FL, Borges L (Massachusetts Gen Hosp, Boston)
J Neurosurg 70:405–410, March 1989   20–12

Recent studies have shown that an anterior approach to decompression and stabilization of spinal metastases for the relief of pain and neurologic deficits is much more effective than laminectomy. However, anterior procedures are often associated with significant morbidity and may require further posterior stabilization. The 1-stage posterolateral approach to decompression and stabilization was used in 9 patients for the treatment of thoracolumbar fractures.

All 9 patients had been diagnosed with primary or metastatic thoracolumbar spinal tumors. Indications for operation included intractable back pain, radiculopathy, progressive thoracic myelopathy, and cauda equina syndrome. Preoperative neurologic deficits were found in 6 patients, 3 of whom were nonambulatory. After decompression, stabilization was accomplished in most patients by Harrington distraction instrumentation and sublaminar wiring. Bone grafting was performed only in those patients whose life expectancy was more than 12–18 months. Each patient underwent aggressive postoperative physical therapy.

All 6 patients who had neurologic deficits before operation were improved after operation, and all 3 nonambulatory patients had become ambulatory. The 2 patients who had required assistance when walking were able to walk unassisted after operation. None of the patients had neurologic deterioration during postoperative follow-up; 4 with severe preoperative back pain and radicular symptoms were definitely improved after operation. Of the 5 patients who were working before operation, 4 were able to return full-time to their occupations. However, 3 patients had serious postoperative complications, including 1 who had a cardiac arrest and died.

Although the patient population in this study was small, the findings indicate that the posterolateral approach to decompression and stabilization is a valid alternative in the treatment of spinal epidural neoplasia.

▶ This report demonstrates that 1-stage posterolateral decompression and stabilization may be successfully performed in the thoracolumbar area. Neurologic deterioration postoperatively was not observed, and a number of patients had improved pain status. There is substantial risk in this situation, as witnessed by the postoperative death, but these patients are, of course, quite ill from their tumor in the first place.

Brief Notes on Spinal Tumors

EXTRADURAL

Magnetic resonance imaging in multiple myeloma may demonstrate spinal lesions as fatty replacement of normal marrow, focal areas of reduced signal intensity, and focal areas of decreased signal intensity on T1 and T2 after previous radiation (Fruehwald FXJ et al: *Invest Radiol* 23:193–199, 1988).

Magnetic resonance imaging can diagnose vertebral hemangiomas associated with spinal cord compression (Marymont JV, Shapiro WM: *Br Med J* 81:1586–1587, 1988).

Gadolinium MR images do not improve the detection of tumors of the epidural space in the spine; nonetheless, in some cases these images were helpful in differentiating disk herniation from tumor, indicating regions of more active tumor for biopsy and demonstrating tumor response to therapy (Zsze G et al: *Radiology* 167:217–223, 1988).

EXTRAMEDULLARY

Cerebral ependymoma may metastasize to the spine (Liote HA et al: *Chest* 94:1097–1098, 1988).

An intramedullary and extramedullary schwannoma may be difficult to diagnose even with MRI, and open biopsy may be required to guide treatment (Garen PD et al: *Pathology* 20:296–298, 1988).

Dural arteriovenous fistulas may cause reversible acute and subacute myelopathy (Criscuolo GR et al: *J Neurosurg* 70:354–359, 1989). ·

Gadolinium MR may detect spinal dural arteriovenous fistulas (Terwey B et al: *J Comput Assist Tomogr* 13:30–37, 1989).

INTRAMEDULLARY

Cavernous hemangiomas of the spinal cord on MR appear as mixed subacute and chronic hemorrhage, suggested by mixed high and low signal intensity (Fontaine S et al: *Radiology* 166:839–841, 1988).

Six intramedullary cavernous malformations were removed from the spinal cord without morbidity. The natural history of 1 lesion is not perfectly known, but MRI is diagnostic (McCormick PC et al: *Neurosurgery* 23:459–463, 1988).

Hemangioblastoma of the conus medullaris was reported associated with cutaneous hemangioma (Michaud LJ et al: *Pediatr Neurol* 4:309–312, 1988).

In 25 patients with spinal cord lesions, gadolinium-enhanced MRI was extremely useful in diagnosis (Dillon WP et al: *Radiology* 170:229–237, 1989).

Magnetic resonance imaging was crucial and spinal angiography useless in planning excision of 2 intramedullary spinal cavernous angiomas (Zenter J et al: *Surg Neurol* 31:64–68, 1989).

A review of spinal ependymomas appears in the *Cleveland Clinic Journal of Medicine* (55:163–170, April 1988). Vijayakumar (a radiation therapist) and his neurosurgery, pathology, and radiology colleagues begin by saying ependymoma is a rare tumor. One does not get this impression from the volumes on neurosurgery by Schneider and co-workers from Michigan (chapter by J. L. Mc-Cauley), nor from those by Schmidek and Sweet, wherein the appropriate chapter is by Post and Stein from Columbia University. It would appear that ependymomas are at least as common as the astrocytomas (so far as intramedullary tumors are concerned); of course, spinal tumors (not metastatic) are probably only a tenth as common as cerebral tumors, and neurofibromas and meningiomas are much more common than the gliomas. So none of the gliomas are common; for a "rare" tumor, the ependymoma certainly has excited a great deal of discussion. The Cleveland group has put together from their own experience and that of others a knowledgeable discussion which leads to the conclusion that the ependymoma within the spinal canal should be totally removed if possible. In the past, total removal has been possible in approximately 50% of cases, but possibly in many more than this with the new equipment available such as intraoperative electrical recording, microscope, laser, ultrasound location during operation, ultrasonic aspirators, etc. If total removal is not possible, postoperative radiation therapy should be given (45 Gy as local field irradiation of the tumor with margins of 1 to 2 vertebral bodies above and below). Craniospinal axis irradiation can be considered with poorly differentiated tumors and when cerebrospinal fluid cytologic findings are positive for tumor cells.—Oscar Sugar, M.D. [Professor Emeritus and Former Head of the Department of Neurosurgery, University of Illinois College of Medicine at Chicago; Clinical Professor of Neurosurgery, University of California at San Diego; and Editor of the Neurosurgery section of the YEAR BOOK OF NEUROLOGY AND NEUROSURGERY from 1953 to 1985.]

Syringomyelia

Treatment of Syringomyelia With a Syringosubarachnoid Shunt
Tator CH, Briceno C (Univ of Toronto)
Can J Neurol Sci 15:48–57, February 1988   20–13

Because of the multifactorial pathogenesis of syringomyelia, there is still no agreement on when surgical intervention is warranted. However, it is the authors' opinion that all patients with signs of deteriorating neurologic function should undergo operation. The case reports of 42 patients with syringomyelia who underwent operation during an 18-year study period were reviewed.

Of 42 patients treated, 24 had idiopathic syringomyelia, 13 had posttraumatic syringomyelia, and 5 had syringomyelia secondary to spinal arachnoiditis. Twelve of the 24 patients with idiopathic syringomyelia had tonsillar ectopia. Symptoms and signs at presentation included pain in 25 (59.5%) cases and motor weakness in 41 (98.0%) cases. Muscle wasting in the upper extremities was present in 95% of the patients. Significant neurologic deterioration was the principal indication for operation in all cases. The duration of preoperative symptoms ranged from 5 weeks to 35 years. A syringosubarachnoid shunt (SS) procedure was performed in 35 patients. Follow-up ranged from 6 months to 15 years; the average follow-up was 4.6 years.

Of the 40 patients for whom adequate follow-up data were available, 19 (47.5%) had excellent postoperative results, 10 (25.0%) had good results, and 11 (27.5%) had poor results. Twenty-six (74.3%) of 35 patients who underwent SS had good or excellent results. The best clinical results were obtained in patients with idiopathic syringomyelia without tonsillar ectopia and in those with posttraumatic disease. All patients with syringomyelia secondary to spinal arachnoiditis had poor results. Eight patients who underwent posterior fossa decompression as an initial surgical procedure required reoperation to attain neurologic improvement or stabilization. No symptoms or signs were identified as being predictive of surgical outcome, but a short duration of preoperative symptoms seemed to favor a better outcome.

These findings support the recommendation by others that early surgical treatment in patients with progressive symptomatic syringomyelia is warranted.

▶ This careful report presents data regarding several forms of syringomyelia treated primarily with syringosubarachnoid shunting procedures. The authors report 29 good or excellent results in 40 cases with adequate follow-up. Patients with syringomyelia related to spinal arachnoiditis had poor results, and results may reflect poor absorption by the spinal arachnoid and may suggest utilization of a syringoperitoneal shunt in such cases.

Another interesting point of this study was the failure of posterior fossa decompression in patients with tonsillar descent to produce long-lasting good results. This failure, coupled with substantial morbidity and even mortality from the literature, has persuaded the authors to reserve posterior fossa decompression for a group of patients with clear-cut evidence of brain stem compression. The experience is at variance with that of Menezes and others who have reported excellent results after posterior fossa decompression with opening of the IV ventricle into the subarachnoid space, this latter perhaps providing an explanation for the superior results. Further long-term follow-up data will be required to elucidate the best management for these cases, which will undoubtedly be related to the specific pathology in individual patients.

Chiari I Malformation With Syringomyelia: Evaluation of Surgical Therapy by Magnetic Resonance Imaging
Batzdorf U (Univ of California, Los Angeles)
J Neurosurg 68:726–730, May 1988   20–14

Chiari I malformation with syringomyelia is being diagnosed more frequently. Current surgical treatment is based on the concept of dissociation of the cranial and spinal pressures. Five patients with Chiari I malformation and syringomyelia beginning in adulthood underwent magnetic resonance imaging (MRI) before and after suboccipital craniotomy with laminectomy of C1 and part of C2, arachnoid retraction, and duraplasty. The posterior arch of the atlas was resected along with part of the posterior arch of C2 if the tonsils extended below the C1 level. The

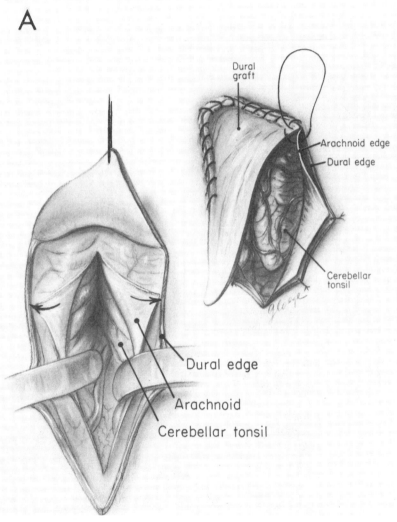

Fig 20–8.—**A, left,** dissection of the arachnoid away from the cerebellar tonsils. **A, right,** closure of the suboccipital wound, showing placement of a dural graft and suture that incorporates the free edge of the retracted arachnoid. (continued.)

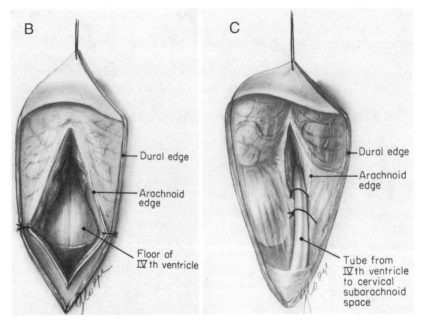

Fig 20–8, cont.— B, separation of the cerebellar tonsils and direction of arachnoid suture in cases where the arachnoid is adherent to the tonsils. C, placement of a tube from the fourth ventricle to the cervical subarachnoid space in cases where the arachnoid is adherent and the tonsils cannot be widely separated. (Courtesy of Batzdorf U: *J Neurosurg* 68:726–730, May 1988.)

cerebellar tonsils were retracted to make sure that the cerebrospinal fluid paths were open (Fig 20–8). Autologous fascia lata is used for dural grafting.

Postoperative MRI in 4 cases showed collapse of the syringomyelic cavity, even when this extended into the thoracic region. The process of collapse appeared to take place over several weeks. One patient had had a cervical cyst-to-subarachnoid shunt several months earlier, and further collapse of the syrinx was observed after hindbrain decompression. A more recent patient had collapse of the syrinx after fenestration of the obstructed fourth ventricle into the cisterna magna.

This operation collapses the syrinx without direct cyst shunting, thereby avoiding the risks of myelotomy and tube implantation. Brain stem symptoms and signs often are dramatically relieved, but relief of direct pressure on the brain stem is difficult to assess with imaging.

▶ The Chiari malformation and syringomyelia may now be easily recognized in the MRI depiction. When there is hydrocephalus, a ventriculoperitoneal shunt is the best treatment. There is mounting evidence that, for the patient without hydrocephalus, a Gardner procedure as described in this report is the best approach. By opening the IV ventricle to the spinal subarachnoid space, the pathophysiologic problem may be reversed, with appropriate follow-up by MRI. Whether obex plugging is important remains a point of some discussion, and it may well not be needed. Direct syringoperitoneal shunting, especially for apparently septate lesions, probably is not as effective and may carry more risks.

Brief Notes on Syringomyelia

In 13 patients undergoing MRI, 12 had abnormal studies corresponding to syringohydromyelia (Houang MTW et al: *Austral Radiol* 32:172–177, 1988). The low signal on T_1 is attributed to the pulsatile nature of the fluids within the cavity.

In 6 cases of posttraumatic syringomyelia treated by syringoperitoneal shunting, 5 cases had sustained neurologic improvement (Lahaye PA, Batzdorf U: *West J Med* 148:657–663, 1988).

Magnetic resonance imaging provides enough information, according to N. Tamaki and colleagues of Kobe, Japan *(Neurol Med Chir [Tokyo]* 27:848–855, September 1987), to allow decision making in Chiari types I and II malformations. If there is no syringohydromyelia, bony and dural decompression is sufficient therapy. If there is cavitation, separation of the tonsils and wide opening of the fourth ventricle is added, providing the syrinx is smooth and cylindrical. Syringotomy appears not to be indicated if the cavity is fusiform with transverse septa or narrow tubular interconnecting segments. In this study, the ages ranged from neonate (6 cases) to 30 in 19 patients with Chiari type II, and from 8 to 52 in 14 patients with the type I malformation.

Of the 19 children with syringomyelia studied by T. Isu and co-workers from Sapporo, Japan, 14 had spina bifida. Of these, 8 had meningomyeloceles with Chiari malformations. Six patients had lipomas, 4 had untyped Chiari malformations, and 1 had idiopathic syringomyelia. Syringomyelia appears not to be as rare in children as was believed before the advent of MRI. This type of imaging is particularly useful in studying children with pes cavus and scoliosis who may have otherwise unsuspected syringomyelia. For children with Chiari malformations and a large syrinx with swollen cord, subarachnoid shunting is effective *(Neurol Med Chir [Tokyo]* 27:973–978, October 1987). Full-length sagittal scans of the spinal cord from C1 to the midlumbar area show the disappearance of long and large syringes in 1 operated case.

Neither group of neurosurgeons were inclined to do the plugging of the upper end of the central canal/syringe as advocated by Gardner, which was so successfully used by Hoffman's group in Toronto (abstracted in *KEY Neurology and Neurosurgery* (3)1, 1988).—Oscar Sugar, M.D.

21 Trauma

Introduction

Evaluation of head injury was the subject of several communications. A review of boxing-related injuries in the U.S. Army from 1983 to 1985 revealed 1 death, 1 incidence of blindness, and 67 hospitalizations (Abstract 21–1). The authors question the advisability of continuing boxing in the U.S. Army. A population-based study of skull fracture indicates that skull fractures do indeed correlate with severity of neurologic deficit and mortality (Abstract 21–2). Undoubtedly magnetic resonance imaging has added refinement and power to the correlation. The Galveston group reports disproportionately severe memory deficit in relation to normal intellectual functioning after closed head injury (Abstract 21–3).

Surgical therapy has undergone further development. The group at the University of Bern reports on subcranial surgery of 395 combined frontobasal-midface fractures with cosmetically rewarding results and a minuscule complication rate (Abstract 21–4). Japanese surgeons have described transfrontal intradural microsurgical decompression for traumatic optic nerve injury in selected cases with good results (Abstract 21–5).

Adjunctive therapy has undergone further development. A large, carefully done multicenter trial provides solid evidence supporting the use of barbiturates in the control of elevated intracranial pressure after severe head injury (Abstract 21–6). Hypertonic saline solution administered early in resuscitation after multiple injuries appears to enhance cerebral perfusion and may benefit head injury patients in hemorrhagic shock (Abstract 21–7).

Spine injury has received attention. According to Hadley and co-workers (Abstract 21–8), isolated C2 fractures are rather stable, and initial management consists of external immobilization. Surgery followed by immobilization is preferred in cases of cervical spine fracture and fracture dislocation (Abstract 21–9). With regard to thoracolumbar spinal injuries, a three-column concept is proposed, including the bodies anteriorly, the facets posteriorly, and as the middle column, the posterior longitudinal ligament, posterior anulus, and posterior vertebral body (Abstract 21–10). This interesting concept needs further clinical verification. Conservative management of thoracolumbar "burst" fractures without neurologic deficit leads to excellent outcome (Abstract 21–11). Surgical intervention appeared to improve outcome in a controlled study of surgical treatment for thoracolumbar spinal fractures (Abstract 21–12). For acute penetrating injuries of the spine, a retrospective analysis comparing surgical and nonsurgical cases showed no significant difference with a trend toward more complications in the surgical group (Abstract 21–13). In a study of 88 patients with gunshot injuries of the terminal spinal cord and cauda equina, good results were obtained after laminectomy (Abstract 21–14).

Other specialized central nervous system injuries were the subject of several communications. In 43 cases of vertebral artery trauma, direct surgical ligation of the vertebral artery was frequently carried out, but this can now be accomplished with balloon catheter technique in stable patients (Abstract 21–15). Compartment syndromes in the limbs must be suspected on clinical grounds, confirmed by pressure measurements, and treated promptly with decompressive surgical techniques (Abstract 21–16).

Head Injury

EVALUATION

Boxing-Related Injuries in the US Army, 1980 Through 1985
Enzenauer RW, Montrey JS, Enzenauer RJ, Mauldin WM (Fitzsimons Army Med Ctr, Aurora, Colo)
JAMA 261:1463–1466, March 10, 1989   21–1

Competitive boxing is currently promoted in the U.S. military. Interunit matches are common on most large installations, and interservice competition is typical at many overseas duty stations. The extent of morbidity and mortality directly related to participation in military boxing was assessed.

The records of hospitalizations for boxing-related injuries in the U.S. Army medical treatment facilities around the world from 1980 to 1985 were reviewed. An average of 67 hospitalizations annually were attributable to military boxing matches. Injured men spent an average of 5.1 days in bed and 8.9 days disabled and unfit for duty. One man died of serious head injury, and another suffered unilateral blindness from ocular trauma requiring enucleation. Sixty-eight percent of all injuries were head injuries, occurring most often in the younger and presumably less experienced boxers.

Evidence that boxing can result in irreversible brain damage is now as indisputable as the link between cigarette smoking and lung cancer. Serious head and eye injuries can be especially devastating sequelae of this competitive sport. Although any sport can result in injury, the main goal of boxing is to cause potentially life-threatening damage. The advisability of continuing to promote boxing in the U.S. military should be addressed.

▶ This compelling communication documents disability, blindness, and death caused by competitive boxing in the U.S. Army. The data presented provide clear statistical documentation of the dimensions of injuries caused by boxing. Now that the risk of military boxing is known, it may be weighed against the perceived benefits of this activity. Only in this way can its advisability in the military be assessed. This communication adds to the very substantial body of evidence that boxing is dangerous, disabling, and sometimes fatal.

Short-Term Outcomes of Skull Fracture: A Population-Based Study of Survival and Neurologic Complications

Wiederholt WC, Melton LJ III, Annegers JF, Grabow JD, Laws ER Jr, Ilstrup DM (Univ of California, San Diego; Univ of Texas, Houston; Mayo Clinic and Found, Rochester, Minn)

Neurology 39:96–102, January 1989   21–2

Most studies of survival and neurologic injury after head trauma involve selected subgroups of hospitalized patients, patients with certain neurologic deficits, or those with specific types of injury. Because such data may not be generalizable, a more thorough description of survival and neurologic morbidity in a population-based cohort of head-injured patients was undertaken.

Residents of Olmsted County, Minnesota, who sustained brain injury between 1935 and 1979, were studied. Their medical records were reviewed for survival and neurologic outcome. To be included in the analysis, residents must have had loss of consciousness or posttraumatic amnesia or neurologic evidence of brain injury or skull fracture. Of 4,660 patients identified, 28% had suffered skull fractures. More than half of the brain-injured patients who died did so within 24 hours of suffering the trauma. Among 1-day survivors, subsequent survival was moderately impaired, particularly in older patients. Death rates were lowest in patients without skull fracture and rose with fracture severity. Related neurologic morbidity, complications, and deficits tended to be more common in patients with skull fractures than in patients without skull fractures and were much more frequent among those with more severe skull fractures. Types of neurologic deficits were comparable in those with and without skull fracture, except that patients with complicated skull fractures had higher proportions of special sensory deficits and multiple deficits.

In this cohort study, short-term survival was inversely related to severity of the brain injury. The 30-day case fatality rate ranged from 4% among those with no skull fracture and 7% among those with linear fractures to 42% and 44% of patients with depressed/comminuted or basilar skull fractures, respectively.

▶ This important population-based study indicates that skull fractures do correlate with severity of deficit and mortality. This counters previous reports denying such a correlation (1). Undoubtedly the addition of MRI to the diagnostic approach will give a greater refinement and power to the correlation of radiographic findings and outcome.

Reference

1. Jennett et al: *Neurosurgery* 4:283–289, 1979.

Disproportionately Severe Memory Deficit in Relation to Normal Intellectual Functioning After Closed Head Injury

Levin HS, Goldstein FC, High WM Jr, Eisenberg HM (Univ of Texas Med Branch, Galveston)

J Neurol Neurosurg Psychiatry 51:1294–1301, October 1988   21–3

It is not clear whether memory impairment is an expression of global cognitive disturbance after closed head injury or a relatively specific sequela. Memory and intellectual functioning were assessed in 87 survivors of moderate or severe closed head injury, aged 18–30 years at the time of injury.

About one fourth of patients, evaluated 5–15 or 16–42 months or both after injury, had defective memory on both auditory and pictorial measures despite Wechsler verbal and performance IQ values within the range of average. Memory-impaired patients did appear to have poorer intellectual functioning after injury than unimpaired patients at both test intervals. Only 1 memory-impaired patient had evidence of a temporal lobe lesion.

Some survivors of moderate or severe closed head injury have a disproportionately marked memory deficit that persists. The disorder resembles some amnesic disturbances of other causes such as that of alcoholic Korsakoff syndrome. The effects of residual memory disorder on everyday function remain to be ascertained.

▶ This study documents with careful neuropsychologic techniques a selective memory deficit after closed head injury. This kind of information is obviously of great importance in establishing disability status and restoring the patient to maximal function and appropriate integration into the community. This particular communication is part of an ongoing series from Eisenberg and colleagues in Galveston regarding the problems of mild to moderate head injury.

SURGERY

Subcranial Management of 395 Combined Frontobasal-Midface Fractures

Raveh J, Vuillemin T, Sutter F (Univ of Berne; Inst Straumann AG, Waldenburg, Switzerland)

Arch Otolaryngol Head Neck Surg 114:1114–1122, October 1988   21–4

Patients with severe traumatic craniofacial injuries often have concomitant injuries involving the basal anterior and middle cranial fossa planes with associated dural tears and optic nerve compression. With the conventional approach to treatment, patients first undergo primary urgent neurosurgical exploration with local repairs as needed and reconstruction of the craniofacial lesions is deferred for 2–3 weeks.

An early, primary, 1-stage operation that has been performed by a team of specialists since 1978 for the treatment of such multiple injuries is described. Operation is usually performed within the first 24–48 hours after trauma. For this 1-stage approach, the classic transethmoidal rhino-surgical approach, which is limited to the median-paramedian skull base region, has been modified by extending exposure over the entire frontal region, including the roof of the orbit to the apex and the lateral orbital walls (Fig 21–1). This approach enables subcranial exposure of all anterior fossa planes, including the sellar-sphenoidal region and avoids the need for retraction of the frontal lobes with its potential for iatrogenic damage to the olfactory filaments.

From 1978 through 1987, 395 patients with midface fractures and concomitant frontobasal fractures have been treated by the extracranial approach. Five patients died, but none of the deaths was directly attributable to the surgical procedure. No cases of postoperative meningitis, postoperative infection, osteitis, or rejection of bone or cartilage transplants were observed. However, 30% to 50% graft resorption was observed in 15.5% of the patients. Only very few patients required secondary corrections because of insufficient primary fracture reduction. Most patients could be discharged from the hospital 11–12 days after operation.

Early 1-stage reconstruction of severe craniofacial injuries by the

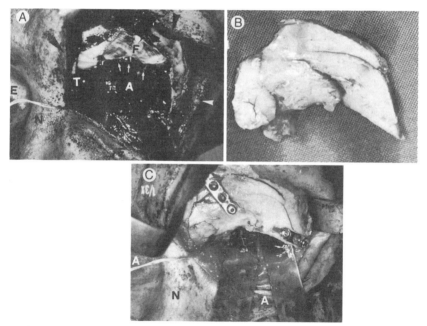

Fig 21–1.—Subcranial exposure and redressment of major dural tears. **A,** eyebrow incision noted by *arrowheads.* Borders of removed fronto-orbital segment indicated by *short arrows.* Closure of dural tears at fronto-orbital and ethmoidal *(T)* roof region performed with fascia lata *(F). A* indicates apex or orbit; *long arrows,* distal orbital roof border; and *E,* upper eyelid. **B,** fronto-orbital segment. **C,** Replaced fronto-orbital sement with miniplates *(long arrow). N* indicates nose. (Courtesy of Raveh J, Vuillemin T, Sutter F: *Arch Otolaryngol Head Neck Surg* 114:1114–1122, October 1988.)

extracranial-subcranial approach is associated with an extremely low morbidity rate when compared with conventional procedures.

▶ This enormous series of frontobasal-midface fractures has been treated with an early repair through a supraorbital wide exposure. The results are cosmetically rewarding, and the complication rate has been minuscule. With results like these, it is difficult to recommend a transcranial approach for the majority of these lesions.

Transfrontal Intradural Microsurgical Decompression for Traumatic Optic Nerve Injury
Waga S, Kubo Y, Sakakura M (Mie Univ, Tsu, Mie, Japan)
Acta Neurochir (Wien) 91:42–46, 1988   21–5

The incidence of optic nerve injury among patients with traumatic head injuries ranges from 0.5% to 5.2%. It has not yet been determined whether surgical decompression of the injured optic nerve gives better results than conservative management. The outcome was reviewed in 26 patients who sustained traumatic optic nerve injuries during a 9-year period.

Twenty-three (88%) patients had incurred optic nerve injuries in traffic accidents; the other 3 patients were injured in falls. All had bruises around the affected eye, 19 (73%) had no direct light reflex, and 7 (23%) had a sluggish or indirect light reflex. None of the patients had bilateral involvement. Twenty-two patients underwent microsurgical decompression of the optic nerve through a transfrontal intradural approach. The operation included a standard frontal craniotomy, unroofing of the optic canal with diamond drills, and opening of the optic nerve sheath and falciform ligament. Follow-up ranged from 8 months to 9 years. Significant improvement was defined as a gain in visual acuity of 0.1 or more, and nonsignificant improvement, as a visual acuity of more than 0.01 but less than 0.1.

Four (18%) of the 22 operated-on patients who were blind before operation did not improve, 11 (50%) had significant improvement, and 7 (32%) had nonsignificant improvement. All 11 patients with significant improvement had been operated on within 21 days after injury, including 8 (73%) who were operated on within 14 days of the event. There were no operative deaths, and only 2 patients had transient cerebrospinal fluid rhinorrhea. Two patients who had postoperative seizures responded well to anticonvulsant therapy.

The results obtained in this group of optic nerve injury patients can be considered acceptable. The data clearly demonstrate that patients with a preoperative visual acuity of 0.01 or more have a reasonable chance of visual improvement after surgical decompression.

▶ The results indicate that, for patients with some preserved vision after optic nerve injury, decompression may be rewarded with improved vision in up to 50%. Certainly, all patients with no vision from the outset should not be considered for such surgery.

ADJUNCTIVE THERAPY

High-Dose Barbiturate Control of Elevated Intracranial Pressure in Patients With Severe Head Injury
Eisenberg HM, Frankowski RF, Contant CF, Marshall LF, Walker MD, the Comprehensive Central Nervous System Trauma Centers (Univ of Texas Med Branch, Galveston)
J Neurosurg 69:15–23, July 1988   21–6

A 5-center randomized clinical trial assessed the effect of addition of high-dose phenobarbital to aggressive conventional management of elevated intracranial pressure (ICP). Conventional management included head elevation, hyperventilation, morphine, pancuronium, mannitol, and ventricular drainage.

Analysis of the 73 patients included in this study indicated a twofold therapeutic advantage among those receiving phenobarbital (table). When patients with cardiovascular complications were excluded, this advantage increased to fourfold. Multiple regression analysis indicated that barbiturate therapy and time from injury to treatment randomization were significant variables in the control of elevated ICP. After failure of treatment, 26 patients crossed over to barbiturate therapy. The response rate of the crossover patients was similar to that of the initial barbiturate group.

The results suggest that high-dose phenobarbital added to conventional management can help control elevated ICP.

▶ This large, carefully done, multicenter trial provides solid evidence supporting the use of barbiturate in the control of elevated ICP after severe head injury. Note that only a small subset of patients with severe head injury is involved here, and in effect only patients with failure of conventional therapy have been demonstrated to warrant this form of treatment.

Control of Intracranial Pressure (ICP) in Study Patients by Treatment Group

Control of ICP	Conventional Treatment	Barbiturate Treatment	Total
yes	6	12	18
no	30	25	55
total cases	36	37	73
% controlled	16.7	32.4*	24.7

*Difference statistically significant ($P = .12$).
(Courtesy of Eisenberg HM, Frankowski RF, Contant CF, et al: *J Neurosurg* 69:15–23, July 1988.)

Head Injury and Hemorrhagic Shock: Studies of the Blood Brain Barrier and Intracranial Pressure After Resuscitation With Normal Saline Solution, 3% Saline Solution, and Dextran-40

Gunnar W, Jonasson O, Merlotti G, Stone J, Barrett J (Univ of Illinois, Chicago)
Surgery 103:398–407, April 1988   21–7

An increase in intracranial pressure in head-injured patients is predictive of poor neurologic outcome and long-term disability. Conventional fluid resuscitation using isotonic crystalloid or colloid solutions has been shown to increase the intracranial pressure acutely in head-injured patients, whereas the use of hypertonic (3%) saline solution (HS) early in resuscitation maintains the pressure at baseline. The effects of fluid resuscitation using normal saline solution (NS), dextran-40 (D-40), and HS on cerebral edema, intracranial pressure, and blood-brain barrier function were compared in hypotensive dogs with simulated head injury.

After anesthetization, 40% of the dogs' blood was shed via left femoral artery catheters over a 5-minute period and was collected in citrated blood bags. After 1 hour of shock, half the shed blood was retransfused over a 15-minute period. Resuscitation was then continued by infusion of either NS, D-40, or HS in quantities equal to the amount of shed blood. Evans blue solution was infused intravenously, and intravascular volume

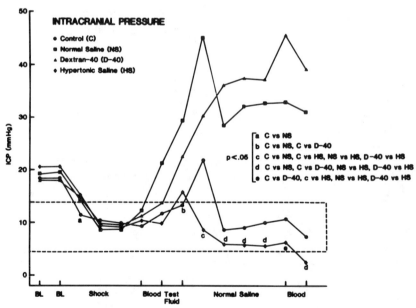

Fig 21–2.—Intracranial pressure measurements with intracranial epidural balloon inflated. Resuscitation was initiated with one half shed blood volume followed 15 minutes later by a volume of test fluid, either *NS, D-40,* or *HS* equal to the amount of shed blood. Control *(C)* did not undergo shock state but received equal volumes of NS. Infusion of NS and the remaining shed blood over 90 minutes completed the study period. (Courtesy of Gunnar W, Jonasson O, Merlotti G, et al: *Surgery* 103:398–407, April 1988.)

was maintained with NS. All dogs were killed after 2 hours of resuscitation.

The average baseline intracranial pressure after epidural balloon inflation was 18.6 mm Hg. During the shock state, the average intracranial pressure decreased equally in the 3 study groups to an average of 10.8 mm Hg at the end of the shock state (Fig 21–2). Fluid resuscitation markedly increased the intracranial pressure to a maximal 46.6 mm Hg in the NS group and to a maximal 45.3 mm Hg in the D-40 group. In contrast, fluid resuscitation with HS increased the intracranial pressure only to a maximal 15.8 mm Hg. Analysis of coronal sections of fixed brains of animals resuscitated with HS showed that the deep Evans blue-staining of the left cortical surface and gray matter on the side of the balloon injury was the most extensive of all 3 study groups, suggesting improved cerebral perfusion to areas of brain injury. Blood-brain barrier function was not restored by HS resuscitation.

Hypertonic-saline solution administered early in resuscitation after head injury appears to enhance the return of cerebral perfusion and cell membrane function, which may benefit head-injured patients in hemorrhagic shock with concomitant neurologic trauma.

▶ This nice study documents the superiority of hypertonic solution early in the resuscitation of patients after head injury. Clearly increased intracranial pressure was more of a problem in normal saline and dextran-40 resuscitation. Further data will be required before clinical utilization of this approach.

Brief Notes on Head Injury

Neurologic injuries in equestrian sports can be minimized by the use of adequate protective headgear and avoidance of horseback riding by patients with temporary paralysis or posttraumatic epilepsy (Brooks WH, Bixby-Hammett DN: *Physicians Sports Med* 16:84–91, 1988).

Among children who sustain injuries on stairs, those younger than 4 years are more likely to sustain head injuries than older children. Among 363 consecutive patients, no patient had life-threatening injuries and no patient required intensive care, whereas 3% required admission (Joffe, Ludwig: *Pediatrics* 82:457–461, 1988).

Bachulas and associates (*Am J Surg* 155:708–711, 1988) report among 367 motorcycle injuries an incidence of severe brain injury 600% higher for patients without helmets. Facial fractures were twice as common in nonhelmeted riders. Helmet laws would help us utilize our limited neurosurgical capacity more effectively.

The incidence of cervical spine injury among patients with craniocerebral injury is 1.8% and not statistically significantly different from that among patients without trauma to the head (O'Malley KF, Ross SE: *J Trauma* 28:1476–1479, 1988).

CLINICAL STUDIES

After head injury, lesions visualized with MRI are important for neurologic-neuropsychologic outcome and may become fully apparent only on late scanning (Wilson JTL et al: *J Neurol Neurosurg Psychiatry* 51:391–396, 1988).

Cerebral dysfunction after trauma may be caused by acute epidural hematoma, depending on its volume. Ikeda and associates from the University at Kanazawa, Japan (*Neurol Med Chir [Tokyo]* 28:321–326, April 1988) describe their use of semiautomatic analysis of CT scans of 54 patients who developed symptomatic acute epidural hematoma within 3 days of trauma. The volume estimate was based on a formula that included thickness of the clot. Starting 6 hours after trauma, there was little or no disturbance of consciousness with a hematoma volume less than 55 ml. Descending tentorial herniation was demonstrable by CT with hematomas larger than 50 ml, and with those greater than 150 ml, herniation was advanced. Nearly all with uncomplicated hematoma showed good recovery within 6 months: poor outcome was related to hematomas of more than 140 ml.—O. Sugar, M.D.

Small epidural hematomas with a fracture overlying a major vessel or sinus or those diagnosed within 6 hours are associated with subsequent deterioration; such hematomas should be evacuated (Knuckey NW et al: *J Neurosurg* 70:392–396, 1989).

Compression and obliteration of the third ventricle and basal cisterns have a close correlation with raised intracranial pressure and poor prognosis (Colquhoumir, Burrows EH: *Clin Radiol* 40:13–16, 1989).

Metabolic studies after severe head injury demonstrate total dependence on aerobic and anaerobic metabolism of glucose without the utilization of β-hydroxybutyrate and acetoacetate (Robertson CS et al: *J Trauma* 28:1523–1532, 1988).

Isolated severe head injury seems to induce a full response in the secretion of catabolic hormones comparable with that encountered in patients with multiple injury and associated with marked increase in protein catabolism (Chiolero R et al: *JPEN J Parenter Enteral Nutr* 13:5–12, 1989).

A cognitive evoked potential (T300) was abnormal after concussion in 20 cases with minor head injury and returned to normal during the follow-up period (Pratap-Chamd R et al: *Acta Neurol Scand* 78:185–189, 1988).

Helling and associates (*J Trauma* 28:1575–1577, 1988) report that, among 319 patients with head trauma, an infectious complication, most often respiratory, developed in half of 82 patients with long-term hospitalization.

Posttraumatic low pressure headaches may be associated with CT evidence of very small ventricles and tight basal cisterns. Management is bed rest and fluid administration (Duerst UN et al: *Wochenschr Med* 118:1448–1452, 1988).

Labetalol helps reduce blood pressure and heart rate after trauma (Harrier HD: *Crit Care Med* 16:1159–1160, 1988).

Among 159 head-injured patients, the presence of visual field defects during the long-term period may be indicative of increased neuropsychologic deficits after injury (Uzzell BP et al: *Arch Neurol* 45:420–424, 1988).

Gennsemer and associates (*Ann Emerg Med* 18:9–12, 1989) report psychologic consequences of blunt head trauma as documented with a battery of psychologic tests.

Psychiatric factors in postconcussion syndrome are reviewed by W. A. Lischman (*Br J Psychiatry* 153:460–469, 1988).

Krus and Nourjahp describe the epidemiology of mild uncomplicated brain injury (*J Trauma* 28:1637–1643, 1988). Among 3,358 San Diego county residents with brain trauma in 1981, 72% of injuries were considered mild, for an incidence rate of 130.8 per 100,000 per year. The proportion of mild brain injury among all hospitalized cases was 82%. In-hospital treatment cost for this group of patients exceeded $6 million in 1981.

EXPERIMENTAL STUDIES

Endogenous opioids may mediate secondary damage after experimental brain injury (McIntosh TK et al: *Am J Physiol* 253:e565–e574, 1987).

Near-infrared spectrophotometry was used to evaluate autoregulation after closed head injury in cats and demonstrated a substantial failure of autoregulation (Proctor HJ et al: *J Trauma* 28:347–352, 1988).

Scanning electron microscopy and transmission electron microscopy show morphological changes in the endothelium of the microvasculature after brain injury (Maxwell WL et al: *J Pathol* 55:327–335, 1988).

Primate studies of head injury indicate that an early response to brain injury is astrocytic swelling followed by morphological changes in the endothelium (Maxwell WL et al: *J Pathol* 155:327–335, 1988).

The kallikrein-kinin system appears to be a mediator of brain edema and secondary brain damage in experimental and clinical settings (Baethmann A et al: *Crit Care Med* 16:972–976, 1988).

In experimental rat brain injury, data is compatible with a theoretic position that brain injury induces a shift in dominance of functional neural systems (Chappell ET, Levere TE: *Behav Neurosci* 102:778–783, 1988).

Spine Injury

Acute Traumatic Atlas Fractures: Management and Long Term Outcome
Hadley MN, Dickman CA, Browner CM, Sonntag VKH (Barrow Neurological Inst, Phoenix)
Neurosurgery 23:31–35, July 1988   21–8

Fractures of the atlas, a ring of bone between the skull and the remainder of the cervical spine, are almost always treated nonsurgically. The fractures may be of the isolated C1 type or combination C1–C2 fractures. Investigators review the diagnosis, treatment, and results of 57 fractures of the atlas.

The 32 isolated fractures were treated with some form of immobilization, depending on the degree of C1–C2 lateral mass dislocation. All recovered without neurologic injury or instability, although 3 patients experienced intermittent neck pain. Combination fractures were treated according to the type of C2 fracture found. Four of the 25 patients with combined fractures required early open reduction and internal fixation, and 1 underwent operative wiring and bone graft fusion. Six patients with C1–C2 fractures experienced neck pain or limited head and neck motion at follow-up. Of the 3 patients with C1–C2 fractures and neurologic deficits upon admission, 2 recovered and 1 died of multiple injuries.

A halo vest for 10 to 14 weeks is recommended in treating patients with isolated C1 fractures having a 6.9-mm or greater dislocation of the lateral masses. A less rigid cervical support can be used when dislocation is less than 6.9 mm. Management of combination fractures is more complicated. Thorough follow-up is required and late surgical therapy may be necessary. In both isolated and combined fractures of the atlas, thin section computed tomography is the diagnostic method of choice.

▶ In essence, isolated C1 fractures are rather stable, and initial management consists of external immobilization. It's not clear whether the halo vest is absolutely essential with lateral displacement of 7 mm or greater. Management of combined C1 and C2 fractures is determined for the most part by the nature of the fracture of the axis.

Management of Post-traumatic Cervical Spine Instability: Operative Fusion Versus Halo Vest Immobilization. Analysis of 49 Cases
Bucci MN, Dauser RC, Maynard FA, Hoff JT (Univ of Michigan)
J Trauma 28:1001–1006, July 1988   21–9

Traumatic cervical spine injuries associated with neurologic deficit can be treated in several ways. Immobilization with a halo vest alone has been found to cause complications. To compare this method with that of early operative fusion, investigators reviewed 49 cases of lower cervical spine fracture (C3–C7) seen over a 5-year period at 1 institution.

The patients' average age was 30.3 years, and most had complex fractures. The second most common injury was compression fracture. In 28 cases, immobilization in halo vests or hard cervical collars followed cervical spinal fusion. Twenty patients had the halo vest treatment only. One patient who refused treatment was given a Philadelphia collar. Immobilization continued for an average of 3 months.

Spinal instability was found in the patient with the collar, in 2 (7%) of the fusion patients, and in 8 (40%) of the halo vest group. In 1 case, that of a 25-year-old man, the halo vest provided good alignment immediately after its application (Fig 21–3). But repeat x-ray examinations after 2 days showed loss of reduction at the C6–C7 level. Posterior cervical fusion was carried out immediately, and normal alignment returned. One other patient in a halo vest also experienced worsening of his existing neurologic deficit. Emergency fusion was unsuccessful, and the patient remains with C6-spared quadriplegia.

In response to these cases, the authors recommend surgery followed by immobilization in cases of cervical spine fracture and fracture dislocation. The halo vest does not completely immobilize the spine or protect patients from neurologic injury.

▶ The authors present well-documented cases of instability after cervical injury despite treatment with the halo vest. This provides important support for the contention that surgery followed by immobilization is preferred in cases of cervical spine fracture and fracture-dislocation.

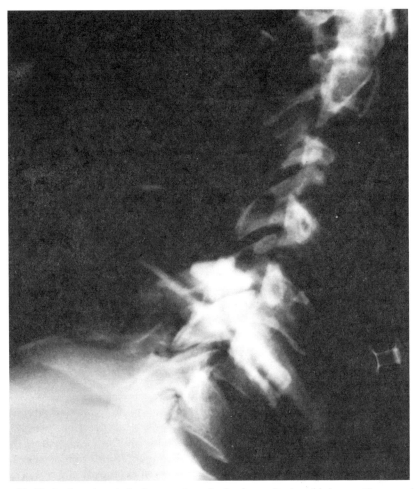

Fig 21–3.—Lateral cervical spine x-ray immediately after application of halo vest. (Courtesy of Bucci MN, Dauser RC, Maynard FA, et al: *J Trauma* 28:1001–1006, July 1988.)

Thoraco-Lumbar Spinal Injuries: Classification

Denis F (Minnesota Spine Center, Minneapolis)
Curr Orthopaed 2:214–217, October 1988   21–10

Holdsworth's spinal injury classification, based on subdividing the spine into 2 columns, has been useful. It was believed originally that rupture of the posterior column was enough to produce instability of the spine. However, recent evidence indicates that instability or the ability to subluxate or dislocate a spinal motion segment is possible only after additional rupture of the posterior longitudinal ligament and anulus fibrosus. Therefore, a new classification, based on a 3-column concept, was proposed.

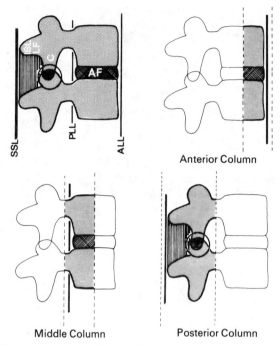

Anterior Column

Middle Column

Posterior Column

Fig 21–4.—The 3-column spine classification. (From Denis F: *Curr Orthopaed* 2:214–217, October 1988. Courtesy of Denis F: *Spine* 8:817–831, 1983.)

In the new classification, the third column is represented by structures that must be torn in addition to the posterior ligamentous complex to produce instability. The middle column structures consist of the posterior longitudinal ligament, posterior anulus fibrosus, and posterior half of the vertebral body. The pedicles, facet joints, laminae, spinous processes, interspinous ligaments, and supraspinous ligaments comprise the posterior column. The anterior column includes the anterior longitudinal ligament, anterior anulus fibrosus, and anterior half of the vertebral body (Fig 21–4 and table).

This 3-column classification for thoracolumbar spinal injuries is proposed as a replacement for Holdsworth's 2-column classification system.

► This is an interesting idea based on experimental evidence. However, before this convenient classification can be accepted, clinical validation will be required.

Thoracolumbar "Burst" Fractures Treated Conservatively: A Long-Term Follow-Up
Weinstein JN, Collalto P, Lehmann TR (Univ of Iowa)
Spine 13:33–38, January 1988

21–11

Type of fracture	Fractures Occurring in Anterior, Middle, and Posterior Column		
	Column		
	Anterior	Middle	Posterior
Compression	Compression	None	None or distraction (severe)
Burst	Compression	Compression	None
Seat-belt type	None or compression	Distraction	Distraction
Fraction dislocation	Compression rotation shear	Distraction rotation shear	Distraction rotation shear

(Courtesy of Denis F: Carr Orthopaed 2:214–217, October 1988.)

Comparable neurologic recovery has been reported in patients with burst fractures of the thoracolumbar spine who are managed conservatively rather than operated on. The late outcome was reviewed in 42 patients with traumatic burst fractures involving T10–L5. Management ranged from immediate ambulation in a body cast or brace to bed rest for 3 months. The average age at injury was 25 years, and at follow-up, 43 years. The most frequent area of injury was T12–L2.

The average patient had minimal to mild back pain at follow-up, but only 4 were free of pain. Neurologic status had improved in 7 patients.

Nearly 90% of patients were able to work at their preinjury level after injury. A majority of patients were blue collar or skilled laborers. Most patients had some kyphosis at the fracture site on radiography. The average translation was 2.45 mm. Neither kyphosis nor the degree of translation was correlated with symptoms. Five patients were operated on, 2 in relation to the initial injury.

Patients with burst fracture of the thoracolumbar spine and no neurologic deficit usually can expect an acceptable long-term outcome after conservative management. Kyphosis was not related to pain or disability in the present patients. Late surgery may be considered in patients with persistent pain related to spinal stenosis or progressive deformity that does not respond to conservative measures.

▶ Long-term follow-up in thoracolumbar "burst" fractures without neurologic deficit demonstrates excellent outcome, with ability to return to preinjury level of work in 90% and minimal to mild back pain. Follow-up radiographs showed remodeling and widening of the canal in some cases. Light surgery may be considered for pain or progressive deformity. In the patient without neurologic deficit, a conservative approach with prompt mobilization in a stabilization device is a reasonable therapy option.

In a related study, among 21 patients with thoracolumbar burst fractures who were neurologically intact with kyphosis less than 35 degrees, a total contact orthosis was applied with excellent results, irrespective of retropulsion or spinal canal narrowing (Reid DC et al: *J Trauma* 28:1188–1194, 1988).

The Neurological Outcome Following Surgery for Spinal Fractures
Gertzbein SD, Court-Brown CM, Marks P, Martin C, Fazl M, Schwartz M, Jacobs RR (Sunnybrook Med Ctr, Toronto; Univ of Kansas, Kansas City)
Spine 13:641–644, 1988   21–12

Management of patients with spinal cord injuries secondary to fractures of the thoracic and lumbar spine remains controversial. To determine the relationship between bony encroachment in the spinal canal and neurologic deficit, to assess neurologic recovery after surgery, and to compare anterior and posterior approaches, 60 patients—14 females and 46 males aged 14–58 years—with more than 20% bony encroachment of the spinal canal were evaluated.

Twenty-nine patients underwent anterior decompression with or without instrumentation and 31 underwent only posterior operation. All patients were graded neurologically according to the Frankel classification system. Follow-up ranged from 1 to 4 years.

Although in some patients the neurologic condition deteriorated immediately after operation, none were worse at the time of follow-up. The rate of improvement in neurologic function was 83% for patients with incomplete lesions who underwent posterior surgery and 88% for patients who underwent the anterior operation. The difference was statistically not significant. There was a positive correlation between the level of

Resulting Frankel Grades With Posterior vs. Anterior Surgery

	Posterior n = 31		Anterior n = 29	
Frankel grade	Preoperative (%)	Follow-up (%)	Preoperative (%)	Follow-up (%)
A	32	29	14	7
B	0	0	21	0
C	6	3	14	3
D	29	13	41	45
E	32	55	10	45

(Courtesy of Gertzbein SD, Court-Brown CM, Marks P, et al: *Spine* 13:641–644, 1988.)

injury and Frankel grades. Cord lesions tended to be associated with more severe neurologic deficits, whereas cauda equina lesions were associated with a less severe deficit. No apparent difference was found between degree of bony encroachment of the spinal canal and initial Frankel grade, nor between patients undergoing anterior versus posterior operations, regardless of the level of injury (table).

The degree of spinal encroachment appears unrelated to the initial neurologic presentation, as 39% of patients with Frankel grade E had more than 50% encroachment, whereas 29% of patients with less than 50% encroachment were Frankel grade A.

▶ In comparing reports of surgical intervention of cases of incomplete neurologic deficit with reports of nonsurgical intervention, surgical intervention appears to improve the outcome. No clear difference between anterior versus posterior surgery was demonstrated. Because the numbers are small, firm conclusions are impossible. However, the correlation of clinical grades and cord encroachment with outcome is a commendable approach. Use of this kind of analysis in a larger number of patients, with operative compared with nonoperative treatment, could more firmly establish the indications for this kind of surgery.

Treatment of Acute Penetrating Injuries of the Spine: A Retrospective Analysis
Simpson RK Jr, Venger BH, Narayan RK (Baylor College of Medicine, Houston)
J Trauma 29:42–46, February 1989   21–13

All battlefield spinal injuries since the Korean conflict have been treated with decompressive laminectomy and intradural exploration. The benefit of surgery has been questioned in civilian cases of penetrating spinal injury, in which neurologic outcome after surgical treatment has been disappointing. Indications for surgery include wound débridement, deteriorating neurologic status, presence of a foreign body, or visceral perforation. The benefits and risks of operative treatment for penetrating injuries of the spine in civilians were evaluated.

One hundred sixty cases were reviewed. One hundred forty-two patients had gunshot wounds, and 18 had stab wounds. Laminectomy, with or without intradural exploration, was performed in 23% of the patients. There were no significant differences in outcome between patients treated surgically and those treated conservatively. Meningitis, cerebrospinal fluid leakage, and wound infections occurred in 22% of the surgically treated group, compared with only 7% in the conservatively managed group.

No clear benefit from surgical decompression and exploration could be found in this retrospective study of penetrating spinal injury in an acute-care civilian hospital. The short-term goals of neurosurgical intervention in such cases—neurologic improvement and prevention of complications—appear to be difficult to achieve. However, if clinical variables are better controlled, subgroups of patients with penetrating injuries of the spine who would benefit from surgery may be identified. Also, the long-term benefits of operative treatment have not been established.

▶ The results of this retrospective study indicate no greater benefit (and in fact a trend toward greater complications) among surgically treated patients than among conservatively treated patients. These results would speak against surgery for gunshot wounds or stab wounds of the spine. Unfortunately, the results are not presented in terms of the location of the lesion: it is possible that the cauda equina injuries could present a special opportunity for surgical benefit. Further information is needed to guide a rational approach to this important neurosurgical problem.

Outcome of Laminectomy for Civilian Gunshot Injuries of the Terminal Spinal Cord and Cauda Equina: Review of 88 Cases
Cybulski GR, Stone JL, Kant R (Cook County Hosp, Chicago)
Neurosurgery 24:392–397, March 1989   21–14

Previous studies on the optimal treatment for civilian gunshot injuries of the terminal spinal cord and cauda equina have reported variable findings. The effect of laminectomy on gunshot injuries of the lower spine was assessed.

Between 1969 and 1987, 83 men and 5 women aged 6–61 (average, 24.7) were treated for gunshot injuries of the terminal spinal cord and cauda equina. Treatment consisted of laminectomy, exploration and débridement of foreign material from the spinal canal, and repair of the dura by dural patch grafting or primary dural closure. Of these 88 patients, 61 (69%) were operated on within 72 hours of injury, and 27 (31%) underwent laminectomy after an average delay of 12 days because of associated injuries which required thoracotomy or laparotomy.

There were no perioperative deaths, and none of the patients had postoperative cerebrospinal fluid fistula or late spinal instability. Postoperative pain relief and improved neurologic function were accomplished in 29 (47.5%) of the 61 patients who underwent early operation and 13 (48.1%) of the 27 patients who underwent late operation. Of 29 patients with complete paraplegia before operation 10 had a partial recovery of motor strength or sensation after operation, but only 2 of these patients had significant functional recovery. Of 7 patients with preoperative paraparesis, 5 and 11 of 19 patients with monoparesis had partial motor recovery. Only 3 of 20 patients with preoperative monoplegia of a lower extremity or complete loss of dorsiflexion or plantar flexion had complete recovery. Among the patients in whom laminectomy was delayed for more than 2 weeks, 15% had arachnoid adhesions and 17% had occult abscesses. The overall improvement rate was 47.7%.

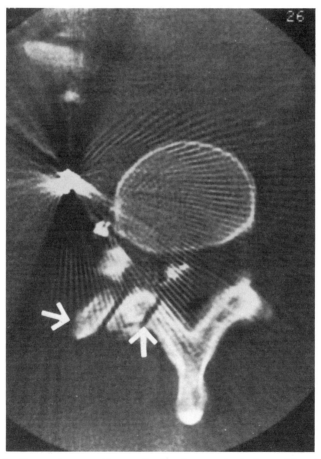

Fig 21–5.—Computed tomographic scan of patient demonstrating laminar and facet fractures *(arrows)* as well as intracanalicular bullet fragments. (Courtesy of Cybulski GR, Stone JL, Kant R: *Neurosurgery* 24:392–397, March 1989.)

Plain anteroposterior and lateral radiographs of the spine demonstrated fractures in 64.5% of the patients. Computed tomographic scanning of the spine has now become the main radiographic modality for investigating spinal gunshot injuries (Fig 21–5). Myelography was used only when indicated.

The timing of laminectomy for gunshot injuries of the thoracolumbar and lumbosacral spine is not essential to neurologic recovery. However, adequate débridement performed as soon as the patient has stabilized from associated injuries may help lower the incidence of such late sequelae as arachnoiditis, infection, and pain syndromes in the lower extremities.

▶ This excellent study demonstrates that good results can be obtained after laminectomy for gunshot wounds of the cauda equina. As the authors point out, it is difficult to know whether this is better than the natural history of the condition in that good studies of natural history are unavailable and each injury is slightly different. The authors demonstrate the utility of computed tomography in the analysis of these cases preoperatively.

Brief Notes on Spine Injury

CLINICAL STUDIES

Stauffer prefers wiring for treatment of traumatic instability of the cervical spine (*Orthopedics* 11:1543–1548, 1988).

Gakim and Sweet (*J Bone Joint Surg [Br]* 70B:728–729, 1988) report a case of transverse fracture through the body of the axis, which was considered unstable but was successfully managed conservatively.

For patients with unstable thoracolumbar fractures, a combined anterior decompression with interbody graft followed by posterior Harrington rods is effective, safe, and recommended if anterior instrumentation is unavailable (Gertzbein SD et al: *Spine* 13:892–895, 1988).

Recurrence of spinal deformity was noted after removal of Harrington rod fixation for spinal fracture in a study of 76 cases (Myllynen P et al: *Acta Orthop Scand* 59:497–502, 1988).

Apparently stable thoracolumbar fractures may develop instability in a delayed fashion. All types of spine fractures in the thoracolumbar region can produce such chronic pain from instability and poor results predominate in wedge compression fractures operated on more than 13 months after injury (Keene JS et al: *J Orthop Trauma* 2:202–211, 1988).

Chylothorax after fracture of the thoracolumbar spine is best treated with thoracotomy drainage and total parenteral nutrition (Gartside R, Hebert JC: *Injury* 19:363–364, 1988).

In a protocol-driven radiologic evaluation of suspected cervical spine injury, a single nondisplaced transverse process fracture of C7 was detected (less than 1% of asymptomatic patients). The combined cost was $59,000. These results call into question the cost and clinical efficacy of routine or protocol-driven cervical spine images for patients with trauma (Mirvis SE et al: *Radiology* 170:831–834, 1989).

After conus medullaris injuries in 18 cases, all patients could walk, but 4 required external support; all patients had regular bladder function, but none had normal sensation; 11 of 16 males were potent, but function was incomplete (Taylor TKF, Coolican MJR: *Paraplegia* 26:393–400, 1988).

An intramedullary gunshot wound with incomplete deficit may cause local compression, with the implication that removal of the bullet could be helpful (*J Trauma* 28:1600–1608, 1988).

Spinal cord injury may lead to reflex hypertension with intracranial hemorrhage (Hanowell LH, Wilmot C: *Crit Care Med* 16:911–913, 1988).

Unilateral facet dislocation in the lower cervical spine may present with quadriplegia (Gideon DE, Mulkey JC: *JAMA* 88:1223–1230, 1988).

Gilgoff and co-workers (*Pediatrics* 82:741–745, 1988) report effective voluntary respiration with neck musculature in otherwise ventilator-dependent quadriplegic children.

Myoclonus in a patient with spinal cord transection may be involved with the spinal stepping generator (Bussel B et al: *Brain* 111:1235–1245, 1988).

EXPERIMENTAL STUDIES

West and Collins (*J Neuropathol Exp Neurol* 48:94–108, 1988) report on cryogenic spinal cord injury in the rat. Electron microscopic studies demonstrate morphological evidence of continuing cellular activity, even 60 days after injury, in axons, astrocytes, and myelinating cells. These studies suggest that damaged axons may be capable of regeneration within the CNS.

The opiate receptor antagonist nalmefene improves neurologic recovery after spinal cord injury in rats (Faden AI et al: *J Pharmacol Exp Ther* 245:742–748, 1988).

Anatomical studies do not demonstrate transsynaptic neuronal degeneration of anterior horn cells after complete transection of the human spinal cord (Kaelan C et al: *J Neurol Sci* 86:231–237, 1988).

Other Topics

Forty-Three Cases of Vertebral Artery Trauma
Reid JDS, Weigelt JA (Univ of Texas Health Science Ctr, Dallas)
J Trauma 28:1007–1012, July 1988   21–15

Injuries to the vertebral artery have been considered rare, but with the available modern diagnostic techniques, vertebral artery injuries are now reported more frequently. Whereas mortality associated with this type of injury once was 90%, the advent of rapid, aggressive resuscitation has significantly improved the survival rate. However, there is still much controversy over the choice of interventional treatment and the role of nonoperative therapy. An 11-year experience with 43 vertebral artery injuries was reviewed.

Thirty-three men and 10 women with a mean age of 27.6 years had trauma, mostly from gunshot or stab wounds to the vertebral artery. Twenty-eight (65%) patients were hemodynamically stable, and 38 (88%) had normal Glasgow Coma Scales. Thirty-two (74%) patients had

Vertebral Artery Trauma:
Operative Findings

Negative	0
Intimal injury	2
Occlusion	8
Disruption	21
Spasm (only)	0
Arteriovenous fistula	2
Total	33

(Courtesy of Reid JDS, Weigelt JA: *J Trauma* 28:1007–1012, July 1988.)

no clinical findings other than a penetrating neck wound or a stable hematoma; the other 11 had expanding hematomas in the neck. Thirty-one (72%) patients had associated cervical injuries. Arteriography was performed in 35 patients; the others were taken directly to the operating room. Six patients were first seen with a neurologic deficit at the level of the cervical spinal cord.

Occlusion was seen on arteriography in 20 (57%) patients. Although the site of injury was accurately identified with arteriography in 34 of the 35 studies, the specific arteriographic diagnosis was not very accurate. For only 13 (50%) of the patients was the specific arteriographic diagnosis confirmed at operation; a disrupted artery was found at operation in 9 patients for whom the preoperative diagnosis had been occlusion.

Forty-one of the 43 patients underwent operation as the initial treatment (table). Thirteen patients underwent proximal ligation, and 28 had proximal and distal ligation. None of the patients underwent arterial reconstruction. The remaining 2 patients were initially observed only, but 1 of these patients required proximal and distal ligation of the artery on day 6 of hospitalization. Two (15%) of the 13 patients who received treatment with proximal vascular control alone had postoperative vascular complications. Three (7%) patients had nonvascular complications. Five (12%) patients died in the hospital, but only 2 (4.7%) deaths were directly related to the vertebral artery injury. The other 38 (88%) patients were discharged from the hospital after a median stay of 7.7 days.

Accurate diagnosis and prompt operative intervention significantly reduces the mortality associated with vertebral artery injuries.

▶ The complications, including the 2 deaths, may have been averted by the use of balloon catheter technique in these patients. Certainly proximal ligation is readily accomplished in most cases by detachable balloon occlusion. In a number of patients distal occlusion could also be accomplished with this methodology.

Compartment Syndromes

Mubarak SJ, Pedowitz RA, Hargens AR (Univ of California, San Diego; VA Med Ctr, San Diego)
Curr Orthop 3:36–40, January 1989   21–16

The compartment syndrome, a condition in which high pressure in a closed fascial space decreases capillary blood perfusion below the level needed for tissue viability, occurs in acute and chronic forms and may be secondary to various causes. An extended period of increased intramuscular pressure may result in irreversible tissue injury and Volkmann's contracture. Knowledge of the pathophysiology, etiology, diagnosis, and treatment of the acute compartment syndrome was reviewed.

The compartments of the musculoskeletal system, containing muscles, nerves, vessels, bones, and connective tissue, are confined by fairly inelastic osseofascial boundaries that normally function to improve the strength and efficiency of the enclosed muscle groups (Fig 21–6). Studies suggest that significant pathophysiologic changes occur when intracompartmental pressures exceed 30–40 mm Hg. Other studies suggest that long-term morbidity does not occur unless pressure exceeds 45 mm Hg or is elevated to within 10–30 mm Hg of the diastolic pressure or within 30–40 mm Hg of the mean arterial blood pressure.

The many causes of the syndrome are all related to either decreased compartmental size or compliance, or both, or to increased intracompart-

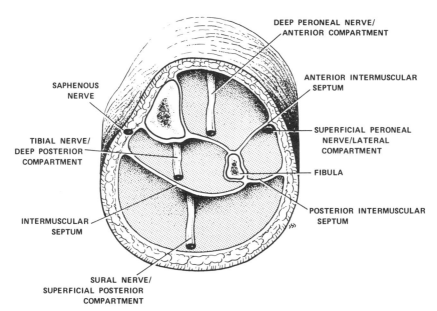

Fig 21–6.—Cross section at the junction of middle and distal thirds of the leg, illustrating the 4 compartments and their respective nerves. (From Mubarak SJ, Pedowitz RA, Hargens AR: *Curr Orthop* 3:36–40, January 1989. Courtesy of Mubarak SJ, Owen CA: *J Bone Joint Surg* 59-A:184–187, 1977.)

mental contents. Decreased compartment size can result from constrictive dressings and casts, closure of fascial defects, and thermal injury or frostbite. Increased intracompartmental contents may be related to bony or soft tissue hemorrhage or edema or both caused by trauma, postischemic reperfusion, burns, a crush injury, or muscle hyperemia and swelling associated with exercise. The most important single factor in correctly diagnosing the syndrome is an adequate clinical index of suspicion. The early findings include pain, pressure, pulses, paresis, parasthesia, and pink color. The goals of treatment are to reduce intracompartmental pressure and improve tissue perfusion.

The compartment syndrome is a condition in which high intracompartmental pressure decreases capillary perfusion, thereby threatening tissue viability. A high index of suspicion is needed to correctly diagnose the syndrome.

Brief Notes on Other Trauma Topics

Clipping of the vertebral artery above and below the site of injury is recommended as an effective technique for hemostasis (Hatzitheofilou C et al: *Br J Surg* 75:234–237, 1988).

For cervical vessel injury after blunt trauma, direct operative repair for accessible lesions is recommended. For surgically inaccessible lesions, intravenous heparin can be started with follow-up studies to determine further therapy (Fakhry SM et al: *J Vasc Surg* 8:501–508, 1988).

Marked flexion of the neck during wrestling caused bilateral vertebral occlusion and sudden death (Rondoyannis GP et al: *Int J Sports Med* 9:353–355, 1988).

Among 64 patients with traumatic brachial artery injury, vascular patency was maintained at 97%, but limb loss resulted from severe soft tissue injury, and functional disability resulted from nerve injury (McCroskey BL et al: *Am J Surg* 156:553–555, 1988).

Weight lifting may be a cause of bilateral upper extremity compartment syndrome (Segan DJ et al: *Physician Sports Med* 16:73–77, 1988).

22 Pediatrics

Introduction

Pediatric tumors attracted considerable attention in 1988. Gadolinium-enhanced magnetic resonance imaging (MRI) is extremely useful for the identification and sizing of central nervous system tumors (Abstract 22–1). A long-term study of juvenile pilocytic astrocytoma indicates that radiation therapy, although not required for completely resected tumors, should be offered to patients aged more than 3 years with incompletely resected juvenile pilocytic astrocytoma (Abstract 22–2). Flow cytometry can be used for prognosis of medulloblastoma (Abstracts 22–3 and 22–4). Suprasellar germinomas in childhood seem best treated by biopsy with subtotal resection, followed by radiation therapy (Abstract 22–5). Dysembryoplastic neuroepithelial tumors appear to have a slow progression with intractable partial seizures and a substantial chance for surgical cure (Daumas-Duport et al, Abstract 22–6). For pineal region tumors in children, open biopsy is suggested with low morbidity (Edwards et al, Abstract 22–7). Preirradiation chemotherapy for pediatric brain tumors permits delay of possibly curative radiotherapy until the child's brain can tolerate radiation (Abstract 22–8).

Radiation leads to growth hormone deficiency but is not the reason for growth retardation in these young patients (Abstract 22–9). Radiotherapy can actually cause intracranial tumors as conclusively demonstrated by extensive statistical study of 10,834 patients who had x-ray treatment for tinea capitis (Ron et al, Abstract 22–10).

Vascular lesions in children have received attention. Cerebral aneurysms during childhood and adolescence are characterized by the posterior fossa location and the high frequency of giant lesions (Abstract 22–11). Endovascular treatment can be offered in some instances. Serial angiograms in moyamoya disease show a shift of flow from internal carotid to posterior cerebral artery over time (Abstract 22–13).

Hydrocephalus remains an important pediatric problem. Ventriculopleural shunts for hydrocephalus may be performed with low morbidity if an antisiphon device is utilized (Abstract 22–14). Epstein and colleagues describe the etiology and treatment of "slit ventricle syndrome" (Abstract 22–15). The key point is the differentiation between shunt malfunction and slit ventricle syndrome. Radionuclide patency scans may assist in the differential diagnoses.

Magnetic resonance imaging after closed head injury affords anatomical evidence of cerebral injury correlating with the severity of clinical findings (Abstract 22–16). Preliminary experience with brachial plexus exploration in children was encouraging, but some children will begin to recover many months after the initial injury, making it difficult to establish clear indications for surgery (Piatt et al, Abstract 22–17).

Tumors

Central Nervous System Lesions in Pediatric Patients: Gd-DTPA-Enhanced MR Imaging

Powers TA, Partain CL, Kessler RM, Freeman MW, Robertson RH, Wyatt SH, Whelan HT (Vanderbilt Univ, Nashville)

Radiology 169:723–726, December 1988   22–1

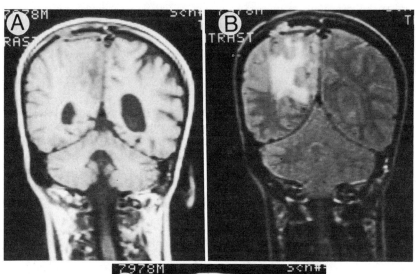

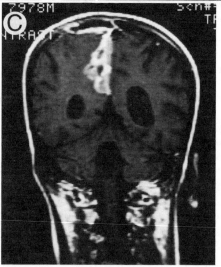

Fig 22–1.—Metastatic medulloblastoma. Precontrast coronal T_1- (A) and T_2-weighted (B) images show a parasagittal area of low signal with surrounding edema. Postoperative changes are present at the vertex. The surgeon saw nodular deposits along the falx but did not perform biopsy of these lesions. Postcontrast T_1-weighted image (C) shows intense enhancement of the metastatic foci as well as the dura overlying the vertex; the latter was due to recent surgery. (Courtesy of Powers TA, Partain CL, Kessler RM, et al: *Radiology* 169:723–726, December 1988.)

Magnetic resonance (MR) imaging has significant advantages over computed tomography in the assessment of lesions of the central nervous system (CNS). However, some lesions are not adequately defined with the usual MR imaging protocols. Gadolinium diethylenetriaminepentaacetic acid (Gd-DTPA) dimeglumine has been under investigation for several years as an MR imaging contrast agent. The efficacy of Gd-DTPA in the evaluation of pediatric patients with known or suspected CNS lesions was studied.

Twenty patients aged 2–18 years were examined with MR imaging at 0.6 tesla with and without 0.1 mmole/kg Gd-DTPA. The multisection, multiecho imaging mode was used. Masses imaged that were later surgically proved included astrocytomas in 6 patients, medulloblastoma in 2 (Fig 22–1), ependymoma in 1, craniopharyngioma in 1, oligodendroglioma in 1, germinoma in 1, and fibrosarcoma in 1. Presumptive diagnoses were made for astrocytomas in 3 cases, arachnoid cyst in 1, tuberous sclerosis in 1, cryptic vascular malformation in 1, and normal in 1. Dramatic enhancement was noted in 11 of 20 patients, with improved definition of the presence and extent of tumors in 6 cases. There was no adverse effect in any of the patients.

For the imaging of a number of lesions, Gd-DTPA has been shown to be useful. This study extended the use of Gd-DTPA to the pediatric population. It was concluded that Gd-DTPA is useful in delineating the presence, extent, and number of certain CNS lesions in children.

▶ This report indicates the utility of gadolinium-enhanced MRI in pediatric patients with intracranial lesions. Substantial enhancement was present in 11 of 20 cases, and improved definition of the presence and extent of tumors was provided for 6 patients. The precise meaning of gadolinium enhancement, however, cannot be established by such a study. Recent correlation between MRI and pathologic findings suggests that the enhancement is not confined simply to the area of the tumor.

Treatment Results of Juvenile Pilocytic Astrocytoma
Wallner KE, Gonzales MF, Edwards MSB, Wara WM, Sheline GE (Univ of California, San Francisco)
J Neurosurg 69:171–176, August 1988   22–2

Juvenile pilocytic astrocytoma (JPA) is usually seen in young children, although patients aged more than 18 years account for about 25% of the cases. The need for radiation after surgery and incomplete removal of the tumor is a matter of some debate. The results of treatment of JPA in 36 patients from 1942 through 1985 were presented.

Twelve of the patients were thought to have complete removal of the tumor, and only 2 of these were given postoperative radiation. None of these 12 experienced a tumor recurrence. All but 1 of those with incomplete removal had a course of irradiation.

Overall, the 10- and 20-year survival rates were 83% and 70%, re-

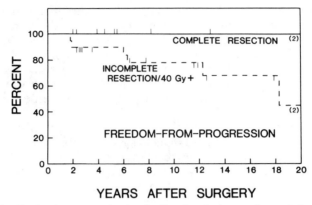

Fig 22-2.—Freedom-from-progression data for 10 patients having complete surgical excision versus those for 21 patients with incomplete excision followed by postoperative irradiation (≥ 40 Gy). *Ticks* represent censored patients; number in parentheses indicate number of patients at risk at that time. (Courtesy of Wallner KE, Gonzales MF, Edwards MSB, et al: *J Neurosurg* 69:171–176, August 1988.)

spectively. Survival rates for those with incomplete resection and treatment with at least 40 Gy was 81% at 10 years and 54% at 20 years. In this group, freedom from progression of the tumor was 74% and 41% at 10 and 20 years (Fig 22–2). All 9 patients who failed treatment were found to have local recurrence.

The data presented here show that complete removal of a JPA offers a survival rate of close to 100%. But those with incomplete resection are at considerable risk for recurrence. The authors recommend adjuvant radiation therapy for all such patients aged more than 3 years. Children aged less than 3 with incomplete removal of a JPA should be carefully monitored and perhaps given chemotherapy if tumor growth is noted.

▶ The results of this long-term study indicate clearly that radiation therapy, although not required in completely resected tumors, should be offered to patients over 3 years of age with incompletely resected juvenile pilocytic astrocytoma. Freedom from progression and actuarial survivorship are presented according to the powerful method of Kaplan and Meier. Figure 22–2 demonstrates graphically the remarkable difference between patients with complete and incomplete resection.

Flow Cytometric DNA Analysis of Medulloblastoma: Prognostic Implication of Aneuploidy
Tomita T, Yasue M, Engelhard HH, McLone DG, Gonzalez-Crussi F, Bauer KD (Northwestern Univ)
Cancer 61:744–749, Feb 15, 1988   22–3

Multiple clinical and therapeutic factors have been described to predict the outcome of patients with medulloblastoma, but the prospective outcome in individual patients remains difficult to predict. Flow cytometric

(FCM) DNA studies that allow a rapid assessment of cellular DNA content are now used in clinical oncology in an effort to link cellular DNA content with the clinical course for various forms of cancer. Because the identification and clinical implication of aneuploidy in patients with medulloblastoma haven not yet been carried out, FCM DNA analysis was used to examine paraffin-embedded surgical medulloblastoma specimens.

The surgical specimens had been obtained from 12 girls and 14 boys, aged 4 months to 14 years at histologic diagnosis, who had undergone a posterior fossa craniotomy between 1972 and 1981. All patients had received radiotherapy, but chemotherapy was not used. Flow cytometric DNA analysis revealed that 13 children had aneuploid medulloblastomas, 12 had diploid medulloblastomas, and 1 child had a tetraploid medulloblastoma.

No correlation was found between the patient's sex and DNA ploidy. The patient's sex and age at diagnosis were not related to survival. More than 5 years after undergoing craniotomy, 16 of the 26 patients were still alive without recurrence of the tumor. The other 10 patients died of recurrences of medulloblastoma, 9 of whom died between 4 and 66 months after operation. One patient survived for more than 5 years. The overall 5-year survival rate among the 26 patients was 65%.

The patients who died included 2 (15.4%) of the 13 patients with aneuploid tumors, 7 (58.3%) of the 12 patients with diploid tumors, and the patient with a tetraploid tumor. Thus, aneuploidy versus diploidy of the medulloblastoma significantly influenced outcome. The extent of tumor resection was also significantly associated with outcome, as only 2 (15.4%) of 13 patients who underwent total resection died, compared with 8 (61.5%) of 13 patients who underwent subtotal resection.

This retrospective FCM DNA analysis of paraffin-embedded surgical specimens indicates that DNA ploidy and extent of surgical resection are the most important determinants of survival in patients with medulloblastoma, provided they were treated with adequate radiation therapy.

▶ This important contribution indicates that patients with diploid or tetraploid medulloblastomas do worse than those with aneuploid tumors. If confirmed by other investigators, this observation could be very useful in selecting cases for especially vigorous adjunctive therapy. The report also confirms once again the superior results for patients undergoing total resection.

Prognostic Importance of DNA Ploidy in Medulloblastoma of Childhood
Yasue M, Tomita T, Engelhard H, Gonzalez-Crussi F, McLone DG, Bauer KD
(Children's Mem Hosp, Chicago; Northwestern Univ)
J Neurosurg 70:385–391, March 1989   22–4

The DNA content in the nuclei of neoplastic cells can be analyzed by flow cytometry and may contribute to the management of patients with various malignancies. The technique of using formalin-fixed paraffin-embedded specimens makes it possible to analyze specimens retrospectively from patients whose clinical outcome is known. This technique was recently used to analyze DNA in 26 medulloblastomas and a significant correlation between DNA ploidy and patient outcome was found. The DNA content was correlated with clinical and histologic findings in a larger group of patients.

The DNA content of 53 medulloblastomas was analyzed by flow cytometry. About half of the tumors were diploid, and half were aneuploid. More diploid tumors occurred among young patients, although the difference was not significant. Cellular differentiation of the tumor and DNA ploidy were not related. Chang's T staging system and DNA ploidy were also not correlated, although the M staging did correlate with ploidy. Diploid medulloblastomas had more of a tendency to metastasize than aneuploid medulloblastomas. When 4-year survival was compared with extent of resection and ploidy, the patients with total resection and aneuploid medulloblastoma were found to have a better prognosis than those with subtotal resection and diploid tumor (Fig 22–3). Only 1 of 8 patients with subtotally resected diploid medulloblastomas survived for 4 years, compared with 5 of the 7 patients with subtotally resected aneuploid medulloblastomas. Comparing the G_0/G_1 phase fraction and S phase fraction in the surviving and deceased groups yielded no significant information.

Cellular ploidy is an important prognostic factor in medulloblastoma. Total resection continues to be the mainstay in the treatment of such patients; surgeons should try to resect as much tumor as possible. Patients with totally resected aneuploid medulloblastomas may require radiotherapy only, whereas those with diploid tumors, especially if resected incompletely, would need more vigorous postoperative therapy, including radiotherapy and chemotherapy.

▶ The results of flow cytometry indicate a worse prognosis for diploid medulloblastomas. If the results of this study can be borne out, then more aggressive

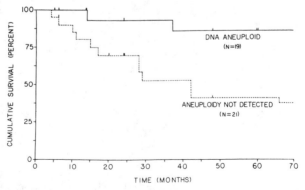

Fig 22–3.—Survival curves of children with medulloblastomas, comparing the aneuploid group with the diploid and tetraploid groups. (Courtesy of Yasue M, Tomita T, Engelhard H, et al: *J Neurosurg* 70:385–391, March 1989.)

treatment protocols involving chemotherapy may be advocated for such patients. These techniques are also being applied to the analysis of other tumors.

Suprasellar Germinomas in Childhood: A Reappraisal

Legido A, Packer RJ, Sutton LN, D'Angio G, Rorke LB, Bruce DA, Schut L (Children's Hosp of Philadelphia; Univ of Pennsylvania, Philadelphia)
Cancer 63:340–344, Jan 15, 1989   22–5

Germinomas account for 0.4% to 9.4% of brain tumors in children and can arise in the suprasellar or pineal region. The best treatment for these tumors has not been established. Although suprasellar germinomas are histologically identical to pineal germinomas, suprasellar lesions appear to have a worse prognosis. The factors that have an impact on outcome were explored.

Between 1976 and 1985, 10 patients with pathologically confirmed suprasellar germinoma were treated with primary surgical debulking and systemic craniospinal axis radiation (CSRT). The outcomes of these patients were compared with those of 4 patients with pineal germinoma treated at the same time and of patient series reported in the literature. The mean age of patients with suprasellar germinoma at diagnosis was 13.9 years. Symptoms had been present for a mean of 18 months and included diabetes insipidus, anterior pituitary dysfunction, decreased vision, headache, vomiting, and diplopia. Staging studies showed dissemination in only 1 case.

Operative treatment involved biopsy in 3 patients, partial resection of the tumor in 5, and total resection in 2. There were no permanent postoperative complications. Tumor sites received a mean radiation therapy dose of 4,953 centigray (cGy). The spine received a mean dose of 3,354 cGy. The patients were followed up for 1.9–10.5 years. In 1 child with suprasellar germinoma who did not receive therapy initially a pineal tumor developed after diagnosis. She was treated with primary surgical debulking and CSRT and was asymptomatic 5 years later. The rest of the children were alive and disease-free at their last follow-up examination.

Primary surgical debulking and CSRT produced excellent results in these 10 patients, all of whom are alive and without disease. This outcome is similar to that achieved in children with pineal germinoma, which is generally considered to have a better prognosis than suprasellar germinoma.

▶ The results of this study indicate good outcome for patients with surgical histologic confirmation and radiation therapy for suprasellar germinoma. Careful review of the data indicated that the 2 patients with total resection both experienced neurologic disturbance, including hypopituitarism, diabetes insipidus, and visual impairment. Because these patients were no worse off than those undergoing biopsy of subtotal resection from the standpoint of effectiveness of therapy, the experience tends to support a careful biopsy and subtotal resection as the preferred surgical approach with the least risk.

Dysembryoplastic Neuroepithelial Tumor: A Surgically Curable Tumor of Young Patients With Intractable Partial Seizures: Report of Thirty-Nine Cases

Daumas-Duport C, Scheithauer BW, Chodkiewicz J-P, Laws ER Jr, Vedrenne C
(Hôpital Ste Anne, Paris; Mayo Graduate School of Medicine, Rochester, Minn)
Neurosurgery 23:545–556, November 1988   22–6

Some complex neuroepithelial tumors develop in patients operated on because of long-standing complex partial seizures, usually starting during early childhood. The term *dysembryoplastic neuroepithelial tumor* (DNT) connotes a probable dysembryogenic origin for these lesions. These tumors are made up of astrocytes, oligodendrocytes, and neurons. Neuronal atypia often is not apparent.

The mean age at the onset of symptoms was 9 years, and at operation, 18 years. All but 3 patients had partial seizures that were consistently drug-resistant and disabling. Most patients had normal neurologic findings interictally. Four patients had a history of head injury. Computed tomography frequently disclosed a hypodense lesion having a cystic appearance (Fig 22–4). All the tumors were supratentorial. Most of them superficially resembled oligoastrocytoma. Foci of cortical dysplasia were frequent observed.

All gross tumor was removed in 22 patients. Thirteen patients received adjunctive radiotherapy. Two deaths were unrelated to tumor. None of the 37 surviving patients had evidence of recurrence during a mean follow-up of 9 years. Seizures were absent in 30 patients and rare in 3; 4 patients have had significantly fewer seizures than before resection. One patient had computed tomographic findings of radionecrosis.

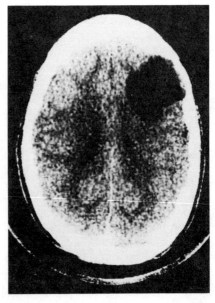

Fig 22–4.—Contrast computed tomography scan. The lesion appears as a well-demarcated low attenuation area with a pseudocystic appearance. The tumor is associated with a deformity of the overlying calvarium. (Courtesy of Daumas-Duport C, Scheithauer BW, Chodkiewicz J-P, et al: *Neurosurgery* 23:545–556, November 1988.)

When DNTs are recognized, aggressive treatment can be avoided, sparing these young patients the adverse long-term sequelae of radiotherapy and chemotherapy. The tumors quite often are the cause of partial complex seizures.

▶ Dysembryoplastic neuroepithelial tumor appears to be a special pathologic determination on the basis of this study of 37 cases. The pathologic diagnosis is important because of the slow progression of the lesions and the possibility of surgical cure. Further pathologic experience will be needed in order to confirm this entity in other centers.

Pineal Region Tumors in Children
Edwards MSB, Hudgkins RJ, Wilson CB, Levin VA, Wara WM (Univ of California, San Francisco)
J Neurosurg 68:689–697, May 1988   22–7

Many pineal tumors are benign or radioresistant. Because even low doses of radiation may impair the developing brain, definitive surgery with histologic diagnosis may be preferable to shunting and radiotherapy. Thirty-six children aged less than 18 years were treated for pineal tumors between 1974 and 1986. Eleven patients had germinomas, 7 had astrocytomas, and the rest had 15 different histologic types of tumors. Levels of β-human chorionic gonadotropin or α-fetoprotein were significantly elevated in 8 of 23 cases (table).

Thirty patients were operated on with no mortality, but 10% of patients had persistent morbidity. On a median follow-up of 4 years, 9 of 11 patients with germinoma were alive without recurrent disease. Six of

Tumor Markers Assayed in 23 Patients With Pineal Tumors

Histology	No. Assayed	Elevated AFP	Elevated β-HCG	Both Elevated	Neither Elevated
germinoma	10	—	3	—	7
malignant teratoma	2	—	—	2	—
endodermal sinus tumor	2	2	—	—	—
pineocytoma	2	—	—	—	2
undifferentiated germ-cell tumor	2	1	—	1	—
pineocytoma/ pineoblastoma	1	—	—	—	1
choriocarcinoma	1	—	1	—	—
embryonal cell tumor	1	—	—	1	—
malignant teratoma/ embryonal cell tumor	1	—	—	1	—
teratoma	1	—	—	—	1

Abbreviations: AFP, α-fetoprotein; β-HCG, β-human chorionic gonadotropin; —, test not performed.
(Courtesy of Edwards MSB, Hudgkins RJ, Wilson CB, et al: *J Neurosurg* 68:689–697, May 1988.)

7 patients with astrocytoma were well after biopsy and radiotherapy. Five of the remaining 18 children (28%) died of progressive tumor.

Histologic diagnosis is suggested in all cases of pineal tumor. These tumors require different approaches to treatment, and modern microsurgery carries low mortality and morbidity. Multidrug chemotherapy may offer a better approach to these tumors than radiotherapy. In any case, careful staging allows treatment to be tailored in individual cases to minimize toxicity.

▶ This report documents low morbidity and no mortality among 36 children with microsurgical exploration of pineal region tumors. Histologic diagnosis is suggested for all cases of pineal tumor. Stereotactic biopsy, however, suffers from sampling problems, which may be especially important in tumors of mixed cell type (8%). Even in the age of accurate localization with MRI and the assist gained from tumor markers, surgical biopsy via open microsurgery appears to be appropriate for the majority of these patients.

Distephani and associates (1) report that among 6 pineocytomas treated with focal radiation (45–54 Gy), 3 were free of disease at 21–84 months, and 1 recurred in local and disseminated areas. Craniospinal radiation is warranted only for dissemination on staging.

Reference

1. Distephani A et al: *Cancer* 63:302–304, 1989.

Feasibility and Efficacy of Preirradiation Chemotherapy for Pediatric Brain Tumors
Horowitz ME, Kun LE, Mulhern RK, Kovnar EH, Sanford RA, Hockenberger GM, Greeson FL, Langston JW, Fairclough DL, Jenkins JJ III (St Jude Children's Research Hosp; Univ of Tennessee, Memphis)
Neurosurgery 22:687–690, 1988   22–8

Preirradiation chemotherapy is potentially an important component of combined therapy for brain tumors. However, concern about side effects and antitumor activity of such therapy has impeded its assessment in clinical trials. A study was done to determine the feasibility of administering such therapy to children.

Thirty-eight children with brain tumors with a median age of 2 years were treated with 12 weeks of combination chemotherapy after surgical resection and before irradiation. Transient myelosuppression occurred in all patients but was not associated with infections or complications of surgical wounds. The ability to perform activities of daily living, as rated with the Karnofsky performance scale, was improved in 14 children and unchanged in 18 children at the end of the evaluation period. In the rest of the group, functional deterioration was obviously related to causes other than drug treatment. Previous chemotherapy did not compromise the delivery of radiotherapy, except for a brief interruption of spinal irradiation in 3 patients.

Objective responses to chemotherapy, which were defined as a greater than 50% decrease in tumor masses, occurred in 16 of the 31 children who had subtotal resections. Only 6 patients showed disease progression during the 12 weeks of drug administration.

The efficacy and safety of preirradiation chemotherapy in children with brain tumors was demonstrated. Chemotherapy of the type used is well tolerated and produces beneficial effects in such patients.

▶ This carefully presented communication demonstrates the safety of preirradiation chemotherapy with objective responses in 16 of 31 children. This could allow for delay of possibly curative radiotherapy until the child's brain has matured to the point of tolerating radiotherapy without serious consequences. In the treatment of malignant intracranial germ cell tumors in children, systematic use of preirradiation chemotherapy for reduction of radiation dose appears to improve prognosis (1).

Reference

1. Deméocg F et al: *Presse Med* 17:2183–2185, 1988.

Brief Notes on Tumors in Children

MEDULLOBLASTOMA

Phenotypic analysis of 4 human medulloblastoma cell lines showed biologic differences (He X et al: *J Neuropathol Exp Neurol* 48:48–68, 1989).

Cerebellar medulloblastoma may be multifocal (Shen WC, Yang CF: *J Comput Assist Tomogr* 2:894–902, 1988).

Primitive neuroectodermal tumor and medulloblastoma may reoccur late, and the period of risk is probably indefinite (Lefkowitz IB et al: *Cancer* 62:826–830, 1988).

Multidrug chemotherapy is at least transiently effective in improving the rate of disease-free survival for children with poor risk medulloblastoma (Packer RJ et al: *Ann Neurol* 24:503–508, 1988).

NEUROBLASTOMA

In neuroblastoma, DNA aneuploidy is a favorable prognosticator, whereas it is a bad indicator for outcome with ganglioneuroma (Taylor SR et al: *Cancer* 62:749–754, 1988).

Histamine may induce intracellular free calcium and electrical changes in neuroblastoma cells (Oakes SG et al: *J Pharmacol Exp Ther* 247:114–121, 1988).

Deferoxamine can inhibit neuroblastoma viability and proliferation (Becton DL, Brylas P: *Cancer Res* 48:7189–7192, 1988).

Congenital cervical neuroblastoma may be associated with Horner's syndrome (Ogita S et al: *J Pediatr Surg* 23:991–992, 1988).

OTHER TUMORS

Elster and Arthur (*J Comput Assist Tomogr* 12:736–739, 1988) report on intracranial hemangioblastomas. In 8 patients, a single tumor was missed with CT, and none were missed with MRI. The tumor nodule when present was identified in every case using MRI, which is found to be the superior study for this problem.

Immunohistochemical studies demonstrate antibodies against substance P and neuropeptide YY in cerebellar hemangioblastomas (Becker I et al: *Am J Pathol* 134:271–275, 1989).

Congenital quadrantanopia is reported with occipital lobe ganglioglioma (Fletcher WA et al: *Neurology* 38:1892–1894, 1988).

In an experience with 15 children with recurrent gliomas treated with lomustine and vincristine, long-term disease stabilization was recorded in the majority of children (Lefkowitz IB et al: *Cancer* 61:896–902, 1988).

Primary central nervous system germ cell tumors are best treated with histologic confirmation and radiation of 5,000 cGy (Kersh CR: *Cancer* 61:2148–2152, 1988).

Brain tumors in infants aged less than a year included astrocytoma, ganglioglioma, and primitive neuroectodermal tumors, radiologically and pathologically similar to analogous lesions in adults (Ambrosino MM et al: *Pediatr Radiol* 19:6–8, 1988).

Glomus tumors can rarely occur in the pediatric age group (Bartels LJ, Gurucharri M: *Otolaryngol Head Neck Surg* 98:392–395, 1988).

EPIDEMIOLOGY

Paternal exposure to ionizing radiation based on industrial codes is positively associated with CNS tumor risks in children (Nasca PC et al: *Am J Epidemiol* 128:1256–1265, 1988).

A mortality-based, case control study of selected risk factors for childhood brain tumors suggests that parental occupation is a potential risk factor (Wilkins JR, Kutras RA: *Am J Ind Med* 14:299–318, 1988).

Epidemiologic studies show a relationship between gliomas and exposure to wood preservatives (Cordier S et al: *Br J Ind Med* 45:705–709, 1988).

Radiation

A Prospective Study of the Development of Growth Hormone Deficiency in Children Given Cranial Irradiation, and Its Relation to Statural Growth
Brauner R, Rappaport R, Prevot C, Czernichow P, Zucker J-M, Bataini P, Lemerle J, Sarrazin D, Guyda HJ (Hôpital des Enfants-Malades; Institut Curie, Paris; Institut Gustave Roussy, Villejuif, France; McGill Univ, Montreal)
J Clin Endocrinol Metab 68:346–351, February 1989   22–9

Cranial irradiation is associated with a high incidence of hypopituitarism. Growth hormone (GH) deficiency is the most common hormonal abnormality occurring after such therapy. The natural course of this complication and its relationship to growth in children were investigated.

Sixteen children, aged 1.7–15 years at the time of treatment, were followed up for 2 years. They had all received cranial and spinal radiation therapy for medulloblastoma or ependymoma. The growth of these children was compared with that of 11 children given similar doses of cranial radiation only. Mean plasma GH responses to arginine-insulin testing

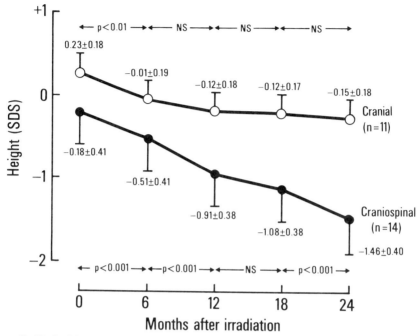

Fig 22–5.—Mean (±SE) changes in height after craniospinal (group 1) or cranial (group 2) radiation. (Courtesy of Brauner R, Rappaport R, Prevot C, et al: *J Clin Endocrinol Metab* 68:346–351, February 1989.)

(AITT) were 9.1 µg/L in the first group and 8.5 µg/L in the second group. After 2 years, 16 of the total 27 children had a peak plasma GH value of less than 8 µg/L after AITT, and 10 had a peak response of less than 5 µg/L. After 2 years, children receiving cranial and spinal radiation therapy had a mean height of 1.46 standard deviations below the normal mean. The children receiving cranial radiation therapy only had a mean height of 0.15 standard deviations below normal (Fig 22–5).

Growth hormone deficiency is an early complication of cranial radiation in children treated for medulloblastoma or ependymoma. No significant growth retardation can be attributed to GH deficiency in the first 2 years. When spinal radiation was included in the treatment, most of the growth failure was related to spinal radiation-induced lesions, with a pattern of progressive height deficiency during the 2-year follow-up. Monitoring growth thus remains essential during the early postirradiation period.

▶ This nice study provides quantitative prospective data regarding the frequency and magnitude of growth hormone deficiency in children given cranial irradiation. Such deficiency is not the reason for growth retardation during the first 2 years after this treatment. These important side effects of cranial irradiation in the young are to be recalled in relation to mental changes that follow cranial irradiation in other patients.

Tumors of the Brain and Nervous System After Radiotherapy in Childhood

Ron E, Modan B, Boice JD Jr, Alfandary E, Stovall M, Chetrit A, Katz L (Chaim Sheba Med Ctr, Tel Hashomer, Israel; Natl Cancer Inst, Bethesda, Md; Univ of Texas, Houston; Israel Cancer Registry, Jerusalem)
N Engl J Med 319:1033–1039, Oct 20, 1988   22–10

In 1974, a significant increase in brain tumors was reported among 10,834 persons who had undergone cranial irradiation in childhood to treat tinea capitis. In an additional 10-year period reviewing individual radiation doses to the brain, data on 10,834 patients who had x-ray irradiation for tinea capitis between 1948 and 1960 were compared with data on 10,834 nonirradiated individuals and 5,392 nonirradiated siblings. All irradiated patients were less than 16 years old when treated. Benign and malignant tumors were identified from the pathology records of all Israeli hospitals and from Israeli national cancer and death registries. Radiation doses to neural tissues were estimated retrospectively.

Sixty of the 73 patients who had neural tumors had been irradiated in childhood; 8 others were from the general population, and 5 were among the siblings. Fifty-six of the 60 neural tumors in the irradiated patients were located in the head and neck, and 16 were malignant. The incidence of tumors was 1.8/10,000 persons per year. After a maximum follow-up of 33 years, the cumulative risk for all neural tumors was only 0.09% for individuals from the general population as compared with 0.84% for the irradiated patients (Fig 22–6). The estimated relative risk in the irradi-

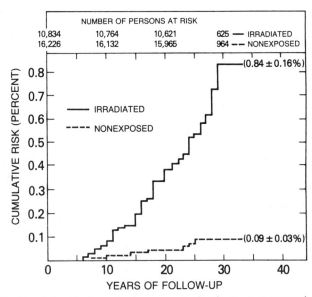

Fig 22–6.—Cumulative risk of neural tumors among irradiated patients, as compared with the combined control groups. (Courtesy of Ron E, Modan B, Boice JD Jr, et al: *N Engl J Med* 319:1033–1039, Oct 20, 1988.)

ated individuals as compared with the general population and siblings was 6.9 for all tumors, with a risk factor of 8.4 when the analysis was restricted to neural tumors of the head and neck. An increased relative risk was observed for meningiomas (9.5), gliomas (2.6), nerve-sheath tumors (18.8), and other neural tumors (3.4). There was a strong dose-response relationship, with the relative risk approaching 20 after estimated radiation doses of approximately 2.5 Gy.

▶ This very important study indicates that exposure to radiation can cause CNS tumors. This long-term side effect of radiation therapy must be borne in mind when considering this form of treatment. Although this complication is unlikely to be encountered in patients undergoing x-ray therapy for intracranial malignancy, it would be more likely in patients undergoing radiation therapy for benign disease, such as inoperable meningioma or other benign tumors. These complications would also lend support to the concept of focused radiation, whereby stereotactically focused beams of radiation are preferentially aimed at a target location with relative sparing of surrounding tissue, which thus would be expected to have a lower risk of later oncogenesis.

Brief Notes on Complications of Radiation Therapy

Two cases of malignant astrocytoma occurred within the radiation field for childhood germinoma and craniopharyngioma. Both of these lesions were not present at the primary site (Kitanaka C et al: *J Neurosurg* 70:469–474, 1989).

Hypothalamic insufficiency and dementia occurred 60 months after irradiation with 54 Gy for pinealoma, and dramatic recovery occurred after hydrocortisone and thyroxine management (Nighoghossian N et al: *Rev Neurol (Paris)* 144:215–218, 1988).

Olfactory acuity may be reduced by radiation exposure of the olfactory mucosa (Ophir D et al: *Arch Otolaryngol Head Neck Surg* 114:853–855, 1988).

Vascular

Cerebral Aneurysms in Childhood and Adolescence
Meyer FB, Sundt TM Jr, Fode NC, Morgan MK, Forbes GS, Mellinger JF (Mayo Clinic, Rochester, Minn)
J Neurosurg 70:420–425, March 1989   22–11

Intracranial aneurysms in children are rare. Such aneurysms have several distinct characteristics in children, suggesting a pathophysiologic entity distinct from aneurysms in adults. The surgical experience with 24 aneurysms occurring in 23 children was reviewed.

The patients had a mean age of 12 years; the youngest was 3 months old. The male-female ratio was 2.8:1. Mycotic lesions and lesions associated with other vascular malformations were excluded from the analysis. Forty-two percent of the aneurysms were found in the posterior circulation. Fifty-four percent were giant aneurysms. In 13 patients the finding on presentation was subarachnoid hemorrhage and in 11, a mass effect. Several of the aneurysms rapidly increased in size over a 3-month to 2-

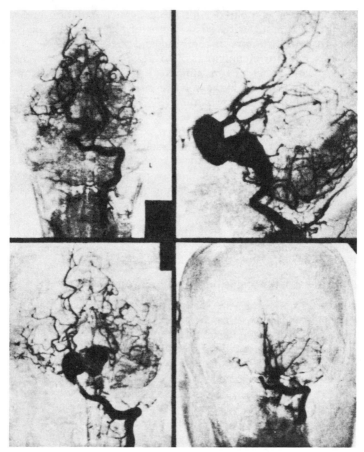

Fig 22–7.—Upper left, left vertebral angiogram obtained during evaluation of giant carotid aneurysm demonstrating mild irregularity and dilatation of both the vertebral and basilar arteries. **Upper right and lower left,** angiograms obtained 2 years later demonstrating progression of the basilar dilatation into a giant bilobed aneurysm. The patient tolerated a 10-minute trial balloon-occlusion of the vertebral artery because of collateral flow from a patent left posterior communicating artery. The base of the aneurysm was clipped from a suboccipital approach with preservation of the left anterior inferior cerebellar artery. **Lower right,** postoperative angiogram demonstrating obliteration of the aneurysm. (Courtesy of Meyer FB, Sundt TM Jr, Fode NC, et al: *J Neurosurg* 70:420–425, March 1989.)

year observation period. All patients were treated surgically. Direct clipping was done in 14 patients, trapping with bypass in 4, trapping alone in 4, and direct excision with end-to-end anastomosis in 2. The outcome was excellent in 87% of the patients, good in 8%, and poor in 1 (Fig 22–7). This patient had only a mild decrease in manual dexterity after the second operation but died 5 months later, probably of a recurrent basilar aneurysm.

Pediatric aneurysms have unique features that make them distinct from aneurysms in adults. Those features include male predominance, a high percentage of giant aneurysms, and an unusual location. Although pediatric aneurysms are rare, physicians should consider them in an initial differential diagnosis. With contemporary microsurgical and neuroanesthetic techniques, an excellent surgical outcome can be achieved in most cases.

▶ In this report from the Mayo Clinic, pediatric aneurysms occurred most commonly in boys, with a high percentage of giant aneurysms often in unusual locations. Histology on a few of these lesions was not different from that found in adult aneurysms. The etiology is thought most consistent with a degenerative theory rather than congenital, and the possibility of traumatic factors is considered by the authors.

Intracranial Arteriovenous Vascular Lesions in Children: Endovascular Techniques Interest About 44 Cases
Rodesch G, Lasjaunias P, Terbrugge K, Burrows P (Hôpital de Bicêtre, Le Kremlin-Bicêtre, France; Toronto Western Hosp; The Hosp for Sick Children, Toronto)
Neurochirurgie 34:293–303, 1988   22–12

The diagnosis and treatment of intravascular cerebral arteriovenous malformations (AVMs) in children present specific technical difficulties not encountered in adults. Although AVMs in children are simpler than those in adults, because they show few or no acquired changes in angioarchitecture, children cannot be treated as miniature adults. The natural history of cerebral AVMs in children has not been well studied. To assess the clinicial manifestations, treatment, and vascular architecture of brain AVMs in children, the records of 25 boys and 19 girls aged 3 days to 15 years were reviewed. Children with undiagnosed AVMs requiring emergency surgery because of acute cerebral hemorrhage were excluded from the study.

Of the 44 children, 20 had AVMs with aneurysmal ectasia of the vein of Galen, 21 had parenchymal or choroid AVMs without vein of Galen abnormalities, and 3 had congenital dural arteriovenous fistulas. Nine (20%) patients had multiple lesions, most commonly arteriovenous fistulas. Thus there was a higher incidence of multiple lesions and a lower incidence of associated arterial aneurysms than commonly found in adult study populations.

Twenty-four (54.5%) patients who underwent intravascular embolization alone had a total of 64 procedures with instruments specially adapted for use in children. Anatomical cure was achieved in 4 (16.6%) of these 24 patients. Significant clinical improvement, including cessation of headaches, improved neurologic signs, and a decrease in epileptic episodes, was achieved in 12 (50%) patients. Embolization had no beneficial effect on clinical symptoms in 4 (16.6%) patients. Anatomical cure was achieved in another 3 patients who underwent intravascular embolization combined with surgical procedures. One newborn infant died during the procedure, 1 child died of thrombosis of the vein of Galen 24 hours after the procedure, and 1 child died after a partial procedure; all 3 deaths occurred in children younger than 5 years of age. Morbidity associated with intravascular procedures was low: of the 64 procedures performed, only 5 (7.2%) complications were directly attributable to the procedure itself, 2 (3.1%) of which were transient neurologic symptoms. Overall, very good clinical results were obtained in 19 (79.2%) of the 24 treated patients, with anatomical cure achieved in 7 (30.4%) cases.

Intravascular embolization in the treatment of congenital intracranial AVMs in children produces good clinical results. The morbidity and mortality associated with the procedure can be considered acceptable.

▶ This communication demonstrates that certain AVMs in children may be treated by an endovascular route. In some cases total obliteration may be obtained; in others, reduction in lesion size for eventual surgical excision is attained. The method is not without some risk, however, in that 3 patients aged less than 5 years died.

Analysis of the Angiographic Findings in Cases of Childhood Moyamoya Disease
Satoh S, Shibuya H, Matsushima Y, Suzuki S (Tokyo Med and Dental Univ)
Neuroradiology 30:111–119, April 1988   22–13

The cerebral angiographic findings in 34 cases of childhood moyamoya disease were reviewed. The mean age was 7.5 years, and the average age at onset was 5.1 years. Thirty patients had transient hemiparesis and multifocal symptoms such as headache and visual disturbance. Five patients had seizures.

Flow to abnormal netlike vessels at the base of the brain was mainly from the internal carotid artery in early cases, whereas later the blood supply was chiefly from the posterior cerebral artery. There was no marked change in volumes of abnormal netlike vessels over the course of illness. However, leptomeningeal collaterals tended to decrease later in the course as posterior cerebral artery stenosis developed. Eighteen occlusive posterior cerebral artery lesions were found, both proximally (Fig 22–8) and distally. Only 2 small aneurysms in the abnormal netlike vessels were discovered.

Abnormal netlike vessels are more extensive in children than in adults with moyamoya disease, but intracranial bleeding and aneurysms are relatively infrequent in children. Bilaterality is a feature of childhood cases; adult disease usually is unilateral. Childhood and adult moyamoya disease may be different entities. In the present series, the angiographic findings were similar in Japanese children and those of other races.

▶ Serial angiograms were used to characterize the temporal evolution of moyamoya disease in childhood. A shift of flow to the abnormal netlike vessels from internal carotid to posterior cerebral artery was demonstrated over time. This sort of careful angiographic temporal profile, combined with clinical observa-

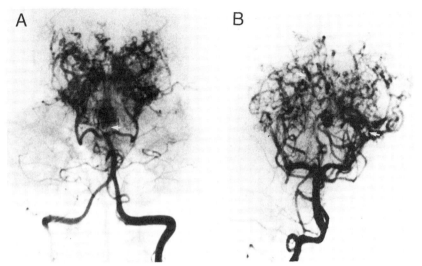

Fig 22–8.—**A,** left vertebral and left internal carotid angiograms, Towne's projection, arterial phase (stage 5). Left posterior cerebral artery (PCA) is occluded at the proximal site *(arrow).* **B,** right vertebral angiogram, Towne's projection, arterial phase (stage 4). Right PCA is irregular *(arrowheads)* and occluded at the distal site *(arrow).* (Courtesy of Satoh S, Shibuya H, Matsushima Y, et al: *Neuroradiology* 30:111–119, April 1988.)

tions, will be necessary to adequately characterize the clinical evolution of this illness. Only such controlled observations will permit eventual evaluation and possible validation of such treatment measures as the encephaloduroarteriosynangiosis.

Brief Notes on Moyamoya Disease

In 11 cases of moyamoya disease treated with indirect nonanastomotic revascularization, recurrent ischemia occurred that was eliminated by subsequent EC-IC bypass (Mujamoto J et al: *J Neurosurg* 68:537–543, 1988).

Maki and Enomoto present an overview of moyamoya disease (*Childs Nerv Syst* 4:204–212, 1988).

Recurrent intracranial hemorrhage occurred in adults with moyamoya disease (Kaufman M et al: *Can J Neurol Sci* 15:430–434, 1988).

Hydrocephalus

Ventriculopleural Shunts for Hydrocephalus: A Useful Alternative
Jones RFC, Currie BG, Kwok BCT (Prince of Wales Children's Hosp, Randwick, Australia)
Neurosurgery 23:753–755, December 1988   22–14

Ventriculopleural shunts are not often used in the treatment of hydrocephalus. Although the pleural cavity has long been considered a suitable site for a short-term shunt, the high incidence of large pleural effusions has dissuaded surgeons from using it in long-term shunting. A group of patients in whom hydrocephalus was well controlled by shunting was described.

Twenty-nine children with progressive hydrocephalus seen from 1969 to 1979 were treated with ventriculopleural shunts. A standard Pudenz pump with a Raimondi catheter was used at that time for all but 1 child, in whom a Holter valve was used. This shunt worked adequately in 7 cases. In the remaining 18 children, however, it had to be changed because of symptomatic pleural effusion. From 1979 to 1982, an additional 52 children were treated with ventriculopleural shunts. At that time, a Portnoy ventricular catheter or a medium- or high-pressure Heyer Schulte pump with an antisiphon device and a Salmon distal catheter was used. Shunt infection developed in 3 children. One child died with the shunt functioning. Four catheters were blocked by adhesions. In only 1 case was a peritoneal shunt substituted because of symptomatic effusion.

In the first group of patients, the problems with pleural shunts were well demonstrated. However, after the differential pressure valve and antisiphon device were used, only 1 in 52 children needed conversion to a peritoneal catheter because of symptomatic hydrothorax. This shunt is a useful long-term alternative to the peritoneal shunt.

▶ This useful communication documents that specially constructed ventriculopleural shunts may produce a good long-term treatment for hydrocephalus. In the hands of this surgical group, a medium- or high-pressure Heyer Schulte valve with an antisiphon device seemed to be effective in avoiding pleural effusion.

"Slit-Ventricle Syndrome": Etiology and Treatment

Epstein F, Lapras C, Wisoff JH (New York Univ Med Ctr; Hôpital Neurologique et Neurochirurgical Pierre Wertheimer, New York)
Pediatr Neurosci 14:5–10, December 1988   22–15

The slit-ventricle syndrome consists of chronic or recurring headache associated with normal or subnormal ventricular volume in shunted hydrocephalic children. The computed tomography (CT) scan has shown that normal or small ventricles are a common entity after a successful shunt and are not related to an increased incidence of shunt malfunction. However, there is a small group of symptomatic children with normal or near normal ventricular volume who may be identified as having slit-ventricle syndrome.

From 1970 to 1986, 20 patients were treated for this syndrome. In 6, intermittent shunt malformation was the underlying problem; in 14, there was increased intracranial pressure not associated with demonstrable shunt dysfunction. In the first group, all children had typical signs and symptoms of the syndrome, including intermittent headache and vomiting. Normal or subnormal ventricular volume during symptomatic remission and slight to moderate ventriculomegaly during symptomatic episodes were disclosed with CT scanning. In all of these children, the

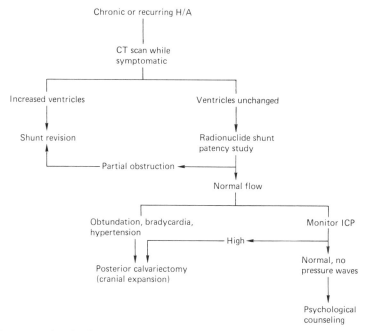

Fig 22-9.—Algorithm for treatment of severe headache *(H/A)* in a child with slit ventricles. (Courtesy of Epstein F, Lapras C, Wisoff JH: *Pediatr Neurosci* 14:5–10, December 1988.)

ventricles returned to normal volume within a few hours of dissipation of symptoms. A malfunctioning ventricular catheter was found in all of these patients. After shunt revision, all became asymptomatic. In the second group, 12 patients with intermittent headache and vomiting included 3 patients with the life-threatening signs and symptoms of obtundation, bradycardia, hypertension, and extensor posturing. Normal function was confirmed by radionuclide shunt patency scans. Treatment in this group consisted of a calvarial expansion procedure (Fig 22–9).

In this series, 6 children had intermittent proximal shunt malfunction, and 14 had increased intracranial pressure with normal shunt function. In the second group, all of the children had a relatively small calvarium. The first group was treated with proximal shunt revision, and the second was treated with a calvarial expansion procedure.

▶ This helpful communication points out that there is a great difference between shunt malfunction and slit-ventricle syndrome. The former may be diagnosed by radionuclide shunt patency scans and treated with revision. The latter, after diagnosis with scanning, will require a cranial depression procedure.

Brief Notes on Hydrocephalus

When to Shunt in Normal Pressure Hydrocephalus?—When extended electroencephalography is carried out in patients with normal pressure hydrocephalus, there may be changes that are difficult to see without computerized analysis. These, in turn, may change when cerebrospinal fluid is partly drained by lumbar puncture. According to Hadeishi and colleagues of Akita, Japan (*Neurol Med Chir [Tokyo]* 28:176–182, April 1988), graphs of time-dependent changes of the EEG with CSF pressures may show changes of prognostic significance. If the magnitude or duration of alpha and beta waves increases, and that of delta waves decreases, in response to reduction of CSF pressure, the patient is a good candidate for CSF drainage. Seven of 9 patients with normal pressure hydrocephalus thus studied improved clinically after ventriculoperitoneal shunting. The authors warn that one should watch for complications of shunting with low-pressure shunt systems, including subdural effusion or hematoma.— O. Sugar, M.D.

Massive peritoneal cyst may occur as a complication of ventriculoperitoneal shunting (Gamao R, Moore TC: *J Pediatr Surg* 23:1041–1042, 1988).

In order to estimate the pressure-volume index in childhood macrocephaly, the ventricle volume rather than cerebrospinal volume should be used (Gooskens RHJN et al: *Childs Nerv Syst* 4:233–236, 1988).

In 34 cases of ventriculostomy with an Ommaya device and external butter-fly needle and shunt valve, drainage was maintained an average of 16 days with no infections (Chan K-H, Mann KS: *Neurosurgery* 23:436–438, 1988).

Stereotactic ventriculocisternostomy is recommended as an effective treatment for triventricular obstructive hydrocephalus (Musolino A et al: *Neurochirurgie* 34:361–373, 1988).

Sudden infant apnea may be associated with insidious hydrocephalus (Bromberger P et al: *Childs Nerv Syst* 4:241–243, 1988).

Pediatric surveys demonstrate that misconceptions about the impact of hydrocephalus in children with myelomeningocele have an impact on pediatricians' decisions about treatment of these patients (Siperstein GN et al: *J Pediatr* 113:835–840, 1988).

Other Topics

Magnetic Resonance Imaging After Closed Head Injury in Children

Levin HS, Amparo EG, Eisenberg HM, Miner ME, High WM Jr, Ewing-Cobbs L, Fletcher JM, Guinto FC Jr (Univ of Texas, Galveston and Houston; Univ of Houston)
Neurosurgery 24:223–227, February 1989   22–16

Recent studies of adults with closed head injury (CHI) have shown that magnetic resonance imaging (MRI) often demonstrates brain lesions that are not detected with computed tomography (CT) in mild to moderate and severe injuries. Neuroimaging of structural changes during cerebral maturation may elucidate substrates underlying neurobehavioral complications of head-injured children with relatively normal CT scans. The MRI findings in 21 children and adolescents who underwent imaging at least 6 months after CHI were reviewed.

Areas of high intensity in the parenchyma were seen in 8 of 11 severely injured patients; MRI findings were normal in all 10 patients with mild to moderate injuries. Lesions involving the subcortical white matter were observed only in severely injured patients whose clinical features were compatible with diffuse axonal injury. Neuropsychologic examination revealed deficits primarily in the severely injured patients. These deficits were significantly associated with persistent lesions seen on MRI.

Areas of high intensity were revealed with MRI in the parenchyma of 73% of children and adolescents studied at least 1 year after severe CHI. Findings of lesions in the subcortical white matter and occipital regions were not seen on early CT examination. Serial MRI and neurobehavioral evaluation after early injury may be useful in documenting cognitive impairment related to structural changes of the young brain.

▶ Serial MRI and neuropsychologic evaluation are likely to be helpful in the evaluation and management of patients with head injury, particularly in the mild and moderate injury categories. These studies provide objective evidence of injury, which is useful to the rehabilitation of these patients.

A related study reports that adolescents with closed head injuries experience pervasive cognitive deficits after injury that may potentially interfere with reentry in the home, school, and social activities (1).

Reference

1. Slater EJ, Bassett SS: *Am J Dis Child* 149:1048–1051, 1988.

Preliminary Experiences With Brachial Plexus Exploration in Children: Birth Injury and Vehicular Trauma
Piatt JH Jr, Hudson AR, Hoffman HJ (Univ of Toronto; Dept of the Army, Fort Sam Houston, Tex)
Neurosurgery 22:715–723, April 1988   22–17

Preliminary experience in the microsurgical treatment of brachial plexus birth injuries was reviewed. Because the patients had had surgical exploration after age 6 months, there was enough time for axonal regeneration to reach most target muscles. Intraoperative evaluation of lesions is based on electrical stimulation of nerve trunks. When stimulation across a lesion in continuity elicits contractions in appropriate muscles, it is assumed that external neurolysis is preferable to resection and reconstruction. Orthopedic reconstruction is postponed for at least 1 year.

Seven brachial plexus explorations were done in 6 birth-injured patients, at an average age of 14 months. Six extremities had weakness chiefly of muscles supplied by the upper part of the plexus, but only 1 patient (2 limbs) had the classical pattern of Erb's palsy. Despite the findings of pseudomeningocele in 4 patients (Fig 22–10), in no case did stimulation of any element of the exposed plexus fail to elicit contractions of appropriate muscles. There were no lesions suitable for grafting or neurotization, and all procedures were limited to neurolysis. Three other children, explored for vehicular trauma, had more marked lesions and

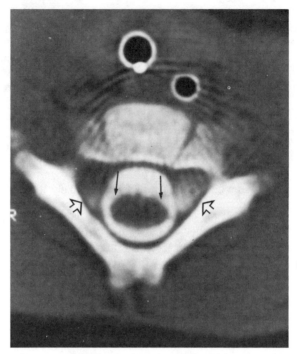

Fig 22–10.—This patient with bilateral Erb's palsies exhibited bilateral pseudomeningoceles from C3–C4 to C6–C7 on CT myelography *(large arrows)*. The preservation of intact ventral nerve rootlets *(small arrows)*, which seem to be entering the pseudomeningocele sacs in this cut, was confirmed by successful intraoperative electrical stimulation. (Courtesy of Piatt JH Jr, Hudson AR, Hoffman HJ: *Neurosurgery* 22:715–723, April 1988.)

electromyographic evidence of ongoing denervation; all of them required reconstruction of the plexus.

Whether nerve stimulation can predict recovery in patients explored late and also whether external neurolysis will allow the eventual recovery of useful neurologic function remain to be learned. Morbidity from exploring the brachial plexus remains very low.

▶ This is a confusing and difficult area. David Kline of New Orleans has seen a number of children who did not begin to recover until aged 6 months or more and yet went on to a satisfactory late result. He believes there is a role for plexus reconstruction in the infant with a birth palsy but only in selected cases, and in some instances surgery may be done later than 6 months. He advocates considering for surgery an infant or young child with persistent complete deficit in the distribution of 1 plexus element, with a meningocele indicating a very proximal nerve injury. Those involved in such surgery need to have a substantial technical and electrophysiologic as well as clinical understanding of these problems. At this time it is not possible to establish indications for brachial plexus exploration in birth injury cases.

Brief Notes on Developmental Defects

According to Oi and colleagues (*Neurol Med Chir [Tokyo]* 28:562–567, June 1988), congenital anomalies of the central nervous system are not so frequently found in Japan as in western countries. Genealogies were obtained for at least 3 generations from 7 pairs of siblings with congenital anomalies, including 3 examples of craniosynostosis, 2 of hydrocephalus, 1 of lissencephaly, and 1 of arachnoidal cyst. Four sibling pairs were female-male, 2 pairs were female, and 1 pair was male. With the exception of the pair with arachnoidal cysts, the inheritance mode suggested something other than sex-linked. For at least 3 generations, only siblings have been affected. The data after chromosome analysis and family tree investigation strongly suggest that genopathic processes were more important than gametopathic factors in the embryogenesis of central nervous system anomalies. Genetic syndromes in Japan may be relatively mild, and their transmission may be predominantly autosomal recessive.—O. Sugar, M.D.

Among the items listed by A. N. Guthkeich (*BNIQ* 4:21–23, Fall 1988) as associated with dysraphism are myelodysplasia, occult meningocele, lipomeningocele, diastematomyelia, dermal sinus, dermoid tumor, hydromyelia, enteric cyst, and tight filum terminale. Most of the time there are combinations of congenital and acquired deficits. Among the latter is pain. The tight filum terminale, often a part of the syndrome of "tethered cord" is among the syndromes that may give symptoms and signs in adult life, a fact that appears not to be widely known by neurosurgeons. Release of tethering, which may involve associated conditions such as diastematomyelia or myelocele, may be very important in relief of pain (89% cured, 11% improved) in the author's series. Sensorimotor defects were cured in 7% of patients; 78% improved, and 15% were unimproved. Sphincter loss was reversed (cured) in 13%, improved in 33%, and unimproved in 54%. Division of the tight filum, under magnification, via laminectomy is the important factor in improvement.—O. Sugar, M.D.

In an 11-year-old boy, Klippel-Feil syndrome was complicated by bilateral vertebral occlusion with brain stem infarction (Born CT et al: *J Bone Joint Surg [Am]* 70A:1412–1415, 1988).

In the VL mutant mouse, neural dysraphism is related to failure of apposition in open areas as well as inappropriate association of cells in areas that do actually fuse and possibly also failure of proper alignment of neural fold elements before apposition (Wilson DB, Wyatt DP: *J Neuropathol Exp Neurol* 47:609–617, 1988).

Transalar sphenoidal encephaloceles may be detected on MRI (Elster AD, Branch CL Jr: *Radiology* 170:245–247, 1989).

In a controlled study, Epstein's method of extended craniectomy produced superior results for sagittal synostosis (Kaiser G: *Childs Nerv Syst* 4:223–230, 1988).

23 Infection

Introduction

In a preoperative study of suspected osteomyelitis in the axial skeleton, erythrocyte sedimentation rate and white blood cell (WBC) count were better indicators than In-WBC scanning (Abstract 23–1). A review of 102 cases of bacterial brain abscess over 17 years shows that the introduction of computed tomography scanning provided the most significant recent advance toward a dramatic drop in mortality from 40% to 4% (Abstract 23–2). The infected spinal column may be treated by surgical drainage of the infection and immediate posterior stabilization with rods (Redfern et al, Abstract 23–3). A case of Creutzfeldt-Jakob disease was probably acquired from a cadaver dura mater graft (Abstract 23–4).

Preoperative Indium-Labeled White Blood Cell Scintigraphy in Suspected Osteomyelitis of the Axial Skeleton
Wukich DK, Van Dam BE, Abreu SH (Walter Reed Army Med Ctr, Washington, DC)
Spine 13:1168–1171, December 1988   23–1

Animal studies and clinical trials have shown the efficacy of indium 111-labeled white blood cell (^{111}In-WBC) scintigraphy in detecting infection of the musculoskeletal system. Six patients with suspected osteomyelitis of the axial skeleton who underwent preoperative ^{111}In-WBC scintigraphy were retrospectively reviewed.

All 6 patients complained of back pain. Five had previously had spinal surgery, 3 of whom had wound drainage. Four patients had osteomyelitis proved by culture and histopathologic evaluation. The results of 3 scans were false-negative, and 1 was false-positive. Of the 3 patients whose scans showed false-negative results, 2 patients had posterior spinal instrumentation in place. The third had a fever and staphylococcal bacteremia; his scan showed definite abnormalities, but it was considered negative for infection. The patient with false-positive results had had a staphylococcal wound infection 17 months earlier during a lumbosacral pseudoarthrosis repair. Overall, the sensitivity, specificity, and accuracy of ^{111}In-WBC scintigraphy in detecting osteomyelitis of the axial skeleton were 25%, 50%, and 33%, respectively.

This preliminary experience suggests that ^{111}In-WBC scintigraphy is neither sensitive nor specific enough to predict infection in patients with suspected osteomyelitis of the axial skeleton. Specificity may be increased by interpreting the ^{111}In-WBC and technetium 99-methylene diphosphonate scans together. "Cold" scans should not be considered negative, as they may represent an acute infection.

▶ In this study the ESR and WBC were better indicators than In-WBC scanning in the detection of spinal osteomyelitis. I have also experienced false-positive and false-negative results with this examination. It may well be that MRI, possibly with the addition of gadolinium scanning, will be more specific and sensitive.

Trends in the Management of Bacterial Brain Abscesses: A Review of 102 Cases Over 17 Years
Mampalam TJ, Rosenblum ML (Univ of California, San Francisco)
Neurosurgery 23:451–458, October 1988   23–2

The cases of 102 patients treated for bacterial brain abscess during 1970–1986 were reviewed. Patients with acquired immunodeficiency syndrome (AIDS) or AIDS-related complex were excluded. Forty-six patients had craniotomy with abscess excision; 33 had aspiration of a single lesion through either a craniotomy or burr hole. Seventeen patients received antibiotic therapy. In 6 earlier patients the abscess was missed.

Localized cranial infection was the most frequent predisposing factor, but congenital heart disease and previous intracranial surgery also were frequent factors. Cardiac and pulmonary causes have been less frequent in recent years. In addition, abscesses are smaller, and fewer patients have poor neurologic condition. Neither the type of infecting organisms nor the number of abscesses has changed significantly over the years.

Computed tomography (CT) has been the most prominent factor in reducing mortality from 41% to 4%. Penicillin and chloramphenicol have been used most often. A majority of patients received dexamethasone in conjunction with abscess excision or aspiration. Mortality and reoperation rates were comparable in the various treatment groups. Four of the 8 treated patients who died had congenital cyanotic heart disease.

Surgery remains the definitive management for nearly all brain abscesses. Certain abscesses can, however, be cured nonoperatively. Patients with multiple abscesses can have the most accessible lesion excised or aspirated, and the others are treated with antibiotics. Surgery is mandatory if there is no known predisposing factor.

▶ The authors demonstrate that the introduction of CT scanning is the most significant recent advance in the treatment of brain abscess, with a dramatic drop in mortality, from 40.9% to 4.3%. The authors give useful guidelines for operative versus nonoperative treatment, including consideration of multiplicity, presence of known predisposing factors, and size of lesion. Antibiotics are withheld until operative treatment, when it can be offered promptly, and steroids are recommended only for treatment of intracranial mass.

Stabilisation of the Infected Spine
Redfern RM, Miles J, Banks AJ, Dervin E (Walton Hosp, Liverpool; Bolton Gen

Infirmary, Bolton; Salford Univ, Manchester, England)
J Neurol Neurosurg Psychiatry 51:803–807, June 1988   23–3

Pyogenic spinal osteomyelitis has traditionally been treated with surgical drainage of the abscess, removal of sequestral bone and disk, antibiotic administration, and prolonged immobilization. Although early mobilization using primary anterior spinal fusion with bone grafts is advocated by some, most adhere to protocols involving prolonged bed rest. Previous studies have shown that the Banks Dervin rod effectively relieved pain in patients with metastatic spinal malignancy. Experience with 6 patients with spinal infections in whom this metal stabilizing rod was inserted at the time of surgical drainage of the spinal abscess is reported here.

Four men and 2 women aged 20–77 years with spinal instability secondary to vertebral osteomyelitis underwent simultaneous surgical drainage of the abscess and posterior stabilization using a Dervin rod. At the time of operation, all 6 patients had disabling back pain; 4 also had neurologic deficits. All patients were treated postoperatively with appropriate high-dose antibiotic chemotherapy.

Cultures from operative specimens yielded *Staphylococcus aureus* in 3 patients, *Mycobacterium tuberculosis* in 1 patient, and *Escherichia coli* in 1 patient. A pathogen was never isolated in the sixth patient, but clinical and radiographic evidence suggested a diagnosis of spinal tuberculosis. All patients attained excellent pain relief soon after operation, allowing early mobilization in all cases. Three of the 4 patients with preoperative neurologic deficits showed marked functional improvement after stabilization of the spine. One already critically ill patient died of pneumonia 25 days after operation, and 1 patient died of unrelated cardiac failure. The other 4 patients remained fully mobile and pain free after a follow-up of up to 12 months (Fig 23–1). The rod was removed from 1 patient after spinal fusion was confirmed on radiographs. To date, the rod has been left in place in the other patients.

This experience suggests that the use of a metal stabilizing rod in the treatment of pyogenic spinal infections associated with instability pain is an effective technique that promptly relieves severe back pain and allows early mobilization of these patients.

▶ This experience indicates that unstable osteomyelitis may be effectively treated with 1-stage drainage and rod stabilization for eradication of infection. Further experience will be needed to establish this promising approach.

Creutzfeldt-Jakob Disease Probably Acquired From a Cadaveric Dura Mater Graft: Case Report

Thadani V, Penar PL, Partington J, Kalb R, Janssen R, Schonberger LB, Rabkin CS, Prichard JW (Yale Univ; Ctrs for Disease Control, Atlanta)
J Neurosurg 69:766–769, November 1988   23–4

Creutzfeldt-Jakob disease (CJD) is a fatal transmissible dementing dis-

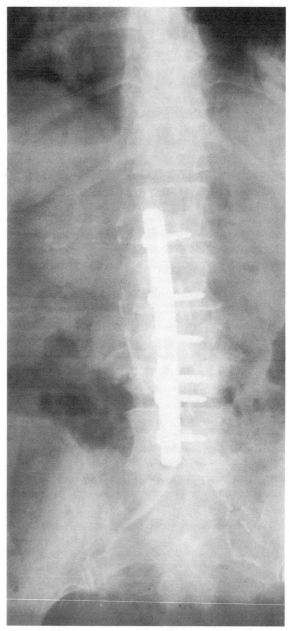

Fig 23–1.—Anteroposterior radiograph 12 months postoperatively showing fusion at L3–L4 and satisfactory position of the prosthesis. (Courtesy of Redfern RM, Miles J, Banks AJ, et al: *J Neurol Neurosurg Psychiatry* 51:803–807, June 1988.)

order. Iatrogenic transmission has apparently occurred through corneal implantation, intracranial electrodes, and human growth hormone extracts from cadaveric pituitary glands. Creutzfeldt-Jakob disease occurred in a woman who had received a cadaveric dural graft 19 months before the onset of neurologic symptoms.

Woman, 28, had resection of a cholesteatoma of the right ear, in which a dural patch graft was placed in the right temporal region. Lyophilized cadaveric dura constituted the graft material. An unsteady gait and slurred speech subsequently developed, and within 1 week, the patient's mental status began to deteriorate. She has paraphasic speech and visual hallucinations. She became unable to walk. Myoclonus developed in all extremities. A computed tomography (CT) scan of the head showed subtle gyral prominence. Electroencephalographic studies revealed generalized slowing, greater over the right hemisphere. Biopsy specimens

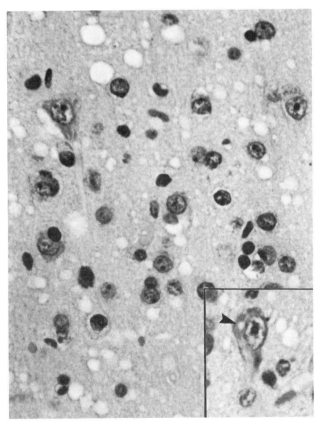

Fig 23-2.—Photomicrograph of temporal lobe cortex showing typical spongiform changes in the neuropil with scattered vacuoles of varying sizes. There is a slight increase in the number of glial cells. Hematoxylin-eosin; original magnification, ×580. **Inset:** A neuron with a cytoplasmic vacuole *(arrowhead)*. Hematoxylin-eosin; original magnification ×650. (Courtesy of Elias Manuelidis, M.D. From Thadani V, Penar PL, Partington J, et al: *J Neurosurg* 69:766–769, November 1988.)

were taken of the right temporal lobe, dural graft, and adjacent native dura. Microscopic assessment revealed numerous vacuoles of varying sizes scattered throughout the neuropil. Rare vacuoles impinged on the neuron cytoplasm (Fig 23–2), and there was slight astrocytic proliferation. Neuronal loss was not evident. Creutzfeldt-Jakob disease was diagnosed. Neurologic deterioration continued, and the patient died 2 months later.

The circumstances of this case suggest that the graft was the most likely source of the disease. Cadaveric dura should be added to the list of materials that may transmit CJD and be very carefully screened, if used at all for grafting. Autologous tissue should be used when possible.

▶ This case certainly alerts the neurosurgical community to the need for great care in the placement of cadaveric dural grafts. Avoidance of dura mater grafts and use of autologous materials is probably the safest course at this time.

Brief Notes on CNS Infections

Computed tomographic diagnosis of spinal infection is dependent on criteria of complete preverterbral soft tissue involvement, diffuse osteolysis, gas in bone or soft tissue, and the process centering on an intervertebral disk (Vanlom K et al: *Radiology* 166:851–855, 1988). Neoplastic disease is characterized by posterior element involvement, partial prevertebral soft tissue swelling, and osteoblastic alterations.

Epidural spinal infection in intravenous drug abusers in 18 cases was most commonly caused by *Staphylococcus aureus,* but in 2 cases *Mycobacterium tuberculosis* was the agent (Koppel VS et al: *Arch Neurol* 45:1331–1337, 1988). Computed tomography was helpful in diagnosis, early treatment improved outcome, but systemic factors also played a role.

Disseminated mucormycosis may cause a cauda equina syndrome (Rozich J et al: *JAMA* 260:3638–3640, 1988).

Saline microbubbles may assist sonography-assisted abscess drainage (Scatamacchia SA et al: *Invest Radiol* 22:868–870, 1987).

Intracranial tuberculoma still occurs in the United States (O'Brien NC et al: *South Med J* 81:1239–1244, 1988).

Intracranial tuberculomas on MRI show central bright signal on T_2-weighted images with peripheral low intensity rims surrounded by high intensity edema (Gupta RK et al: *J Comput Assist Tomogr* 12:280–285, 1988).

A 56-year-old woman became blind during antifungal chemotherapy for cryptococcal neoformans meningitis. The optic disks were pale in spite of raised intraspinal fluid pressure, and the organism was found in the cerebrospinal fluid. In the absence of papilledema, blindness was thought caused by optochiasmatic arachnoiditis. Metrizamide CT cisternography revealed contrast material in the quadrigeminal and interpeduncular cisterns but not in the cistern of the chiasm. Immediate operation allowed removal of thick yellow adhesive arachnoid from around the optic apparatus. Immediately thereafter, the blood vessels on the optic nerves, which had been "rudimentary," became dilated. On the seventh postoperative day pupillary reaction to light returned, and by day 17 she began to see again. Repeat metrizamide cisternography before discharge revealed ready filling of the chiasmatic cistern with metrizamide. A year after discharge she remains free of visual problems. Maruki and associates from Juntendo (*Neurol Med Chir [Tokyo]* 28:695–697, 1988) point to the frequency of visual abnormalities in patients with intracranial cryptococcosis. In this case, optochiasmatic arachnoiditis was blamed for the visual problems, and because this can be helped by surgery (whereas direct invasion of the optic nerves by the organism or angiitis cannot be), the course was set for diagnosis by CT cisternography and subsequent removal of the adhesions. Once the diagnosis has been made, operation is warranted.—O. Sugar, M.D.

Paranasal sinus aspergillosis with intracranial extension may occur without immunologic compromise (Sarti EJ et al: *Laryngoscope* 98:632–635, 1988).

A cerebral hydatid cyst was reported in a 9-year-old boy with cure after puncture and systemic antihelminthic treatment with mebendazole followed by total excision (Braunstorfe W et al: *Childs Nerv Syst* 4:249–251, 1988).

Magnetic resonance imaging appears to be superior to CT in the diagnosis of cysticercosis (Bouilliant-Linete et al: *J Radiol* 69:405–412, 1988).

Nonanthrax bacillus may be isolated from CSF in patients without shunts (Feder HM Jr et al: *Pediatrics* 82:909–913, 1988).

Kartush and co-workers (*Laryngoscope* 98:1050–1054, 1988) report that bacitracin irrigation reduces the incidence of wound infection for translabyrinthine surgery.

24 Functional

Introduction

In the area of *pain,* recurrent glycerol injections into the trigeminal cistern for facial pain have unfortunately led to rather frequent painful dysesthesias, making this repeated injection an undesirable approach (Abstract 24–1). Surgeons from the University of Washington have presented long-term follow-up data after microvascular decompression indicating a powerful beneficial effect (Burchiel et al, Abstract 24–2).

In the field of *epilepsy,* a magnetic field of epileptic spikes agrees nicely with intracranial localization in complex partial epilepsy (Sutherling et al, Abstract 24–3.) Corpus callosum section can reduce seizure disturbance in patients with intractable epilepsy, but there is a significant complication rate (Spencer S, Abstract 24–4). Olivier in 560 procedures achieved remarkable effectiveness in controlling epilepsy by surgery, with a success rate of 80% in psychomotor seizures without an operative death (Abstract 24–5). The extent of psychologic disorder after surgical treatment of seizures is not greater than that in nonoperative cases (Abstract 24–6). Magnetic resonance imaging can provide quantitative evaluation of resection of the temporal lobe for epilepsy (Jack et al, Abstract 24–7).

A study of psychosurgery cases from a defined population indicates that modified leukotomy still has a place in psychiatric therapy and should remain available as a measure of last resort in certain carefully selected cases (Hussain et al, Abstract 24–8). A long-term study indicates that stereotactic thalamotomy can improve neurologic status in patients with cerebral palsy, but in these cases dating back to 1958, the complication rate is high (Abstract 24–9). An important study from a careful group of American investigators indicates modest improvement in patients undergoing medullary adrenal transplantation for parkinsonism (Abstract 24–10).

Robert M. Crowell, M.D.

Pain

Recurrent Trigeminal Cistern Glycerol Injections for Tic Douloureux
Rappaport ZH, Gomori JM (Hadassah Univ Hosp, Jerusalem)
Acta Neurochir (Wien) 90:31–34, 1988   24–1

Trigeminal cistern glycerol injection (TCGI) in the treatment of intractable trigeminal pain is easy to perform and appears to be relatively successful. Although TCGI is increasingly being used in clinical practice, its role as a therapeutic modality is still controversial because high rates of

Complications of Repeat Trigeminal Cistern Glycerol Injection
for Recurrent Trigeminal Neuralgia

	No.	%
New sensory deficit	4	29%
Decreased corneal reflex	1	7%
Increase in previous sensory deficit	2	14%
Dysaesthetic pain	2	14%
Partial pain relief	1	7%
No pain relief	1	7%

Note: No. = 14.
(Courtesy of Rappaport ZH, Gomori JM: Acta Neurochir [Wien] 90:31–34, 1988.)

recurrence and major sensory deficits have been reported. Experience with TCGI was reviewed.

Of 60 patients who were treated with TCGI because of intractable trigeminal pain, 17 (28%) experienced a recurrence of pain after a mean pain-free interval of 14 months. Three of these 17 patients were successfully treated with medication; the other 14 (23%) underwent repeat TCGI. The 10 patients with satisfactory pain relief after the second procedure have remained free of pain during a follow-up period ranging from 2 to 25 months. Painful dysesthesia developed in 2 patients after the second injection. One patient underwent 2 more TCGI procedures, which resulted in pain relief. The remaining patient was unrelieved by the repeat procedure (table).

A comparison of the trigeminal cistern volumes measured at the first and second procedures showed that the cistern volume had decreased from a mean of 0.38 ml at the first treatment to 0.29 ml at the second treatment. Four (29%) patients had evidence of nerve root clumping, which was compatible with local arachnoiditis.

Trigeminal cistern glycerol injection can be recommended as the procedure of choice with elderly patients. However, because of a possibility of deafferentation pain developing after TCGI, the technique should be used with caution for younger patients.

▶ The occurrence of painful dysesthesias in 2 of 14 patients subjected to repeat glycerol injections for tic douloureux is high enough (14.3%) to warrant consideration of another treatment modality such as radiofrequency lesioning in these patients. These painful dysesthesias are of such disturbing nature that the occurrence of this complication must be taken as a very serious problem.

Long-Term Efficacy of Microvascular Decompression of Trigeminal Neuralgia

Burchiel KJ, Clarke H, Haglund M, Loeser JD (Univ of Washington)
J Neurosurg 69:35–38, July 1988

24–2

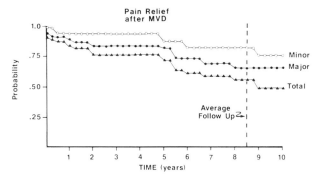

Fig 24–1.—Kaplan-Meier plot of the probability of remaining pain free over time after microvascular decompression *(MVD)*. Thirty-six patients underwent 36 MVD procedures. Patients were censored at the following rate: year 7: 2 patients; year 8: 10 patients; year 9: 25 patients; and year 10: 33 patients. (Courtesy of Burchiel KJ, Clarke H, Haglund M, et al: *J Neurosurg* 69:35–38, July 1988.)

Trigeminal neuralgia that is resistant to medical treatment can be managed by a number of surgical procedures. The operation involving microvascular decompression (MVD) of the trigeminal nerve at the nerve root entry is frequently employed, but long-term follow-up had not been previously reported.

A group of 36 patients were followed for an average of 8.5 years after MVD of the nerve. Of these, 19 were pain-free without antineuralgic medication and 17 experienced some pain during the follow-up period. Eleven patients had major recurrences; their pain was as severe after MVD as it was before surgery (Fig 24–1).

Arterial cross-compression of the trigeminal nerve discovered at the time of surgery was associated with a pain-free outcome. But 4 of 7 patients with venous compression of the nerve had a major recurrence of pain. Prior neurodestructive surgery was significantly associated with minor recurrences of pain. In 8 patients who had repeat or primary rhizotomies, 4 experienced major recurrences, and 1 had a minor recurrence.

Microvascular decompression may not actually cure trigeminal neuralgia, although the effects of the procedure are long-lasting. Investigators, using an annual rate of 3.5% for major recurrences and 1.5% for minor recurrences, predict an expected 10 years of freedom from pain after successful MVD of the nerve. The mechanism of MVD, like that of trigeminal neuralgia itself, remains uncertain, but MVD remains one of the most important treatments for the disorder.

▶ Burchiel and colleagues present important long-term follow-up data after microvascular decompression for trigeminal neuralgia. The results suggest a powerful beneficial effect from MVD, especially for arterial compressions. Venous compression is much less effectively arrested. Technical factors of course could be important in explaining the difference between this series and the more favorable report of Jannetta. The latter is a series of more than 450 patients, unfortunately without long-term follow-up data. The present communication helps to establish a role for MVD but also highlights its limitations.

Brief Notes on Pain

Clonadine worked better than codeine for postherpetic neuralgia in a controlled study (Max MB et al: *Clin Pharmacol Ther* 43:363–371, 1988).

Stellate ganglion block can produce long-lasting relief in postherpetic neuralgia with sympathetic components (Fine PG, Ashborn MA: *Anesth Analg* 67:897–899, 1988).

Encouraging results are reported after implanted epidural stimulation for pain secondary to arachnoiditis in 20 cases (Husson JL et al: *J Chir [Paris]* 125:522–524, 1988).

Injections of epidural morphine produced pain relief but never for more than 1 month during treatment of the postlaminectomy syndrome (Rocco AG et al: *Pain* 36:297–303, 1989).

Tizanidine specifically depresses dorsal horn convergent neurons, probably by postsynaptic inhibitory action. This could explain at least in part the analgesic action of the compound (Villanueval et al: *Pain* 35:187–197, 1988).

Intrathecal somatostatin in rats produces antinociception only when toxic effects are caused (Gaumann NDM, Yaksh TL: *Anesthesiology* 68:733–742, 1988).

Dorsal root ganglion substance P and VIP are affected by diskography (Weinstein J et al: *Spine* 13:1344–1348, 1988).

Metenkephalin levels rose significantly over age with no changes observed in β-endorphin in studies of human CSF (Alessio L et al: *Life Sci* 43:1545–1550, 1988).

Facet joint injection in low back pain led to pain relief in only 29% (Jackson RP et al: *Spine* 13:966, 971, 1988).

Opioid receptor activity in CSF may reflect an abnormality of sensory input in patients with low back pain (Desiderio DM et al: *Life Sci* 43:577–583, 1988).

Radio frequency lesions have been used to interrupt the gray communicating rami for pain relief in failed back patients (Sluijter ME: *Int Disabil Stud* 10:37–44, 1988).

Among psychosocial variables, outcome from low back pain was independently associated with education, previous episodes, and whether the patient "always feels sick" (Deyo RA, Diehl AK: *J Rheumatol* 15:1557–1564, 1988).

Compensated back injury in New Zealand is reviewed by Burry HC (*NZ Med J* 101:542–544, 1988).

Data indicate that workers' compensation patients receiving time-limited financial benefits do not necessarily represent a problem subgroup of chronic pain patients (Jamison RN et al: *J Psychosom Res* 32:277–283, 1988).

Cohen and associates (*Pain* 35:57–63, 1988) suggest that in chronic pain related to a chronic medical catastrophe, aspects of the McGill Pain Questionnaire and Minnesota Multiphasic Personality Inventory assist in assessment of the person's total medical disability, not just of the painful state.

Some evidence suggests that biofeedback-induced self-control of event-related potentials can modify individual pain sensations (Miltner W et al: *Pain* 35:205–213, 1988).

In a series of 595 cases of true trigeminal neuralgia treated at the Mitsui Memorial Hospital, Tokyo, Miyazaki and colleagues found 45 patients with vascular compression by an elongated basilar artery (*Neurol Med Chir [Tokyo]* 27:742–

748, 1987). Enhanced computed tomograms were important in preoperative diagnosis. They visualized the artery as a linear enhancement crossing the prepontine cistern in all instances. In a postoperative follow-up period of 6 to 50 months (mean, 19), complete relief was obtained by decompression in 43 cases (95.6%). Tortuosity, hypertrophy, and sclerosis of the basilar artery made adequate decompression of the nerve difficult. Facial hypesthesia and diplopia due to fourth or sixth cranial nerve palsies were the most permanent neurologic deficits in 5 patients (11%). The technical difficulties should not, in the authors' opinion, deter attempts to carry out microvascular decompression.—O. Sugar, M.D.

Rarely, patients with tinnitus may benefit from vascular decompression of the eighth nerve (Meyerhoff WL, Mickey BE: *Laryngoscope* 98:602–605, 1988).

Vertigo has been caused by basilar artery compression of the eighth nerve, and selective section of the vestibular nerve provided complete relief (Benec KE Jr, Hitselberger WE: *Laryngoscope* 98:807–809, 1988).

Retrolabyrinthine vestibular neurectomy was reported to control completely vertigo in 29 of 31 cases (Monsell EM et al: *Laryngoscope* 98:835–839, 1988).

Epilepsy

The Magnetic Field of Epileptic Spikes Agrees With Intracranial Localizations in Complex Partial Epilepsy

Sutherling WW, Crandall PH, Cahan LD, Barth DS (Univ of California, Los Angeles)
Neurology 38:778–786, May 1988   24–3

Localization of the epileptic focus with the magnetoencephalogram (MEG) generally is simpler than with the EEG because of a relative lack of distortion by the skull. The 2 modalities each are more sensitive to different orientations of intracranial currents. Both the MEG and EEG were measured during interictal epileptic spikes in 9 patients with complex partial epilepsy resistant to medical measures. Seven patients had temporal lobe seizures, and 2, frontal lobe seizures.

Localization with MEG was accurate in all cases; the MEG agreed with both electrophysiologic and structural localizations. Localization estimates consistently were in the same lobe as the interictal spike focus on intracranial recordings (Fig 24–2). Dipolar magnetic field patterns had well-defined peaks of opposite polarity with a relative null point or phase reversal between.

The MEG and a combination of MEG and EEG recordings can improve the noninvasive localization of focal electrical activity in the brain. These methods may aid the selection of surgical candidates.

▶ This communication offers preliminary data correlating good agreement of localization of epileptiform spikes using MEG and intracranial EEG localization. Magnetoencephalography and EEG together may be useful in selecting patients for surgical management.

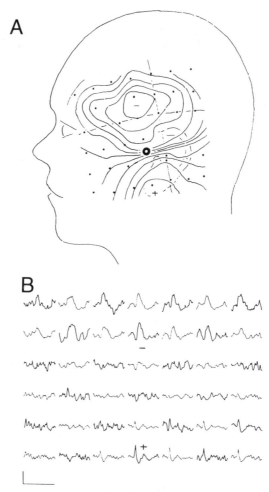

Fig 24–2.—Magnetoencephalogram (MEG) spike map. **A,** isocontour map of averaged MEG spikes shows a dipolar pattern with amplitude peaks at − and +. *Small open circle* is the MEG localization of the center of the spike focus (equivalent dipole), brought out to the surface. **B,** averaged MEG spikes show a dipolar phase reversal between the upper and lower parts of the matrix. Dot spacing is 2 cm. *Crosshairs* centered on midtemporal electrode position T3. Heavy traces are measured data; light traces are interpolated. Calibration: MEG, 750 fT; 1 sec. (Courtesy of Sutherling WW, Crandall PH, Cahan LD, et al: *Neurology* 38:778–786, May 1988.)

Corpus Callosum Section and Other Disconnection Procedures for Medically Intractable Epilepsy

Spencer SS (Yale Univ)
Epilepsia 29(Suppl 2):S85–S99, 1988   24–4

When it is not feasible to resect a focus that initiates seizures, disconnection procedures that limit the clinical expression of severe seizures are an alternative approach. The corpus callosum is the chief structure re-

Response of Specific Etiologies to Corpus Callosum Section

	Elimination of at least one type of generalized seizure	Decreased generalized seizures	No change
Infantile hemiplegia and variants	83%	17%	0
Focal (calcification, tumor)	75%	25%	0
Acquired			
Encephalitis	70%	15%	15%
Trauma	38%	56%	6%
Perinatal injury	43%	38%	19%
Congenitally abnormal	67%	8%	25%
Unknown etiology	59%	22%	19%

(Courtesy of Spencer SS: *Epilepsia* 29[Suppl 2]: S85–S99, 1988.)

quired for generalized 3-Hz spike-and-wave discharge in animal models of generalized epilepsy. Consequently section of the corpus callosum is the most widely practiced disconnection procedure. Stereotactic lesions of the amygdala, globus pallidus, and various thalamic nuclei also have been attempted.

Total section of the corpus callosum and hippocampal commissure, with or without the anterior commissure and fornix, disrupts synchronous spike-and-wave EEG discharges in about half of operated patients. Many severely disabled patients have been helped by the procedure. Results in adults and children are comparable. Some improvement occurs in substantial proportions of patients with a wide range of seizure types (table).

Variable motor deficits, including leg weakness and hand apraxia, occur in about 15% of patients after total section and in fewer patients after partial callosal section. Similar proportions of patients have expressive language and writing deficits, which may be as severe as persistent mutism. Intelligence quotients usually are unchanged after callosal section. Abnormal behavior may be aggravated, but patients have not become aggressive or violent for the first time after the operation. Some patients have substantial improvement in overall function after surgery.

▶ Corpus callosum section can reduce seizure disturbance in patients with intractable epilepsy. However, there is a significant complication rate for this procedure. Moreover it is difficult to know which patients will respond. This method should be confined to use in the specialized epilepsy centers where a team approach to the problem is available.

Risk and Benefit in the Surgery of Epilepsy: Complications and Positive Results on Seizures Tendency and Intellectual Function
Olivier A (Montreal Neurological Inst and Hosp, Montreal)
Acta Neurol Scand [Suppl] 78:114–121, 1988   24–5

In a significant proportion of epileptic patients undergoing surgery, the seizure tendency can be improved markedly with an acceptable rate of complications. In a 10-year period, 526 patients underwent 560 cranial surgery procedures in the management of epilepsy.

Temporal resections were done most frequently: 198 patients had procedures on the left side and 189 on the right. No operative deaths occurred. Complications included persistent hemiparesis plus dysphasia in 1 patient, postoperative hematoma in 2, postoperative myoclonus in 1, meningitis in 1, postoperative brain swelling in 3, subdural abscess in 2, scalp infections in 5, and in some, aseptic meningitis. No patient experienced clinically significant intellectual or memory deficit.

Overall, the success rate was 80%. Patients with right-sided surgical removal of tissue tended to respond better than patients who had left-sided procedures. Removal of the hippocampal formation appeared to improve the outcome significantly. Patients studied with intracerebral electrodes tended to do better than those undergoing surgery without depth electrodes. Anterior temporal resection was followed in most patients by a significant increase in intellectual function when assessed 1 year after surgery.

Resective surgery should be offered to all epileptic patients who have frequent psychomotor seizures and in whom an active temporal focus can be demonstrated.

▶ This careful report from an extremely experienced surgeon operating in the birthplace of epilepsy surgery is a valuable update. In patients with psychomotor seizures, a success rate of 80% was achieved without operative death. A serious lasting deficit rate was 1% or less. Under these conditions, we can confidently recommend surgery for intractable epilepsy. It is important to note that these results were achieved by a highly experienced surgeon with a well-trained team.

Prevalence of Psychologic Disorders After Surgical Treatment of Seizures
Koch-Weser M, Garron DC, Gilley DW, Bergen D, Bleck TP, Morrell F, Ristanovic R, Whisler WW Jr (Rush-Presbyterian-St Luke's Med Ctr, Chicago)
Arch Neurol 45:1308–1311, December 1988   24–6

Surgery for the treatment of refractory epilepsy has become common. However, some researchers suggest that patients who have surgical treatment are at risk for serious psychopathologic disorders. Whether rates of serious psychopathologic disorders were increased after such surgery was investigated in a retrospective study.

Twenty-five previously treated patients were compared with 25 candidates for surgery with comparable demographic and neuroepileptic characteristics. Diagnoses were based on the National Institute of Mental Health Diagnostic Interview Schedule. There were no differences between groups in lifetime or point prevalence rates. The rate of psychosis among the previously treated patients was 8%, about the same as the lower estimates reported in previous studies. Patients with electroencephalographic evidence of temporal lobe foci or tumor as the epileptogenic lesion were more likely to have serious disorders than the other patients. Anxiety disorders were also more prevalent among the total group of patients than in the general population.

Surgical treatment of seizures does not appear to increase the risk of development of serious psychopathologic disorders. Findings of previous studies may reflect increased risk generally in epileptic patients, especially those with resected temporal lobe foci or epileptogenic tumor. Anxiety disorders are prominent among patients with intractable epilepsy and appear to be unaffected by surgical treatment for seizures.

▶ This careful psychologic study indicates that surgical treatment of intractable epilepsy does not increase the frequency of serious psychopathology in these patients.

Use of MR Imaging for Quantitative Evaluation of Resection for Temporal Lobe Epilepsy
Jack CR Jr, Sharbrough FW, Marsh WR (Mayo Clinic, Rochester, Minn)
Radiology 169:463–468, November 1988   24–7

Because magnetic resonance imaging (MRI) is superior to computed tomography (CT) in demonstrating focal structural lesions that cause temporal lobe epilepsy, the postoperative studies of 40 patients having surgery to treat medically resistant epilepsy were reviewed. The goal was to examine the hypothesis that the surgical outcome is dependent on the degree of resection of medial temporal lobe structures. Twenty-six patients had a standard temporal lobectomy. In 14 others an attempt was made to maximize resection of medial temporal structures while limiting resection of the basal and lateral temporal gyri.

Seizure control was correlated closely with at least partial removal of all medial temporal lobe structures (Fig 24–3). However, the total amount of tissue removed did not always relate to the clinical outcome in individual patients. The presence of bilateral independent EEG foci predicted a poorer outcome, as did a history of meningoencephalitis.

It is important to at least partially resect all medial temporal structures. Quantitative MRI is the only objective method other than autopsy for determining the extent of temporal lobe resection. Magnetic resonance imaging may help evaluate postoperative cognitive deficits and also aid in determining whether to reoperate when the patient has a poor result or relapse.

▶ This excellent study demonstrates that excision of medial temporal structures is crucial for relief of medically intractable epilepsy by surgical means. Incidentally, data are provided that suggest that basal and lateral temporal gyri need not be excised for good results. We must add MRI to EEG in the postop-

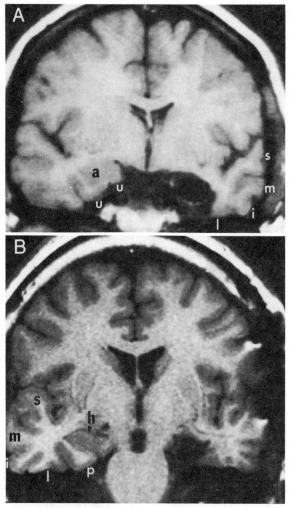

Fig 24–3.—Images obtained in patients who had an excellent outcome after surgical procedures designed to spare the basal and lateral gyri, with extensive medial temporal resection. *i*, inferior temporal gyrus; *l*, lateral occipitotemporal gyrus; *m*, middle temporal gyrus; *s*, superior temporal gyrus. **A**, anterior coronal image through amygdala *(a)* and uncus *(u)* of woman aged 31 years after transsylvian medial temporal resection. Note complete removal of left amygdala and uncus and sparing of superior temporal, middle temporal, inferior temporal, and lateral occipitotemporal gyri. **B**, posterior coronal image through hippocampal gyrus of woman aged 40 years after limited anterior lobectomy with medial temporal resection. Note complete removal of left hippocampal formation *(h, arrowhead)* and parahippocampal gyrus *(p)* and sparing of superior temporal, middle temporal, inferior temporal, and lateral occipitotemporal gyri. (Courtesy of Jack CR Jr, Sharbrough FW, Marsh WR: *Radiology* 169:463–468, November 1988.)

erative evaluation and follow-up of patients undergoing temporal lobe surgery. (Others have already pointed out the importance of preoperative MRI, which detects many minute lesions in the temporal lobe as the source of epileptogenic foci.)

Brief Notes on Epilepsy

Magnetic resonance imaging can demonstrate completeness of callosotomy (Bozen JE et al: *Arch Neurol* 45:1203–1205, 1988).

Corpus callosum surgery causes memory deficits only when there is extra-callosal injury, especially to the fornix (Clark CR, Geffen GM: *Brain* 112:165–175, 1989).

After callosotomy there is reduced side-to-side olfactory memory (Eskenazi B et al: *Yale J Biol Med* 61:447–456, 1988).

The site of anterior temporal lobectomy to control partial complex seizures has a distinguishing effect on cognitive function, with recent memory most susceptible to postoperative impairment (Ivnak RJ et al: *Mayo Clin Proc* 63:783–793, 1988).

Assessment of rate of forgetting after bilateral temporal lobectomy is dependent on the procedures used to assess memory (Freed DM, Corkin S: *Behav Neurosci* 102:823–827, 1988).

Epilepsy with congenital suprasellar arachnoid cyst has been reported in an infant (Giroud M et al: *Childs Nerv Syst* 4:252–254, 1988).

Excitatory amino acids are elevated in human epileptic cerebral cortex (Sherwin A et al: *Neurology* 38:920–923, 1988).

Other Topics

A Cohort Study of Psychosurgery Cases From a Defined Population
Hussain ES, Freeman H, Jones RAC (Greaves Hall Hosp, Southport; Hope Hosp, Salford, England)
J Neurol Neurosurg Psychiatry 51:345–352, March 1988   24–8

The antipsychiatric movement that developed in the mid-1960s has severely attacked the use of psychosurgery. As a result, only few leukotomies are still being performed, even though for some patients who experience intractable distress or disability, such an operation might be the only viable option. The records of all patients in an urban population who underwent psychosurgery in a 20-year period were reviewed to assess the outcome.

Thirty-two women and 12 men were aged 22–69 years at the time of leukotomy; all had previously had severe, disabling, and intractable illnesses. Thirty-three patients were available for a personal follow-up interview; the other 11 patients were assessed by case record review only. The outcome of leukotomy was measured on a 5-point scale that graded patients as recovered, well, improved, unchanged, or worse. The diagnoses of referring psychiatrists were accepted as valid, but all patients had been evaluated by a consultant for a second opinion. The mean follow-up after psychosurgery was 11.02 years. Nonstereotactic operations were performed in 36 patients, and stereotactic, in 6 patients, with 1 having both procedures.

Twenty-five (75.8%) of the 33 interviewed patients and 8 (72.7%) of the 11 patients assessed by case record were graded as recovered or well. The other 8 (24.2%) interviewed patients and 3 (23.3%) patients re-

Comparison of Outcome: Interview vs. Case Records

	I	II	III	IV	V	Total
Records outcome	22	3	5	2	1	33
Interview outcome	19	6	5	2	1	33

(Courtesy of Hussain ES, Freeman H, Jones RAC: *J Neurol Neurosurg Psychiatry* 51:345–352, March 1988.)

viewed from records were graded as improved, unchanged, or worse (table). One death was directly attributable to the operation. The improvement rate for nonstereotactic operations was 85% and that for stereotactice operations, 40%. Fourteen patients experienced adverse effects, but most were not serious.

▶ Modified leukotomy still has a place in psychiatric therapy and should remain available for certain carefully selected patients as a measure of last resort.

Cerebral Palsy and Stereotactic Neurosurgery: Long Term Results
Speelman JD, van Manen J (Academic Med Ctr, Amsterdam)
J Neurol Neurosurg Psychiatry 52:23–30, January 1989   24–9

Stereotactic encephalotomy has been used for the symptomatic relief of dyskinesia, rigidity, and spasticity in patients with cerebral palsy. However, reports on outcomes have been conflicting, possibly because of differences in patient selection, surgical technique, and duration of follow-up. Data on 28 patients with cerebral palsy who had undergone stereotactic encephalotomy and who had been followed up for 12–27 years were reviewed retrospectively.

The patients were divided into 3 groups according to the principal symptom targeted at operation. Of the 28 patients, 9 had painful spasms and hemidystonia, 9 had generalized dystonia, and 10 had hyperkinesia. After a mean postoperative follow-up of 21 years, 18 patients were still alive, 9 had died, and 1 could not be traced. The surviving patients were examined clinically for overall disability and were graded on a Dutch scale of activities of daily living that measures mental function, communication, locomotion, feeding, dressing, and hygiene.

Eight of the 18 reassessed patients had benefited from operation in that the principal symptom targeted at operation was relieved. However, assessment of activities of daily living showed that operation had not reduced the degree of preoperative disability in most patients. Of 16 patients who were living at home before operation, 8 were still living at home at follow-up, 2 of whom were fully dependent on others. Permanent complications that were directly attributable to the operation included paresis in 6 patients and speech impairment in 6 patients. The best results occurred in patients operated on because of hyperkinesia, tremor, and mostly unilateral dystonia. Those with generalized dystonia had a less favorable outcome.

Stereotactic thalamotomy can lessen hyperkinesia in patients with moderate to severe dyskinetic cerebral palsy and is helpful to those with unilateral dystonia caused by a pallidal or thalamic lesion. Patients with severe tetraplegic or diplegic palsy should not have stereotactic surgery. Surgery is not done in patients aged less than 14 years.

▶ This report demonstrates that stereotactic thalamotomy can improve neurologic status and activities of daily living in patients with cerebral palsy. The advantages of this study include follow-up by an independent neurologic observer and extremely long-term results extending up to 48 years. However, it is important to recognize that the last opration was performed in 1958, and present-day operative techniques including localization, stereotactic targeting, and lesion making have been substantially improved since then. Stereotactic complications have decreased remarkably also. These results are likely to be substantially worse than those obtainable today.

Multicenter Study of Autologous Adrenal Medullary Transplantation to the Corpus Striatum in Patients With Advanced Parkinson's Disease

Goetz CG, Olanow CW, Koller WC, Penr RD, Cahill D, Morantz R, Stebbins G, Tanner CM, Klawans HL, Shannon KM, Comella CL, Witt T, Cox C, Waxman M, Gauger L (Rush-Presbyterian-St Luke's Med Ctr, Chicago; Univ of South Florida, Tampa; Univ of Kansas, Kansas City)
N Engl J Med 320:337–341, Feb 9, 1989   24–10

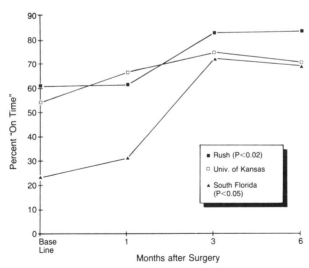

Fig 24–4.—Percent "on time," according to study center. This variable was 1 of the 4 in which improvement occurred in the entire study population. Although improvement followed the same pattern in the 3 centers, when data were analyzed according to center, improvement was significant in only 1 center. The values in this figure are based on 18 patients (Rush, 7 patients; University of Kansas, 6; South Florida, 5). (Courtesy of Goetz CG, Olanow CW, Koller WC, et al: *N Engl J Med* 320:337–341, Feb 9, 1989.)

Parkinson's disease has been successfully ameliorated by a transplantation of the adrenal medulla to the right caudate nucleus. These surgical procedures were replicated to treat 19 patients with severe Parkinson's disease.

Patient function was monitored with the use of standardized scales to determine the amount and quality of "on" and "off" time: the hours of the waking day when the antiparkinsonian medications were effective and ineffective, respectively. Significant improvement was noted in focal areas of motor function. The mean percentage of on time increased from 47.6% to 75% after the operation (Fig 24−4), and the mean percentage of on time without chorea increased from 26.6% to 59.2%. The mean severity of off time decreased, as determined by the Activities of Daily Living subscale of the Unified Parkinson's Disease Scale and the Schwab and England scale. However, dosages of antiparkinsonian medications could not be reduced after the procedure, and postoperative morbidity was substantial.

Although the results at 6 months justify cautious optimism about this procedure, the widespread use of this technique outside research centers is premature. The improvement that resulted in this series was slighter than in cases previously reported.

▶ This important study from a group of careful and critical American investigators indicates modest improvement in patients undergoing medullary adrenal transplantation for parkinsonism. However, it is clear that further investigation of the procedure will be needed before it can be recommended for routine use.

Brief Notes on Other Functional Neurosurgery Topics

Stereotactic subfrontal tractotomy was helpful in the treatment of resistant bipolar affective disorder (Poynton A et al: *Br J Psychiatry* 152:354–358, 1988).

CNS Transplantation

Neural transplants disrupt the blood-brain barrier and allow peripherally acting drugs to assert a centrally mediated behavioral effect (Sandberg PR et al: *Exp Neurol* 102:149–151, 1988).

Striatal grafts provide the brain protection from kainic and quinolinic acid-induced damage (Tulipan N et al: *Exp Neurol* 102:325–332, 1988).

Differential plating of chromaffin cells from the adrenal medulla yielded relatively pure populations of these cells with excellent viability (Hansen JT et al: *Ann Neurol* 24:599–609, 1988).

Experimental adrenal medullary autografts in the basal ganglia of cebus monkeys produced results most consistent with induction of recovery of remaining dopaminergic systems by the implantation procedure (Fiandaca MS et al: *Exp Neurol* 102:76–91, 1988).

Studies of adrenal medullary autografts in the basal ganglia of monkeys show histologic evidence of cellular degeneration but robust spouting of fibers adjacent to the implant site (Hansen JT et al: *Exp Neurol* 102:65–75, 1988).

Transplantation of brain or adrenal medullary tissue into the brains of epileptic rats did not reduce the intensity of seizures (Stevens JR et al: *Epilepsia* 29:731–737, 1988).

Fetal pituitary transplants survive and secrete in the hypothalamic area of hypophysectomized rats (Alexander N et al: *Surg Neurol* 30:342–349, 1988).

Thyrotropin-releasing hormone augments growth of spinal cord transplants in oculo (Henschen A et al: *Exp Neurol* 102:125–129, 1988).

Radiofrequency power can be utilized for millimeter- and submillimeter-sized neuroprosthetic implants (Heetderks WJ: *IEEE Trans Biomed Eng* 35:323–325, 1988).

25 Nerve

Introduction

Ultrasonography can image peripheral nerve tumors and may be regarded as an adjunct to magnetic resonance for diagnosis (Fornage, Abstract 25–1). Neoplasms of the vagus nerve usually appear as asymptomatic masses in the neck (Green et al, Abstract 25–2). Excision is generally warranted, but conservative management may be indicated in older patients. For simultaneous loss of median and ulnar nerves in the forearm, extensive pedicle nerve transfer may improve the final outcome (Greenberg et al, Abstract 25–3). For the management of facial palsy, a combination of techniques may be required, including microsurgery, conventional surgery, dynamic or static slings, and ancillary cosmetic procedures (Mackinnon and Dellon, Abstract 25–4).

Robert M. Crowell, M.D.

Peripheral Nerves of the Extremities: Imaging With US
Fornage BD (Institut Jean–Godinot, Reims, France)
Radiology 167:179–182, April 1988   25–1

Peripheral nerve tumors are rare. They are usually benign and subcutaneous and appear as soft tissue swelling. The ultrasonographic appearance of peripheral nerves of the extremities was evaluated in healthy volunteers and in patients with a mass developed from a peripheral nerve. High-resolution, real-time ultrasound was used. Scanned were the large nerves, including the median nerve in the carpal tunnel and the forearm, the ulnar nerve in the forearm and at the elbow, the sciatic nerve in the thigh, and the external popliteal nerve at the fibular neck.

Normal nerves all had an echogenic fibrillar texture (Fig 25–1). Pathologic findings in 11 patients included 9 benign tumors (4 schwannomas, 3 neurofibromas, and 2 traumatic neuromas); 1 patient had neurilemmitis and 1 had tuberculoid leprosy. All lesions were seen as hypoechoic. Three schwannomas had well-defined contours; 2 of these had typical distal sound enhancement. Neurofibromas and traumatic neuromas were not as sharply delineated. Inflammatory conditions were characterized as a hypoechoic, thickened nerve.

Based on these findings, high-resolution ultrasound appears to detect tumors of the extremities readily.

▶ Ultrasonography can image peripheral nerve tumors and may be regarded as an adjunct to magnetic resonance.

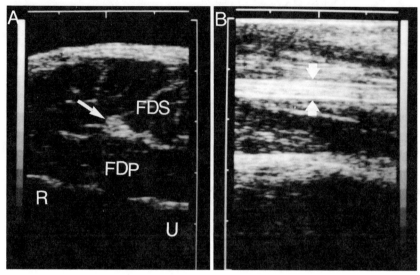

Fig 25–1.—Normal median nerve. **A,** transverse sonogram of the anterior aspect of the mid-third of the forearm shows the round echogenic section of the median nerve *(arrow)* lying between flexor digitorum superficialis *(FDS)* anteriorly and flexor digitorum profundus *(FDP)* posteriorly. *R,* radius; *U,* ulna. **B,** longitudinal sonogram of the median nerve *(arrowheads)* shows the echogenic fibrillar texture resembling that of a tendon. Upper left-hand corner is toward patient's head. (Courtesy of Fornage BD: *Radiology* 167:179–182, April 1988.)

Neoplasms of the Vagus Nerve
Green JD Jr, Olsen KD, DeSanto LW, Scheithauer BW (Mayo Clinic and Mayo Found, Rochester, Minn; Mayo Clinic Scottsdale, Scottsdale, Ariz)
Laryngoscope 98:648–654, June 1988   25–2

The unique physiologic and anatomical features of cranial nerve X require special consideration when neoplasms of the vagus nerve are being treated. All neoplasms of the vagus nerve treated surgically at the Mayo Clinic from 1965 to 1987 were reviewed.

Thirty-six neoplasms were treated in 35 patients. The most frequent finding on presentation was a mass in the upper cervical or parapharyngeal region (Fig 25–2). The masses were usually asymptomatic. Fifty percent of the neoplasms were paragangliomas; 31%, neurilemmomas; 14%, neurofibromas, and 6%, neurofibrosarcomas. When the vagus nerve can be preserved, surgical resection is the treatment of choice. There was no increased incidence of recurrence when the vagus nerve was spared. The surgical approach should be tailored to the size, location, and histologic type of the lesion. Special problems noted in this series were postoperative dysfunction, catecholamine secretion, and intracranial or skull-base extension.

In this series, an upper cervical mass was the most common finding, and in 40%, it was the only finding on presentation. The incidence of preoperative vocal cord palsy was lower than has been reported in other series. The treatment of choice for lesions of the vagus nerve is complete surgical excision. The long survival observed in this series and the slow

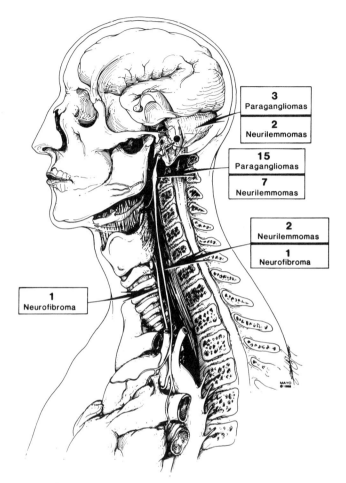

| **3** Paragangliomas |
| **2** Neurilemmomas |

| **15** Paragangliomas |
| **7** Neurilemmomas |

| **2** Neurilemmomas |
| **1** Neurofibroma |

| **1** Neurofibroma |

Fig 25–2.—Distribution of tumors along the vagus nerve. (Courtesy of Mayo Foundation. From Green JD Jr, Olsen KD, DeSanto LW, et al: *Laryngoscope* 98:648–654, June 1988.)

growth pattern of vagal nerve neoplasms underscore the need for long-term follow-up.

▶ These tumors usually present as an asymptomatic mass in the neck. Occasional sarcomatous degeneration can lead to an aggressive course and death. In some patients a complete excision appears warranted. However, there are substantial morbidities to excision, including aspiration in 46% and cranial neuropathies in 44%, thus mandating a less aggressive approach in older patients.

St. Clair Strange Procedure: Indications, Technique, and Long-Term Evaluation
Greenberg BM, Cuadros CL, Panda M, May JW Jr (Harvard Univ)
J Hand Surg 13A:928–935, November 1988   25–3

Simultaneous traumatic loss of the median and ulnar nerves in the forearm poses a difficult reconstructive problem. The St. Clair Strange procedure is a pedicled nerve transfer that preserves the intrinsic blood supply of the pedicle and makes it possible to bridge large defects in relatively avascular scarred wounds.

After complete soft tissue healing the nerve stumps are mobilized for a short distance and the proximal nerve ends are resected. An epineural median nerve repair is done in the forearm using 8-0 nylon sutures. A 1-cm segment of ulnar nerve is removed, and the proximal stump is buried in muscle (Fig 25–3). When the median nerve Tinel sign approaches the divided proximal ulnar nerve above the cubital tunnel, the entire ulnar nerve to be pedicled is exposed and transferred distally. Distal repairs are outside the zone of injury. Median nerve continuity is reestablished through the transposed ulnar nerve distally, by either an epineural or a grouped fascicular repair (Fig 25–4). If feasible, ulnar nerve continuity may be similarly established. The average interval between procedures is 7 months.

Seven patients have had this operation; 5 were observed for a mean of 10 years. All patients achieved protective sensation in the "new" median-innervated tissues, as well as variable return of touch localization. Light-touch sensation returned in the palm and innervated digits, but no patient achieved 2-point discrimination. All patients are able to perform daily activities, using the injured extermity either directly or as an assisting hand.

This operation is especially indicated for combined massive median and ulnar nerve lesions and in a devascularized bed with little donor graft material available.

▶ This communication indicates the complexity and creativity that may be utilized to deal with complex upper limb nerve injuries. The variety of surgical techniques employed also suggests that a simplistic approach, focusing on nerve alone, is unlikely to prevail in the management of these injuries in the future.

St. Clair Strange Procedure

FIRST STAGE

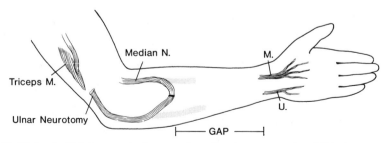

Fig 25–3.—St. Clair Strange procedure, stage 1: median-ulnar nerve repair and high ulnar nerve resection, with proximal ulnar nerve placed in triceps muscle. (Courtesy of Greenberg BM, Cuadros CL, Panda M, et al: *J Hand Surg* 13A:928–935, November 1988.)

St. Clair Strange Procedure

SECOND STAGE

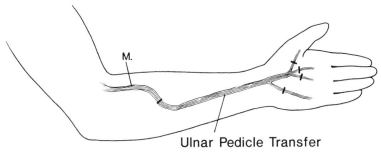

M.

Ulnar Pedicle Transfer

Fig 25–4.—St. Clair Strange procedure, stage 2: the vascularized ulnar nerve is transposed distally, to the wrist (median ulnar nerve) to palm. Common digital nerves (*black bars*, nerve repair sites). (Courtesy of Greenberg BM, Cuadros CL, Panda M, et al: *J Hand Surg* 13A:928–935, November 1988.)

A Surgical Algorithm for the Management of Facial Palsy
Mackinnon SE, Dellon AL (Univ of Toronto; Johns Hopkins Univ)
Microsurgery 9:30–35, 1988   25–4

Facial nerve palsy is difficult to treat, even with advances in microsurgery that allow cross-facial nerve grafting and free muscle transfer (Fig 25–5). Often a combination of techniques are required: microsurgery, conventional surgery, dynamic or static slings, and ancillary cosmetic procedures. The various surgical approaches and stages of surgical reconstruction for rehabilitation of patients with facial nerve injuries are described.

The ideal nerves and muscles for reconstruction are the facial nerves and muscles themselves, and technically demanding microsurgery can be the means of achieving successful reconstruction with normal expression and movement. But much is demanded of the patient in the course of reinnervating facial muscles. Extensive preoperative counseling is needed, and the patient should understand the multistaged nature of the surgery.

Neural input to the facial muscles can be achieved with a repair or graft of the proximal portion of the ipsilateral seventh nerve. The surgeon may also neurotize part of the hypoglossal nerve to the ipsilateral facial nerve. And facial muscles should be salvaged so that fewer free muscle flaps will be needed. Whether or not it is possible to reinnervate the facial muscles, the course of treatment concludes with 1 or more "touch up" operations to achieve balance and symmetry in the face.

▶ This interesting presentation reviews various modern methods for the management of facial palsy. Though substantial results are not presented, nonetheless the importance of considering various alternatives is advanced. The neurosurgeon and plastic surgeon should work together in this important arena.

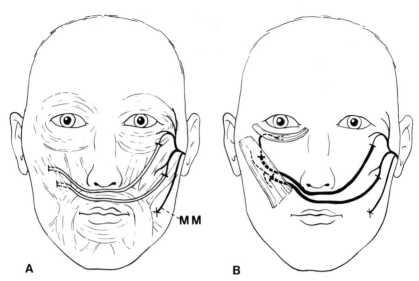

Fig 25–5.—Schematic drawing of a proposed procedure of facial muscles have been denervated for such a prolonged time that they cannot be salvaged. **A,** cross-facial nerve graft(s). Approximately 1 year after this procedure, a free muscle flap will be transferred to the face innervated by the cross-facial nerve graft(s) (**B**). (Courtesy of Mackinnon SE, Dellon AL: *Microsurgery* 9:30–35, 1988.)

Brief Notes on Nerves

TUMORS OF THE NERVE

Labauge and co-workers (*Rev Neurol [Paris]* 144:606–609, 1988) report a neuroma of the vagus nerve with contralateral peripheral facial paralysis.

An intradural, extramedullary mass lesion at C2 spinal level produced quadriparesis and numbness of all 4 extremities in a woman, 38, whose case is reported by Kawaguchi and associates of Osaka, Japan (*Neurol Med Chir [Tokyo]* 27:1190–1194, 1987). Total removal was accomplished with recovery. Typical Antoni type B neurinoma was found, arising from the right spinal accessory nerve trunk. Only 10 previous tumors of the 11th cranial nerve have been reported up to now; this is believed to be the first reported case in which the tumor was confined entirely to the spinal canal.—O. Sugar, M.D.

Melonotic schwannoma rising in the sympathetic ganglia has been reported by Kayano and Katayama (*Arch Pathol* 19:1355–1363, 1988).

Neurilemoma and neurofibroma may occur in the same nerve trunk (Cavallazzi RM et al: *J Hand Surg* 13B:96, 1988).

Facial nerve palsies may develop from facial nerve tumors (Ma KH, Fagan PA: *Aust N Z J Med* 18:613–616, 1988).

MEDIAN NERVE

Severe carpal tunnel syndrome may be caused by gout (Ogilvie C, Kay NRM: *J Hand Surg* 13B:42–45, 1988).

Carpal tunnel syndrome and amyloidosis have been reported in association with continuous ambulatory peritoneal dialysis (Gagnon RF et al: *Can Med Assoc J* 139:753–755, 1988).

Carpal tunnel syndrome may be associated with vascular compression of the median nerve motor branch (Widder S, Shons AR: *J Hand Surg* 13A:926–927, 1988).

Nerve regeneration and adaptation after median nerve reconnection is imperfect when sensory nerves to digits are relocated (Dyck PJ et al: *Neurology* 38:1586–1591, 1988).

Computed tomography of the wrist may be valuable in the evaluation of nonidiopathic carpal tunnel syndrome but is not needed for idiopathic disease (Schmitt VR et al: *Fortschr Roentgenstr* 149:280–285, 1988).

BRACHIAL PLEXUS

Magnetic resonance imaging often provides more information than CT regarding brachial plexus pathology (Rapoport S et al: *Radiology* 167:161–165, 1988).

Electroencephalography, somatosensory evoked potential, and sensory nerve action potential are all useful in the evaluation of brachial plexopathies (Aminoff MJ et al: *Neurology* 38:546–550, 1988).

Among 28 operated patients with complete brachial plexus paralysis, 14 recovered active elbow function of grade 3 or better (Allieu Y et al: *Func Orthop Surg* 2:74–81, 1988).

CRANIAL NERVE

Partial recovery is reported after oculomotor nerve section and repair during tumor excision (Deruty R et al: *Neurochirurgie* 34:287–292, 1988).

According to Politis and associates (*J Trauma* 28:1548–1553, 1988) application of electrical fields may be followed by regeneration of optic nerve.

NERVE SURGERY

In rats, sciatic nerve regeneration across allogeneic nerve grafts was significantly superior in those immunosuppressed with cyclosporin A (Bain JR et al: *Plast Reconstr Surg* 82:1052–1064, 1988).

Neurolysis or transposition for intractable leprous neuritis produced good results in more than 80% of patients (Nores JN et al: *Presse Med* 17:1756–1759, 1988).

Regeneration across a sural nerve graft and a vascularized nerve sheath was similar in experimental studies (Mackinnon SE, Dellon AL: *J Hand Surg* 13A:935–942, 1988).

A vascularized nerve graft compared with conventional yields superior regeneration, better subjective sensory recovery, and better sensibility (Mackinnon SE et al: *Microsurgery* 9:226–233, 1988).

A new technique for end-to-end peripheral nerve anastomosis has been developed utilizing freezing of nerve ends with trimming of the ends and subsequent repair. Functional recovery was 300% to 400% better than that from epineurial repair (Wikholm RP et al: *Otolaryngol Head Neck Surg* 99:353–361, 1988).

Alon and associates (*Clin Orthop* 234:31–33, 1988) report bilateral suprascapular nerve entrapment due to anomalous transverse scapular ligament.

26 Neuroscience

Introduction

Remarkable advances in *developmental* biology have enormous implications for understanding congenital anomalies, regeneration after neural injury, and tumor biology. Modern studies indicate that axons are guided biochemically by extracellular signals to their appropriate targets (Dodd and Jessell, Abstract 26–1). In the cerebral cortex, the radial unit hypothesis focuses on the relevance of glial matrix in cortical parcellation (Rakic, Abstract 26–2). This hypothesis provides a framework for understanding cerebral evolution.

Synapses are viewed in light of new developments. Elegant quantitive studies of transmitter release suggest that different boutons have different likelihoods of transmitter release, thus giving rise to a new model of synaptic transmission (Walmsley et al, Abstract 26–3). According to Nicoll, multiple postsynaptic receptors modulate the same ion channels in the synapse (Abstract 26–4). Recent studies indicate that hippocampal neurons produce nerve growth factor, which in turn maintains cholinergic projections to the hippocampus from other limbic areas, a remarkable trophic feedback loop (Ayer-LeLievre et al, Abstract 26–5).

In the area of *memory,* cellular studies underlie new concepts. Modification of synaptic transmission and calcium channels appears to underlie long-term synaptic potentiation, a strong candidate as mechanism of rapid learning in mammals (Brown et al, Abstract 26–6). Muscarinic cholinergic systems appear to be important in long-term potentiation (Williams and Johnston, Abstract 26–7). Specific medial temporal lobe neurons in patients appear to be the site of encoding of individual words and faces (Heit et al, Abstract 26–8).

Degeneration is also a focus for basic research. Amyloid protein precursor messenger RNAs appear to have differential expression in Alzheimer's disease (Palmert et al, Abstract 26–9).

Robert M. Crowell, M.D.

Development

Axon Guidance and the Patterning of Neuronal Projections in Vertebrates
Dodd J, Jessell TM (Columbia Univ)
Science 242:692–699, Nov 4, 1988   26–1

The functional properties of the vertebrate nervous system are dependent on the network of neuronal connections formed during development. An early step is the projection of axons to their targets through diverse and changing environments. The process can be viewed as a series

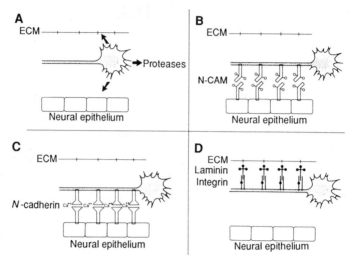

Fig 26–1.—Axons extend on neuroepithelial and ECM substrates. **A,** growth cones may create spaces in their environment by releasing proteases that degrade collagen fibril meshworks and other components of the ECM. **B** and **C,** adhesion between axons and neural-epithelial cells is mediated by homophilic interactions between surface molecules such as N-CAM and *N*-cadherin. This set of molecules contributes to axon extension but may not provide directional cues. **D,** ECM glycoproteins such as laminin promote the extension of axons by interacting with receptor molecules termed integrins located on the axonal surface. (Courtesy of Dodd J, Jessell TM: *Science* 242:692–699, Nov 4, 1988.)

of short-range projections to intermediate targets under the influence of local guidance cues.

Recent interest in axonal guidance focuses on identifying molecules that regulate growth cone extension and navigation (Fig 26–1). General cell adhesion molecules expressed on neural epithelial cells apparently surround the early axons and provide permissive substrates for axonal extension. Other molecules with restricted or graded patterns of expression may provide directional cues by enhancing or inhibiting axonal extension over certain regions. Later selective fasciculation of axons becomes an important guidance mechanism. Growth cones may be guided to their intermediate or final targets by gradients of diffusible factors secreted by restricted cell populations within the target. Once the axons arrive near their targets, formation of highly ordered projections may be dependent on the recognition of positional cues expressed as molecular gradients within either the neurons themselves or their targets.

One means by which axons may adapt to changing cellular environments is spatially regulated transitions in glycoprotein expression on different segments of the same axon. Altered integrin function and changes in neural cell adhesion molecule sialylation also may be involved in the adaptive process.

▶ This clear summary provides a modern picture of how axons are guided biochemically by extracellular signals to their appropriate targets. The extraordinary importance of the extracellular milieu and its matrix components, such as internectin, is now becoming apparent through basic investigation. There are enormous implications for development of congenital anomalies, regeneration after neural injury, and tumor biology. Advances in clinical diagnosis and management may well come from this new arena.

Specification of Cerebral Cortical Areas

Rakic P (Yale Univ)
Science 241:170–176, July 8, 1988
26–2

The human cerebral cortex contains cytoarchitectonic areas with distinct cellular, biochemical, connectional, and physiologic characteristics. These areas govern various motor, sensory, and cognitive functions, and an understanding of their principles would help to explain the evolution of human creativity and the origins of mental disease. The radial unit hypothesis of cortical parcellation, focusing on the relevance of glial scaffolding, is presented.

This hypothesis provides a framework for understanding cerebral evolution. The ependymal layer in the embryonic cerebral ventricle is made up of proliferative units that provide a protomap of the cytoarchitectonic areas. Neurons, in their migration to the cortex, follow glial guides over a lengthy and difficult path across the expanding intermediate and subplate zone (Fig 26–2). Migrating neurons and ingrowing afferents interact in the subplate zone before arriving at the cortical plate. Neurons then enter the cortical plate to form radially oriented columns.

According to the radial unit hypothesis, each proliferative unit produces a corresponding ontogenetic column. Proliferative units produce cohorts of neurons with some degree of area specific competence, and interaction of neurons and afferents in the subplate can further regulate the number of ontogenetic columns devoted to a given area.

Data contributing to this hypothesis are drawn from such advanced neurobiologic techniques as electron microscopy, retrovirus gene transfer, immunocytochemistry, and [³H]thymidine and receptor autoradiography. Experimental and neuropathologic findings suggest that each step—the formation of proliferative units, ontogenetic columns, and cytoarchitectonic areas—can be altered by extrinsic factors or genetic defects.

► Professor Rakic brings together data from a host of modern neuroscience studies in a debatable but useful hypothesis centering on the radial unit. Although it may not be correct in all details, the hypothesis is helpful in understanding modern concepts of neural migration, cytoarchitectonics, and glial functioning.

Synapses

Nonuniform Release Probabilities Underlie Quantal Synaptic Transmission at a Mammalian Excitatory Central Synapse

Walmsley B, Edwards FR, Tracey DJ (Univ of New South Wales, Kensington; Australian Natl Univ, Canberra, Australia)
J Neurophysiol 60:889–907, September 1988
26–3

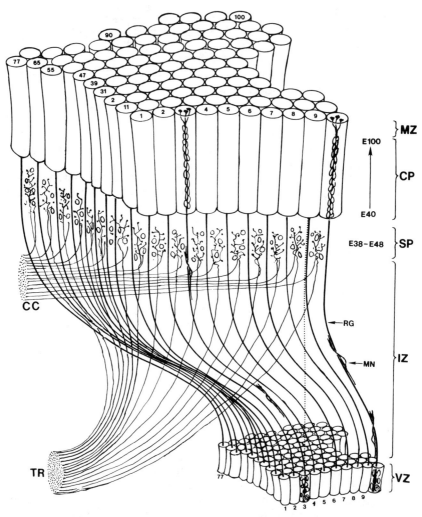

Fig 26–2.—The relationship between a small patch of the proliferative, ventricular zone *(VZ)* and its corresponding area within the cortical plate *(CP)* in the developing cerebrum. Although the cerebral surface in primates expands and shifts during prenatal development, ontogenetic columns (outlined by cylinders) remain attached to the corresponding proliferative units by the grid of radial glial fibers. Neurons produced between E40 and E100 by a given proliferative unit migrate in succession along the same radial glial guides *(RG)* and stack up in reverse order of arrival within the same ontogenetic column. Each migrating neuron *(MN)* first traverses the intermediate zone *(IZ)* and then the subplate *(SP),* which contains interstitial cells and "waiting" afferents from the thalamic radiation *(TR)* and ipsilateral and contralateral corticocortical connections *(CC).* After entering the cortical plate, each neuron bypasses earlier generated neurons and settles at the interface between the CP and marginal zone *(MZ).* As a result, proliferative units 1 to 100 produce ontogenetic columns 1 to 100 in the same relative position to each other without a lateral mismatch (for example, between proliferative unit 3 and ontogenetic column 9, indicated by a *dashed line).* Thus, the specification of cytoarchitectonic areas and topographic maps depends on the spatial distribution of their ancestors in the proliferative units, whereas the laminar position and phenotype of neurons within ontogenetic columns depends on the time of their origin. (Courtesy of Rakic P: *Science* 241:170–176, July 8, 1988.)

Single-fiber excitatory postsynaptic potentials (EPSPs) fluctuate in amplitude between approximately equal, or quantal, increments. The quantal fluctuations could not be described by simple binomial statistics.

The EPSPs evoked by impulses in single group I muscle afferents in dorsal spinocerebellar tract neurons of anesthetized cats were studied.

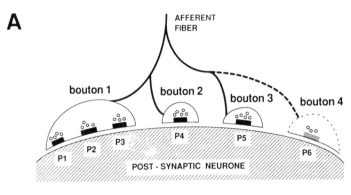

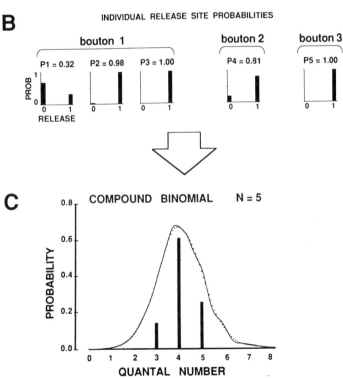

Fig 26–3.—Proposed model of synaptic transmission at the connection between single group I fibers and dorsal spinocerebellar tract neurons. (Courtesy of Walmsley B, Edwards FR, Tracey DJ: *J Neurophysiol* 60:889–907, September 1988.)

Analytic procedures were used to formulate a probabilistic model of transmission.

Each single-fiber EPSP consisted of the sum of 3 to 30 uniform quantal events. The amplitude of single quantal events was quite constant. The quantal fluctuations were described by a compound binomial model in which each event was associated with a particular but independent release probability. The estimated likelihood of transmitter release varied substantially between release sites.

A model of transmission at this connection features a number of "active" release sites with generally high probabilities of release and a number of "reserve" release sites with zero or virtually zero release probability (Fig 26–3). The efficacy of transmission could be modulated by adding or dropping active release sites rather than by a change in release probability for all release sites in a connection. There is ultrastructural evidence that presynaptic inhibition, which lowers the amplitude of the synaptic potential, operates on a selected proportion of synaptic boutons.

▶ These elegant studies of excitatory postsynaptic potentials give rise to a interesting model illustrated in Figure 26–3. In essence, different boutons have different likelihoods of transmitter release, and even within a bouton the sites for transmitter release show remarkable variation in their likelihood of transmitter release. Such quantitative analyses of synaptic transmission seem likely to further elucidate the nature of this extremely important phenomenon. One can imagine further extension of this approach to elements of modulation involving neuropeptide modulators interacting with sites of transmission.

The Coupling of Neurotransmitter Receptors to Ion Channels in the Brain
Nicoll RA (Univ of California, San Francisco)
Science 241:545–551, July 29, 1988
26–4

Hippocampal pyramidal cells respond to so many neurotransmitters that multiple receptors must modulate the same ion channels. This review describes what is currently known about the relationship between receptors and ion channels in these cells.

Serotonin, γ-aminobutyric acid, and adenosine activate a G protein via distinct receptors. This activation opens a common potassium channel. Norepinephrine, histamine, and corticotropin-releasing factor appear to act via cyclic adenosine monophosphate (cAMP) to block a common potassium channel. Acetycholine blocks the same channels but does not utilize cAMP. Protein kinase C activation may be involved. These 2 mechanisms are illustrated in Figure 26–4.

The existence of multiple receptor types in 1 postsynaptic cell permits complex neuronal signaling. The response of the cell can be dependent on the amount of transmitter released and the coupling mechanism between transmitter and response. It is possible that different synapses may activate different receptors.

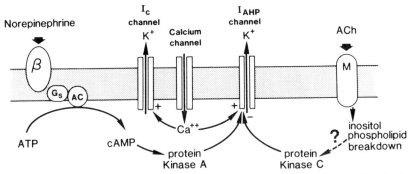

Fig 26–4.—The proposed mechanisms of action of norepinephrine and acetylcholine in blocking the slow Ca^{2+} activated K^+ conductance. (Courtesy of Nicoll RA: *Science* 241:545–551, July 29, 1988.)

Synaptic transmission in the central nervous system is extremely complex. The large number of transmitter molecules and transduction mechanisms that can be used by a single postsynaptic cell allow for much diversity in information processing.

▶ Professor Nicoll summarizes the present complex state of affairs in neural transmission. The essential point is that multiple receptors modulate the same ion channels.

Expression of the β-Nerve Growth Factor Gene in Hippocampal Neurons
Ayer-LeLievre C, Olson L, Ebendal T, Seiger Å, Persson H (Karolinska Inst, Stockholm; Uppsala Univ, Uppsala Sweden; Univ of Miami)
Science 240:1339–1341, June 3, 1988   26–5

Cholinergic neurons of the septum-basal forebrain respond to exogenous nerve growth factor (NGF) by increasing levels of choline acetyltransferase. The target areas of these neurons—the hippocampus and cortex—contain the highest levels of NGF mRNA in the brain. Septumbasal forebrain neurons also carry NGF receptors.

In situ hybridization was performed with cDNA probes for NGF to identify cells containing NGF mRNA in rat and mouse brain. Labeling was most intense in the hippocampus (Fig 26–5), where hybridizing neurons appeared in the dentate gyrus and pyramidal cell layer. With RNA blot analysis, NGF mRNA was found to be reduced in the rat dentate gyrus after a lesion was produced by colchicine. The lesion also reduced Thy-1 mRNA and increased glial fibrillary acidic protein mRNA. Labeled neurons also were present in the cerebral cortex.

These findings strongly suggest that hippocampal neurons produce NGF. The terminal fields of the septohippocampal cholinergic projections may be maintained by a trophic supply of NGF from the target neurons. A disordered balance between the intensity of input from septal to hip-

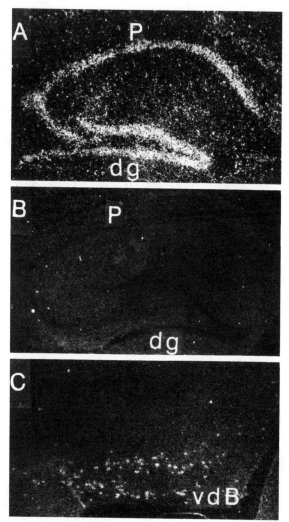

Fig 26–5.—In situ hybridization to sections of rat hippocampus. The DNA probes were labeled with $(\alpha\text{-}^{32}P)$deoxycytidine $5'$-triphosphate (dCTP) by nick translation to a specific activity of approximately 10^9 cpm/µg, and 5–10 ng of probe were added to each section. The conditions for in situ hybridization were as described in original article. The slides were dehydrated and dipped in 50% Ilford K5 nuclear emulsion and exposed for 9 days. The following probes were used: **A,** a 900-bp Pst I fragment from a mouse NGF cDNA clone, and **B** and **C,** a 400 bp Bst EII fragment derived from a rat NGF receptor cDNA clone. **A** and **B,** sagittal sections of rat brain at hippocampus level. **C,** transverse section through the ventral part of vertical limb of diagonal band of Broca *(VDB).* The sections are shown in dark-field illumination (original magnification, × 18). *P* indicates pyramidal cell layer; *DG,* granular cell layer of dentate gyrus. (Courtesy of Ayer-LeLievre C, Olson L, Ebendal T, et al: *Science* 240:1339–1341, June 3, 1988.)

pocampal neurons and the level of NGF provided by the latter may underlie some of the changes involved in aging and brain disease.

▶ These sophisticated basic studies strongly suggest that neurons in the hippocampus produce nerve growth factor. The findings invite speculation that NGF from target neurons may modulate incoming cholinergic projections from other limbic structures. Here we have a nice example of how a well-established transmission system may be altered by a newly described system. Extension of such studies will be important to improved understanding of brain mechanisms in health and disease.

Memory

Long-Term Synaptic Potentiation

Brown TH, Chapman PF, Kairiss EW, Keenan CL (Yale Univ)
Science 242:724–728, Nov 4, 1988   26–6

Long-term synaptic potentiation (LTP) is a strong candidate for a mechanism of rapid learning in mammals. The phenomenon is a lasting increase in synaptic efficacy that is rapidly inducible. In addition to so-called associative LTP, 1 form of potentiation is formally similar to the synaptic memory mechanism postulated some time ago by Donald Hebb. The core concept is a use-dependent synaptic enhancement based on interaction between concurrent presynaptic and postsynaptic activity.

An important aspect of the process of modification involves the *N*-methyl-D-aspartate (NMDA) receptor-ionophore complex. The ionophore permits calcium influx only if the endogenous ligand glutamate binds to the NMDA receptor and if voltage across the channel is sufficiently depolarized to relieve a magnesium block. The resultant increase in intracellular calcium may activate protein kinases that enhance postsynaptic conductance. Maintenance of LTP may depend on conversion of a protein kinase to an activator-independent form. There is no evidence that LTP is associated with generalized changes in excitability of the postsynaptic neuron.

It remains to be demonstrated conclusively that LTP is endogenously generated and how it is involved in the development and organization of behavior. Both pharmacologic studies and studies of whether induction of LTP affects later learning may be informative.

▶ This review points out the current thinking regarding long-term synaptic potentiation and rapid learning. Note that the strategy involves correlation of biochemistry, electrophysiology, and biophysics in a theory of induction maintenance and expression of learned memory. Though there is still a way to go, the LTP theory has much to support it and is a leading contender in this arena.

Muscarinic Depression of Long-Term Potentiation in CA3 Hippocampal Neurons

Williams S, Johnston D (Baylor College of Medicine, Houston)
Science 242:84–87, Oct 7, 1988   26–7

There is evidence from behavioral studies that muscarinic cholinergic systems are important in learning and memory. Because long-term potentiation (LTP), a form of use-dependent synaptic plasticity, may underlie both learning and memory, the effects of the cholinergic agonist mucarine on LTP in the voltage-clamped mossy fiber-CA3 pyramidal cell synapse of the rat hippocampus were studied. Excitatory postsynaptic potentials and currents were measured.

Long-term potentiation was blocked by muscarine (Fig 26–6). Concentrations of 1 μM significantly reduced the probability of induction of LTP and its magnitude while having little effect on low-frequency synaptic stimulation. Voltage clamp studies indicated that muscarine blocked the increase in excitatory synaptic conductance normally associated with LTP.

That muscarine depresses LTP supports a role for cholinergic systems in memory; however, the role may be more complex than previously thought. If LTP is in fact a substrate for learning, its induction probably is carefully regulated.

▶ The authors present evidence that muscarine depresses long-term potentiation, a form of synaptic activity throught to underlie memory. These data, therefore, support the notion that cholinergic mechanisms are important to memory.

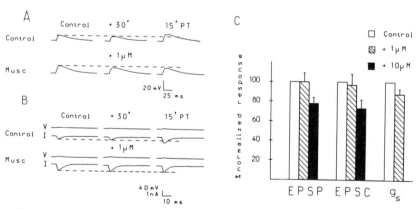

Fig 26–6.—The effects of muscarine on synaptic transmission and LTP. **A,** upper traces show that in a control cell, the excitatory postsynaptic potential (EPSP) is stable for 30 minutes (30'), but that 15 minutes after tetanus (15' PT), an increase in amplitude is seen. The lower traces (*musc,* different cell) show that 1 μM muscarine produced a small depression of the EPSP before tetanus and prevented the development of LTP at 15' PT. **B,** in a similar experiment under voltage clamp (*V,* membrane potential; *I,* clamp current), LTP in the control cell was seen as an increase in the excitatory postsynaptic current (EPSC), but in the muscarine-treated cell, no increase was apparent. **C,** summary of the actions of muscarine (1 and 10 μM) on synaptic transmission. All data were normalized to control. EPSP: 1 μM, n = 10; 10 μM, n = 6. EPSC: 1 μM, n = 8; 10 μM, n = 5. g_s: 1 μM, n = 5. (Courtesy of Williams S, Johnston D: *Science* 242:84–87, Oct 7, 1988.)

Hebb, several decades ago, proposed that the cellular site of learning might involve the interaction of unconditioned stimulus reaching cell body from 1 dendrite and the conditioned stimulus arriving from another. Recent evidence suggests that synapses for these 2 inputs may be anatomically quite close, on the same dendrite, with enzymatic alterations developing in and around cell wall at these sites (Alkon D: *Sci Am* July 1989). Such studies provide an impressive fusion of electrophysiologic and biochemical activities that may underlie memory.

Neural Encoding of Individual Words and Faces by the Human Hippocampus and Amygdala
Heit G, Smith ME, Halgren E (Univ of California, Los Angeles; Stanford Univ; Wadsworth VA Med Ctr, Los Angeles; Hosp St Anne, Paris)
Nature 333:773–775, June 23, 1988   26–8

Lesions in the medial temporal lobe (MTL) produce severe impairment in the ability to recall and recognize words or faces encountered recently. The effect of word repetition on cortical event-related potentials is abolished. Ten patients with refractory complex partial epilepsy undergoing neurosurgery were presented with both abstract words and faces to ex-

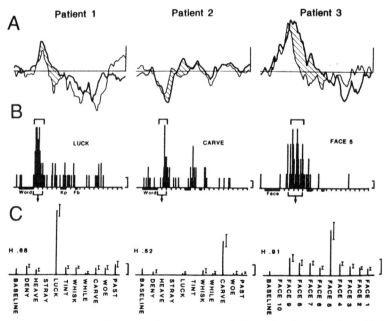

Fig 26–7.—Responses of hippocampal neurons to a particular word or face in 3 patients. Displayed are simultaneous averaged field potentials (**A**), sum histograms of neuronal firing in response to preferred stimuli (**B**), and total number of action potentials in response to all repeated stimuli during a selected time period (**C**), for 3 left anterior hippocampal units. *Abbreviations: Kp,* averaged keypress; *Fb,* feedback tone; *H,* breadth of tuning index. (Courtesy of Heit G, Smith ME, Halgren E: *Nature* 333:773–775, June 23, 1988.)

amine responses of individual MTL neurons to delayed recognition tasks.

Some MTL neurons preferentially fired on sight of a particular word or face. This stimulus-specific firing peaked during the time that neocortical event potenitals were most sensitive to stimulus repetition (Fig 26–7).

The MTL may contribute specific information to the cortex during retrieval of recent memories. The MTL stimulus-specific responses appear to represent the temporary allocation of some MTL neurons to the ensemble encoding of distinct events in a given context. The MTL seems to do more than diffusely modulate the encoding of stimuli in recent memory.

▶ The data indicate that some medial temporal lobe neurons are preferentially activated by specific words and faces. A remarkable specificity of information in these structures in relation to recent memory is suggested.

Degeneration

Amyloid Protein Precursor Messenger RNAs: Differential Expression in Alzheimer's Disease

Palmert MR, Golde TE, Cohen ML, Kovacs DM, Tanzi RE, Gusella JF, Usiak MF, Younkin LH, Younkin SG (Case Western Reserve Univ; Harvard Univ)
Science 241:1080–1084, Aug 26, 1988   26–9

In situ hybridization techniques were used to estimate total amyloid protein precursor (APP) messenger RNA and the subset of APP messenger RNA containing the Kunitz protease inhibitor (KPI) insert in brains from 11 patients with Alzheimer's disease and 7 controls. The 2 groups were matched for age and postmortem interval.

A significant twofold increase in total APP messenger RNA was found in the nucleus basalis and locus coeruleus neurons in Alzheimer brains (Fig 26–8). No such increase was seen in hippocampal subicular neurons or neurons in the basis pontis or occipital cortex. The increase in APP messenger RNA in the former neurons was due solely to APP messenger RNA lacking the KPI domain.

The occurrence of increased APP messenger RNA lacking the KPI domain selectively in nucleus basalis and locus coeruleus neurons could reflect a selective effect of Alzheimer pathology on these neurons. Alternately, increased APP gene expression may be part of a compensatory response that develops uniquely in surviving nucleus basalis and locus coeruleus neurons as other cells in these populations are lost. It is believed that the KPI-free APP may be a substrate that is acted on preferentially by cerebral proteases to generate much of the A4 polypeptide (β-protein) that is deposited as cerebral amyloid in Alzheimer's disease.

▶ This impressive report shows that messenger RNA for amyloid protein precursor is abnormal in several loci of Alzheimer brains. Such biochemical studies bring closer the biochemical understanding of this illness. The story becomes yet more fascinating with the addition of precise genetic data that indicate that,

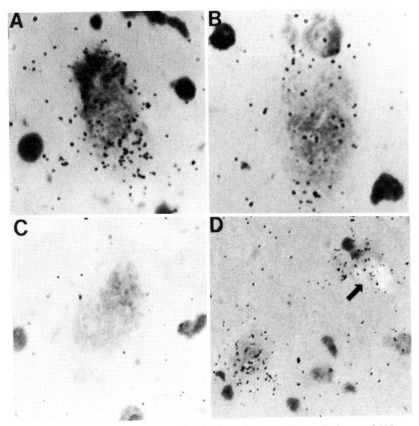

Fig 26–8.—In situ hybridization with a ^{35}S-labeled complementary RNA probe for a total APP messenger RNA. **A**, Alzheimer's disease nucleus basalis of Meynert (nbM). **B**, control nbM. **C**, control nbM, noncomplementary probe matched to the probe for total APP messenger RNA. **D**, Alzheimer's disease subiculum. The *closed arrow* identifies a neurofibrillary tangle within a subicular neuron. Hybridizations were performed with 0.6-nanomolar probe (3 × 10^9 cpm/nmole), and the autoradiographic exposure time was 1 day. Stain: (**A–C**) 0.4% cresyl violet in water; original magnification, ×1,250; (**D**) hematoxylin and Congo red; original magnification, ×900. (Courtesy of Palmert MR, Golde TE, Cohen ML, et al: *Science* 241:1080–1084, Aug 26, 1988.)

at least for certain Alzheimer patients, specific genetic abnormalities can be demonstrated. These leaps forward in the basic biologic understanding of the illness bring us closer to specific methods for diagnosis, genetic counseling, and treatment.

BRIEF NOTES ON NEUROSCIENCE

During embryogenesis in *Drosophila*, specific segmentation genes control neuronal cell fate (Doe CQ et al: *Nature* 333:376–378, 1988).

A target-derived neurotrophic factor in chick embryo can reduce naturally occurring motoneuron death in vivo (Oppenheim RW et al: *Science* 240:919–922, 1988).

Prenatal tetrodotoxin blocks segregation of retinogeniculate afferents (Shatz CJ, Stryker MP: *Science* 242:82–84, 1988).

A bifunctional calmodulin-binding peptide may inhibit calcium 2+/calmodulin-dependent protein kinase-type 2 (Kelly PT et al: *Proc Natl Acad Sci USA* 85:4991–4995, 1988).

Weissmann and associates (*J Pharmacol Exp Ther* 2247:29–33, 1988) report a high density of sigma receptor sites in the cerebellum, nucleus accumbens, and cerebral cortex. The density of sigma binding in these sites suggests applications for the psychotomimetic actions of benzomorphans, which interact at this site. A role for the sigma system is suggested in cognitive or affective disorders or both.

27 Miscellaneous Topics

Introduction

Cerebrospinal rhinorrhea is precisely evaluated with computed tomography with metrizamide (Chow et al, Abstract 27–1) and may be repaired by application of fibrin glue (Ferrante et al, Abstract 27–2). Modern neuroanesthesia can avoid catastrophe during neurosurgery in the malignant hyperthermia-susceptible patient (Wackym et al, Abstract 27–3). Diversion of cerebrospinal fluid is often effective in the treatment of benign intracranial hypertension (Johnston et al, Abstract 27–4). With modern techniques, postoperative intracranial hemorrhage can be minimized (0.8%), and postoperative hypertension appears to be the single most important factor (Kalfas and Little, Abstract 27–5). Decisions to limit care raise troubling legal and moral ramifications, and an ethics committee may be helpful to the treating physician (Brennan, Abstract 27–6).

Robert M. Crowell, M.D.

Evaluation of CSF Rhinorrhea by Computerized Tomography With Metrizamide
Chow JM, Goodman D, Mafee MF (Univ of Illinois, Chicago)
Otolaryngol Head Neck Surg 100:99–105, February 1989   27–1

After the use of metrizamide in conjunction with computed tomography (CT) was introduced, several case reports were published documenting the ability of metrizamide and CT to localize the site of the defect. A later study, however, was not in full agreement with these earlier findings, stating that the technique was useful but could not determine the exact site of leakage in most cases. Investigated was the ability of metrizamide and CT to delineate the site of leakage in patients with cerebrospinal fluid (CSF) rhinorrhea.

From 1981 to 1986, 13 patients underwent metrizamide CT cisternography to localize the site of CSF leakage. Of the 17 examinations performed, 13 (76%) scans identified the site of the CSF leakage, 9 of which were subsequently confirmed during surgery. The other 4 scans were done on patients who refused surgery. Of the 15 scans done on patients with active CSF leaks, 13 (87%) were positive. Of the 2 patients with inactive leaks, neither scan was positive. In 1 case, metrizamide CT cisternography was both diagnostic and therapeutic (Fig 27–1).

Metrizamide CT is an accurate diagnostic imaging technique that can be used to identify the site of leakage in patients with active CSF rhinor-

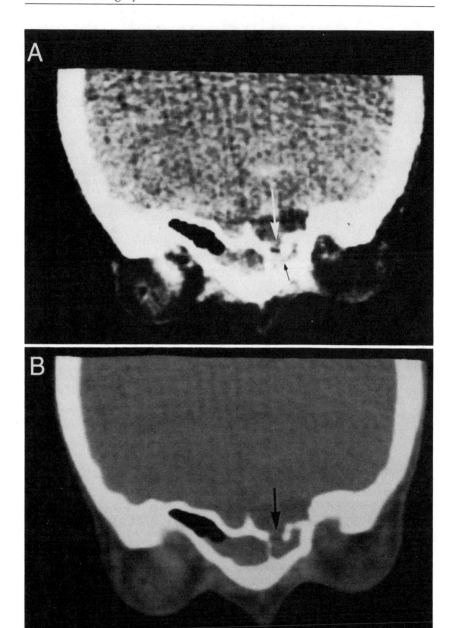

rhea. Minimal morbidity was associated with its use. It was most useful in patients with active leaks at the time of radiologic assessment.

▶ This report documents the great effectiveness of metrizamide CT cisternography in identifying the site of leakage. It should be pointed out that the success of the technique is directly related to the experience of the radiologist and his involvement in the precise performance of these studies. Having worked directly with Dr. Mafee, I can attest to his extraordinary helpfulness in planning the study and interpreting the films.

Endaural Extracranial Repair for Cerebrospinal Otorrhea With Human Fibrin Glue: Technical Note

Ferrante L, Palatinsky E, Acqui M, Matronardi L (Univ "La Sapienza" of Rome)
J Neurol Neurosurg Psychiatry 51:1438–1440, November 1988   27–2

Cerebrospinal otorrhea usually is treated operatively except for post-traumatic cases. A simple repair based on fibrin glue was used in 2 recent patients, 1 with a glomus jugulare chemodectoma and 1 with a giant eighth nerve neurinoma. Both patients had cerebrospinal otorrhea postoperatively that did not cease despite continuous lumbar drainage for 10 days and the use of diuretics. Neither patient had hydrocephaly.

After drying the middle ear by drawing off cerebrospinal fluid (CSF) through a lumbar tap, a speculum is used to examine the tympanic perforation and the medial wall of the tympanic cavity (Fig 27–2). Human fibrin glue is injected through the breach to fill the cavity, and after 3 minutes another 0.5 cc is dropped into the external auditory meatus against the tympanic membrane. Continuous CSF drainage is maintained for 1 week.

Both patients were free of otorrhea after 20 and 24 months, respectively. This nontraumatic procedure can be repeated if necessary or replaced by another method. If the middle ear is exposed to contamination or infection, the method is contraindicated.

▶ This is a clever application of fibrin glue for closing otorrhea leaks. Because the indications are rather narrow and exclusions are substantial, it seems unlikely that this will be frequently required. Success of the method suggests that use of fibrin glue may well be helpful in the sealing of other CSF leaks, including the open neurosurgical correction of CSF fistulas.

Fig 27–1.—**A,** semicoronal CT (soft tissue windows) shows a bony defect *(long arrow)* along the posterior left frontal sinus and metrizamide in the left frontal sinus *(short arrow)*; **B,** semicoronal CT (bone windows) shows the bony defect *(arrow)* and metrizamide with a fluid level in the frontal sinuses. (Courtesy of Chow JM, Goodman D, Mafee MF: *Otolaryngol Head Neck Surg* 100:99–105, February 1989.)

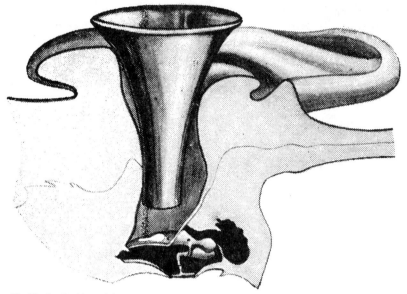

Fig 27–2.—Position of the speculum in the external auditory meatus and canal and break in the eardrum through which the glue was injected. (Courtesy of Ferrante L, Palatinsky E, Acqui M, et al: *J Neurol Neurosurg Psychiatry* 51:1438–1440, November 1988.)

Neurosurgery in the Malignant Hyperthermia-Susceptible Patient

Wackym PA, Dubrow TJ, Abdul-Rasool IH, Peacock WJ (Univ of California, Los Angeles)
Neurosurgery 22:1032–1036, June 1988   27–3

Malignant hyperthermia (MH) is a rare, often fatal complication of general anesthesia that is triggered in the presence of a genetic myopathy. After exposure to inhaled anesthetics or depolarizing muscle relaxants such as succinylcholine, susceptible persons have hyperpyrexia and a hypermetabolic crisis, which causes fatal multiple organ failure. Because of the extraordinary risk of death in susceptible patients, neurosurgeons are often reluctant to operate on these patients. Three case reports of patients susceptible to MH who had been referred for surgical and anesthetic management after aborted neurosurgical procedures secondary to episodes of MH are presented.

The referred patients included a 10-year-old boy and a 37-year-old woman who required craniotomy procedures and a 51-year-old woman who needed a L5-S1 laminectomy and diskectomy. None of the patients had any other risk factors for myopathy. A modified version of a previously described anesthetic management protocol was used, consisting of anesthesia induction with sodium thiopental and anesthesia maintenance with nitrous oxide, opiates, tranquilizers, and nondepolarizing muscle relaxants. Intravenous dantrolene was not given before anesthesia induction. After completion of the neurosurgical procedures, all 3 patients underwent vastus lateralis muscle biopsy. Susceptibility to MH was confirmed by a positive response to the caffeine and halothane contracture test performed on the muscle biopsy specimens for all 3 patients. Preoperative, intraoperative, and postoperative assessment of rectal temperature, cardiac activity, and muscle tone showed no sign of impending MH crisis, and none of the patients had any clinical signs of MH.

Patients with known or suspected MH can safely undergo general anesthesia, provided a specific protocol designed for such cases is strictly adhered to.

▶ This important communication outlines an effective technique for neurosurgery in the malignant hyperthermia susceptible patient. It is important for surgeons to recognize the susceptibility of patients for this problem on the basis of family history, congenital neuromuscular disorders, or other myopathies as well as previous episodes of malignant hypothermia.

Cerebrospinal Fluid Diversion in the Treatment of Benign Intracranial Hypertension
Johnston I, Besser M, Morgan MK (The Children's Hosp; Royal Prince Alfred Hosp, Sydney, Australia)
J Neurosurg 69:195–202, August 1988   27–4

The disease mechanism underlying benign intracranial hypertension (BIH) has not been elucidated, and treatment of this disorder has been largely empirical. In recent years there has been increasing support for an increase in cerebrospinal fluid (CSF) volume as the underlying cause of BIH. If this theory is true, shunting would be the most rational form of treatment for BIH. A few case reports have documented a rapid resolution of BIH with shunting, but no larger studies have as yet been published. This study was done to assess the effectiveness of CSF shunting in the treatment of BIH.

The study population comprised 41 patients with BIH, including 5 patients who were not treated with shunting, 12 patients who were treated with shunting as the first line of treatment, and 24 patients who were treated with shunting only after other forms of treatment had failed. Two of the 5 patients who received no shunt had improvement without treatment, 2 had improvement with steroid therapy, and 1 had improvement with a course of acetazolamide. Reasons for selecting shunting as a primary option for 12 patients included severe deterioration of vision in 9 cases, and a concern about possible side effects of steroids in 3 cases. All 12 patients had rapid and complete resolution of BIH, although the shunts had to be kept in place in 8 patients. All 24 patients in whom a shunt was inserted when other forms of treatment had failed also had rapid and complete resolution of BIH, but the shunts were kept in place in 20 patients.

Unfortunately, the revision rate was high, with 50 revisions required in 18 (50%) of the 36 shunted patients, 2 of whom had a total of 15 revisions. In addition, the continuing treatment in 28 of 36 shunted patients after a mean period of 3.5 years compared unfavorably with a reported 87% cure rate with steroid therapy. Evaluation of the various types of shunts showed that the percutaneous lumboperitoneal shunt was associated with the lowest revision rate and the least complications. Cisternal shunting to either the atrium or pleural cavity was the next most effective shunt, whereas valved lumboperitoneal shunts inserted via a laminectomy were the least effective of all. Ventricular shunts were used in only 2 patients.

Shunting is indeed effective in the treatment of BIH, but its significant complication rate and the possibility of inducing shunt dependence should be recognized.

▶ This report confirms that CSF diversion is effective in the treatment of benign intracranial hypertension, but unfortunately there is a significant complication rate and the possibility of inducing shunt dependence.

Postoperative Hemorrhage: A Survey of 4,992 Intracranial Procedures
Kalfas IH, Little JR (Cleveland Clinic Found)
Neurosurgery 23:343–347, September 1988   27–5

Postoperative hemorrhage can be a fatal neurosurgical complication. A series of 4,992 intracranial procedures (table) performed over an 11-year period were reviewed for the occurrence of postoperative hemorrhage.

In this series of patients, 0.8% had postoperative hemorrhaging. Of these hemorrhages, 60% were intracerebral, 28% were epidural, 7.5% were subdural, and 5.0% were intrasellar. The majority of the hematomas occurred at the operative site. Hemorrhages were more common among female patients. Of the patients in whom a clot developed, 56% were operated on for intracranial tumor. Meningioma was the most common tumor associated with these hemorrhages. The use of a sitting position for the operation was not asssociated with increased incidence of hemorrhage. However, disturbances in coagulation and hypertension appeared to be risk factors. An altered level of consciousness was detected in all patients. The postoperative hemorrhage was detected within 12

Intracranial Procedures: 1976–1986

Procedure	No. Cases	No. Hematomas (%)
Craniotomy/craniectomy	3355	33 (1.0)
Minor procedure[a]	1378	5 (1.1)
Transsphenoidal procedure	259	2 (0.8)
Total	4992	40

[a]Ventricular shunting, brain biopsy, Ommaya reservoir placement.
(Courtesy of Kalfas IH, Little JR: *Neurosurgery* 23:343–347, September 1988.)

hours in 35% of the patients. However, there was no discernible relationship between the time of hemorrhage recognition and clinical outcome. Parenchymal clots had the worst prognosis.

In this series of neurosurgical patients, there was an approximately 1% rate of postoperative intracranial hemorrhage. The relationship between hematomas and preexisting hypertension requires further study.

▶ This exhaustive review of an important topic is likely to be the landmark reference on the subject for years to come. The low incidence of postoperative hemorrhage (0.8%) is commendable. Postoperative hypertension appears to be the single most important factor. One wonders whether aspirin therapy or other disruption of the clotting system may have played a role as well. Many surgeons routinely use brief hypertension or Valsalva maneuver to check hemostasis at the occlusion of the procedure. Hemorrhage at a distance from the operative site may be related to extensive drainage of cerebrospinal fluid and lessening of intracranial pressure.

Ethics Committees and Decisions to Limit Care: The Experience at the Massachusetts General Hospital
Brennan TA (Brigham and Women's Hosp, Boston; Harvard Univ)
JAMA 260:803–807, Aug 12, 1988   27–6

Physicians have started to study empirically the ethically controversial limitations on care, with particular attention to do-not-resuscitate (DNR) orders. During the past 13 years, the Optimum Care Committee (OCC) of the Massachusetts General Hospital in Boston has provided consultation to 73 patients. The records of these patients were reviewed and compared with those of 113 patients who were accorded limited-care status or DNR status without OCC input during a 3-month period.

Each OCC patient was classified into 1 of 6 broad categories based on the type of decision made by the OCC and the attending physician. These categories were not used by the OCC but were assigned only for the purpose of this study. Analysis of each of the categories showed that during the previous 3 years, 80% of the consultations provided by the OCC pertained to patients who were incompetent and critically ill and whose prognosis was very poor, but whose families demanded that everything be done. On the other hand, the number of cases in which the patient was accorded DNR status according to the family's wishes has remained constant.

A comparison of the OCC experience with data obtained from the 113 patients accorded DNR status without OCC input showed that the OCC is asked to review only a very small percentage of all patients with limited-care orders, as only 6 of the 113 patients were interviewed by the OCC. In most cases, the physicians, patients, and the patients' families do not disagree on the limiting of care. Of the 6 types of recommendations made by the OCC, that of DNR for an incompetent and moribund patient made despite the wishes of the patient's family to resuscitate was the most controversial, as this type of case has the most troubling legal and moral ramifications.

The experience of the OCC at the Massachusetts General Hospital provides a model for an ethics committee's role in limited care cases and illustrates the complexity of the problems associated with such decisions.

▶ Dr. Brennan's communication illustrates the difficulty of decisions to limit care and the usefulness of ethics committees in helping the physician grapple with these difficulties. In the same issue of *JAMA*, Field and co-workers state that, in certain selected cases, there may be medical and ethical bases for the maintenance of a brain-dead mother until the newborn can be expected to thrive. The cost may be high: in 1 case, $217,784 (Field DR et al: *JAMA* 260:816–822, 1988).

Brief Notes

CSF LEAKAGE

Primeau and associates (*Clin Nucl Med* 13:701–703) report demonstration of a lumbar CSF leak by radioisotopic cisternography.

Studies of rabbits show no significant neurotoxicity for autologous fibrin tissue adhesive for CSF leaks (Feldman MD et al: *Am J Otol* 9:302–305, 1988).

Fibrin glue enhances the results of muscle packing alone for the treatment of cerebrospinal fluid rhinnorhea in an experimental setting (Lishihira S, McCaffrey TV: *Laryngoscope* 98:625–627, 1988).

A porcine peritoneal biomembrane used in canine dural repair is nontoxic, given to watertight closure, dispensable, and free of adhesions to the brain (Bang-Zong X et al: *J Neurosurg* 69:707–711, 1988).

CRANIOFACIAL SURGERY

A team approach can be effective for wide resection of skull base tumors via a combined orbital and intracranial approach, with primary reconstruction of the skull with a musculocutaneous flap (Goignard RM et al: *Eur J Plast Surg* 11:169–174, 1988).

Repeated tissue expansion may be helpful for reconstruction of very extensive scalp-forehead avulsion injuries (Wieslander JB: *Ann Plast Surg* 20:381–385, 1988).

A pericranial flap may be utilized for reconstruction of anterior skull base defects (Price JC et al: *Laryngoscope* 98:1159–1164, 1988).

For orbital-cranial disorders, 3-dimensional imaging, cranial bone grafts, a free composite flap, and a computer-generated implant may be helpful adjuncts (Toth BA et al: *Ophthalmology* 95:1013–1026, 1988).

Titanum is an excellent inert material for cranioplasty. It has been used by Ban and co-workers from Kobe, Japan (*Neurol Med Chir [Tokyo]* 27:984–989, October 1987), when acrylic plates have broken. In 114 cases, followed for up to 11 years, infection developed in only 2; tissue reaction was insignificant. Subgaleal fluid collection was rare. This metal does not prevent proper interpretations of angiograms, computed tomograms, electroencephalograms, or magnetic imaging. It is economical and easy to handle.—O. Sugar, M.D.

Craniofacial surgery is associated with complications in 22% with a mortality of 1% and an infection rate of 1% (Poole MD: *Br J Plast Surg* 41:608–613, 1988).

Porous hydroxyapatite has been used as a bone graft substitute in cranial reconstruction in the canine laboratory model (Holmes RE, Hagler HK: *Plast Reconstr Surg* 81:662–671, 1988).

OTHER TOPICS

Among the more subspecialized forms of neurosurgery, fetal neurosurgery is the most apt to cause outcries about ethical behavior. An excellent review of experimental and human work in this field has been put together by Kim Manwaring, pediatric neurosurgeon in Phoenix (*BNIQ* 4:26–33, 1988). Long after the first intentional destructions in utero to facilitate delivery (c. first century A.D.), human fetal operations were begun with transperitoneal infusions of erythrocytes for Rh incompatibility. When it became evident that transperitoneal cephalocentesis for ventricular enlargement was not helpful, transperitoneal placement of a valved silicone catheter was done under ultrasound control, terminating in the amniotic cavity (1982). Such operations are being monitored via the International Fetal Treatment Registry. Review of patient selection, timing of intervention, and reports of outcome indicate that this type of treatment for prenatally diagnosed hydrocephalus may be producing better viability and postnatal growth than waiting until after birth for treatment. The extension of animal experimental work with hysterotomy and return of the fetus to the uterus after ventriculoperitoneal shunt remains for the future, although animal experiments show the technical feasibility of such procedures.—O. Sugar, M.D.

Among 38 patients with intracranial mass lesions undergoing spinal puncture, none deteriorated (Zisfein J, Tuchman AJ: *Mt Sinai J Med [NY]* 55:283–287, 1988).

From the Acute Spinal Cord Injury Unit at the University of Toronto comes a report by Meguro and Tator on the interaction of spinal cord or cauda equina injury and multiple injuries elsewhere in the body (*Neurol Med Chir [Tokyo]* 28:34–41, 1988). The additional injuries included cerebral contusion, hemothorax, major intra-abdominal bleeding, and femoral fracture. In a series of 27 patients with multiple injuries, hypotension on admission was present in 59%, compared with only 7% in 117 patients with only spinal cord (or cauda) injuries. The first group with multiple injuries had more severe initial neurologic deficits, poorer neurologic recovery, and a higher mortality than those with only neurologic injuries. The authors believe that the greater incidence of hypotension among the patients with multiple injuries may play a significant role in the different end results so far as neurologic function is concerned. Obviously, other factors producing hypoxia also play a role. The authors also suggest that the concomitant presence of spinal cord and abdominal injuries may mask the physical findings in the latter. They therefore support the performance of routine minilaparotomy when spinal cord injury occurs during significant impact, as in motor vehicle accidents.—O. Sugar, M.D.

Review of 579 posterior fossa operations at the Mayo Clinic revealed no substantial advantage for either a horizontal or sitting position (Black S et al: *Anesthesiology* 69:49–56, 1988).

Extravascular migration of a central venous catheter was reported to cause hydromediastinum and secondary Horner's syndrome (*Chest* 94:1093–1094, 1988).

Fernandes (*S Afr Med J* 74:280–282, 1988) reported successful management of intractable vasorhinitis treated with transnasal vidian neurectomy.

Cerebrospinal fluid and plasma levels of mannitol varied greatly after intravenous infusions of the drug in 12 neurosurgical patients under general anesthesia (Anderson P et al: *Eur J Clin Pharmacol* 35:643–649, 1988).

A randomized controlled trial indicates that graduated compression stockings (TED stockings) alone or in combination with intermittent pneumatic compression are effective methods of preventing deep venous thrombosis in neurosurgical patients (Turpie AGG et al: *Arch Intern Med* 149:679–681, 1989).

Perforation of the gastrointestinal tract is not uncommon in patients receiving steroids for neurologic disease (Fadul CE et al: *Neurology* 38:348–352, 1988).

Gastrointestinal bleeding was noted in 9.3% of 518 patients after craniotomy (Muller P et al: *Can J Neurol Sci* 15:384–387, 1988). Twenty-one percent of patients with a score on the Glascow Coma Scale of less than 10 had gastrointestinal bleeding, whereas only 7% of patients with a score greater than 10 had such bleeding.

Oxygen can be carried in the blood by substitutes for red blood cells; both hemoglobin solutions and fluorocarbon emulsions can do this, maintaining normal oxygen consumption, CO_2 production, and circulatory dynamics in the virtual absence of the red blood cell. The perfluorochemicals, which are so effective in carrying oxygen, are unfortunately not water miscible, and the emulsion forms are perforce of lower concentrations than optimal for oxygen transport. Clinical trials have been carried out by S. A. Gould and colleagues at Michael Reese Hospital in Chicago (*Surgical Rounds* March 1988, pp 37–46). Of 23 patients studied, 15 had no physiologic evidence of need for increased arterial oxygen content despite hemoglobin levels of 7.2 gm/dl. Fourteen of those who did not receive Fluosol survived. Mortality is high among severely anemic patients who refuse red blood cell therapy in spite of receiving Fluosol-DA therapy. Overall, the authors contend, Fluosol-DA is unnecessary when anemia is moderate and ineffective when it is severe. Fluosol-DA is an inadequate red cell substitute and should not be considered by neurosurgeons who may well run into severe blood loss in removing meningiomas and arteriovenous malformations in patients who refuse red-cell transfusions or for whom compatible blood is not available.—O. Sugar, M.D.

Reduced levels of vitamin A and E in plasma are associated with weight reduction (Szwiauerk et al: *Acta Pediatr Scand* 77:760–761, 1988).

A population study estimates that, in Maryland hospitals in 1983, charges related to injury were $109 million, with 43% incurred by individuals with a principal injury to 1 or more of the extremities (MacKenzie EJ et al: *JAMA* 260:3290–3296, 1988).

Subject Index

A

Abscess (*see* Brain abscess)

Abuse
  cocaine, neurovascular complications, 158

Acromegaly
  preoperative SMS 201–995 for, 266

ACTH
  in multiple sclerosis, results, 140
  -secreting pituitary microadenoma, 237

Acyclovir
  in herpes zoster with encephalitis, 149

Adenoma
  microadenoma (*see* Microadenoma)
  pituitary
    GH-secreting, microsurgery results in, 253
    large, transsphenoidal surgery, 254
    MRI of cavernous sinus in, 239

Adolescence
  cerebral aneurysms during, 373

Adrenal (*see* Transplantation, adrenal)

Age
  reaction time and, simple, decade differences, 27

Aged
  with depression, major, medical evaluation, 22
  dizziness in, 13
  neurofibrillary tangles and senile plaques (in aged bear), 86
  symptomatic, carotid endarterectomy in, 273

Aging
  rabbits, learning of, and nimodipine, 28

Alcohol
  consumption
    moderate, coronary disease and stroke risk in women and, 33
    seizures and, new-onset, 103
    smoking and ischemic stroke risk, 32
    withdrawal and new-onset seizures, 103

Alcoholic
  pellagra encephalopathy, case pathology analysis, 167

Alcoholism
  with autonomic neuropathy, mortality in, 129

Algorithm
  surgical, for facial palsy, 413

Alzheimer's disease
  amyloid protein showing protease inhibitor activity, 87
  genetic linkage studies in, 25

RNA in, amyloid protein precursor messenger, 428

Alzheimer's type senile dementia
  psychotic symptoms in, 26

Amines
  vasoactive, in cerebral vasospasm after subarachnoid hemorrhage, 38

Amitriptyline
  for central post-stroke pain, 55

Amnesia
  transient global, case study, 182

Ampicillin
  -chloramphenicol in bacterial meningitis in children, 67

Amygdala
  neural encoding of individual words and faces by, 427

Amyloid protein
  Alzheimer's disease, showing protease inhibitor activity, 87
  precursor messenger RNA in Alzheimer's disease, 428

Amyotrophic lateral sclerosis
  no association with cancer, 125
  parkinsonism dementia and, 91

Anabolic
  androgenic steroids and stroke in athlete, 34

Analgesia
  rebound headache, 71

Androgenic
  anabolic steroids and stroke in athlete, 34

Aneuploidy
  DNA analysis of medulloblastoma and, 362

Aneurysm(s), 189, 269
  basilar artery
    circulatory arrest, hypothermia and barbiturate cerebral protection in, 285
    surgical approaches, 283
  carotid-ophthalmic, bifrontal interhemispheric approach, 282
  cavernous sinus, surgical management, 220
  cerebral
    in childhood and adolescence, 373
    giant, endaneurysmal microendarterectomy in, 287
  clips and MRI, 195
  intracranial
    intraarterial digital subtraction angiography of, 280
    large, MRI of, 197
  poor-grade aneurysm patients, nimodipine for, results, 289

Author Index

A

Abdullah, A.F., 317
Abdul-Rasool, I.H., 434
Abrahamsson, P., 82
Abreu, S.H., 385
Abu El Ella, A.H., 67
Acqui, M., 433
Adams, H.P., 273
Adams, H.P., Jr., 281
Agid, Y., 117
Aikawa, M., 320
Al-Aska, A.K., 152
Alavi, A., 207
Alavi, J.B., 207
Albers, J.W., 161
Alberts, M.J., 25
Alessi, A.G., 161
Alfandary, E., 372
Allen, D., 157
Allen, M.C., 68
Allison, S., 27
Al-Mefty, O., 219, 222
Alvarez, L.A., 63
Aminoff, M.J., 15, 104, 173
Ammirati, M, 221
Amparo, E.G., 380
Andermann, F., 105
Andersen, B., 52
Andersen, E.D., 52
Anderson, V.E., 107
Annegers, J.F., 337
Anthony, M., 76
Anzalone, N., 182
Arbit, E., 209
Arbuckle, J.D., 133
Asai, M., 280
Atkinson, J.L.D., 273
Ausman, J.I., 220, 300
Austin-Seymour, M., 243
Ayer-LeLievre, C., 423

B

Baba, H., 311
Badger, G.J., 169
Baerentsen, D.J., 133
Baggoley, C.J., 73
Baghurst, P.A., 162
Bahemuka, M., 152
Bamford, J.M., 36
Ban, S., 324
Banks, A.J., 386
Barkan, A.L., 266
Barmada, M.A., 60
Barnett, C.M., 262
Barnett, P.A., 266
Barrett, J., 342
Barth, D.S., 397
Bartlett, R.J., 25
Baskerville, J., 144

Bass, B., 144
Bass, N.M., 40
Bataini, P., 370
Batz, U., 35
Batzdorf, U., 330
Bauer, K.D., 362, 363
Baughman, R., 290
Beaumier, P., 266
Bedford, R.F., 209
Beevers, G., 31
Beitins, I.Z., 266
Bello, J.A., 255
Benoit, B.G., 289
Benson, D.F., 90
Bentzen, L., 175
Berg, S.Z., 65
Bergen, D., 400
Berger, J.R., 9
Berginer, V.M., 35
Bergman, I., 60
Berkel, I., 85
Bertalanffy, H., 310
Bertsch, L., 263
Besser, M., 435
Bhagavati, S., 151
Bigner, D.D., 232
Bigner, S.H., 232
Biller, J., 273
Bird, C.R., 198
Black, P.G., 178
Black, P.M., 254
Blair, C.J., 169
Blazer, D., 13
Bleck, T.P., 400
Blitzer, A., 172
Bocci, L., 137
Boder, E., 85
Boerman, J., 169
Boesel, C.P., 11
Bognanno, J.R., 241
Bohlman, H.H., 315, 321
Boice, J.D., Jr., 372
Boivie, J., 55
Boller, F., 26
Bolte, R.G., 178
Bondesson, L., 82
Bonnet, A.-M., 117
Book, W.J., 120
Borges, L., 327
Bornstein, N.M., 42, 48, 54
Bouche, P., 125
Bowers, R.S., 178
Boysen, G., 52
Bradley, W.G., 169
Braedt, G., 85
Brand, J., 74
Brandt, L., 195
Brauner, R., 370
Bregman, D.J., 129
Brennan, T.A., 437
Briceno, C., 329
Brin, M.F., 172
Bromberg, M.B., 161
Brooke, M., 122

Brooke, M.H., 123
Brown, G.W., 145
Brown, R.H., 122
Brown, T.H., 425
Brownell, A.-L., 11
Browner, C.M., 345
Bruce, D.A., 365
Brunberg, J., 60
Brust, J.C.M., 103
Bucci, M.N., 346
Buge, A., 167
Bulas, R., 11
Bunke, J., 198
Burchiel, K.J., 394
Burger, P.C., 232
Burnstine, T.H., 102
Burrows, P., 375

C

Cahan, L.D., 397
Cahill, D., 405
Call, G.K., 38
Callaham, M., 147
Callen, P.W., 58
Calne, D.B., 148
Cameron, G.S., 289
Campi, A., 140
Candia, G., 254
Canini, F., 168
Cannon, M., 101
Caputo, A.J., 68
Caroscio, J.T., 125
Carreras, M., 123
Carriere, W., 144
Carroll, R., 243
Carter, C.M., 62
Carter, J., 320
Carter, J.R., 321
Carter, L.P., 285
Cascino, T.L., 273
Caskey, C.T., 122
Castaigne, P., 167
Castle, R.L., 230
Cathala, H.P., 125
Cedarbaum, J., 169
Chadwick, L.G., 48
Chaine, P., 125
Chakeres, D.W., 11
Challa, V.R., 240
Chamberlain, J., 122
Chamberlain, K., 177
Chamberlain, S., 88
Chan, R., 289
Chancellor, A.M., 40
Chandler, W.F., 266
Chapman, L.J., 165
Chapman, P.F., 425
Charman, C.E., 65
Charmley, P., 85
Chawluk, J., 207
Chehrazi, B.B., 38

461

TO ORDER: DETACH AND MAIL

Please enter my subscription to the journal(s) and/or Year Book(s) checked below:
(To order by phone, call **toll-free 800-622-5410**. In IL, call **collect 312-726-9746**.

	Practitioner (approx.)	Resident	Institution
Current Problems in Surgery® (1 yr.)	___$57.95	___$34.95	___$78.50
Current Problems in Pediatrics® (1 yr.)	___$46.95	___$34.95	___$65.00
Current Problems in Cancer® (1 yr.)	___$54.95	___$29.95	___$71.50
Current Problems in Cardiology® (1 yr.)	___$57.95	___$34.95	___$75.50
Current Problems in Obstetrics, Gynecology, and Fertility® (1 yr.)	___$49.95	___$29.95	___$65.00
Current Problems in Diag. Radiology® (1 yr.)	___$57.50	___$29.95	——$75.50
Current Problems in Dermatology® (1 yr.)	___$49.95	___$29.95	___$65.00
Disease-A-Month® (1 yr.)	___$46.95	___$34.95	___$65.00
	Binder ___$14.95		
1989 Year Book of Anesthesia® (AN-89)	___$49.95	___$29.95	
1989 Year Book of Cancer® (CA-89)	___$51.95	___$29.95	
1989 Year Book of Cardiology® (CV-89)	___$51.95	___$29.95	
1989 Year Book of Critical Care Medicine ® (16-89)	___$49.95	___$29.95	
1989 Year Book of Dentistry® (D-89)	___$49.95	___$29.95	
1989 Year Book of Dermatology® (10-89)	___$51.95	___$29.95	
1989 Year Book of Diagnostic Radiology® (9-89)	___$51.95	___$29.95	
1989 Year Book of Digestive Diseases® (13-89)	___$51.95	___$29.95	
1989 Year Book of Drug Therapy® (6-89)	___$49.95	___$29.95	
1989 Year Book of Emergency Medicine® (15-89)	___$49.95	___$29.95	
1989 Year Book of Endocrinology® (EM-89)	___$51.95	___$29.95	
1989 Year Book of Family Practice® (FY-89)	___$49.95	___$29.95	
1989 Year Book of Geriatrics and Gerontology (GE-89)	___$49.95	___$29.95	
1989 Year Book of Hand Surgery® (17-89)	___$51.95	___$29.95	
1989 Year Book of Hematology® (24-89)	___$49.95	___$29.95	
1989 Year Book of Infectious Diseases® (19-89)	___$49.95	___$29.95	
1989 Year Book of Medicine® (1-89)	___$51.95	___$29.95	
1989 Year Book of Neurology and Neurosurgery® (8-89)	___$51.95	___$29.95	
1989 Year Book of Nuclear Medicine® (NM-89)	___$51.95	___$29.95	
1989 Year Book of Obstetrics and Gynecology® (5-89)	___$49.95	___$29.95	
1989 Year Book of Ophthalmology® (EY-89)	___$51.95	___$29.95	
1989 Year Book of Orthopedics® (OR-89)	___$51.95	___$29.95	
1989 Year Book of Otolaryngology-Head and Neck Surgery® (3-89)	___$51.95	___$29.95	
1989 Year Book of Pathology and Clinical Pathology® (PI-89)	___$54.95	___$29.95	
1989 Year Book of Pediatrics® (4-89)	___$49.95	___$29.95	
1989 Year Book of Perinatal/Neonatal Medicine (23-89)	___$49.95	___$29.95	
1989 Year Book of Plastic and Reconstructive Surgery® (12-89)	___$51.95	___$29.95	
1989 Year Book of Podiatric Medicine and Surgery®(18-89)	___$49.95		
1989 Year Book of Psychiatry and Applied Mental Health® (11-89)	___$49.95	___$29.95	
1989 Year Book of Pulmonary Disease® (21-89)	___$49.95	___$29.95	
1989 Year Book of Rehabilitation® (22-89)	___$49.95	___$29.95	
1989 Year Book of Sports Medicine® (SM-89)	___$49.95	___$29.95	
1989 Year Book of Surgery® (2-89)	___$51.95	___$29.95	
1989 Year Book of Urology® (7-89)	___ $51.95	___$29.95	
1989 Year Book of Vascular Surgery (20-89)	——$51.95	___$29.95	

*The above Year Books are published annually. For the convenience of its customers, Year Book enters each purchaser as a subscriber to future volumes and sends annual announcements of each volume approximately 2 months before publication. The new volume will be shipped upon publication unless you complete and return the cancellation notice attached to the announcement and it is received by Year Book within the time indicated (approximately 20 days after your receipt of the announcement). You may cancel your subscription at any time. The new volume may be examined on approval for 30 days, may be returned for full credit, and if returned Year Book will then remove your name as a subscriber. Return postage is guaranteed by Year Book to the Postal Service.

Prices quoted are in U.S. dollars. Canadian orders will be billed in Canadian funds at the approximate current exchange rate. A small additional charge will be made for postage and handling. Illinois, Massachusetts and Tennessee residents will be billed appropriate sales tax. **All prices quoted subject to change.**

NAME_____ ACCT.NO._____

ADDRESS_____

CITY_____STATE_____ZIP_____

Printed in U.S.A.

DF1

Year Book Medical Publishers
200 North LaSalle Street Chicago, Illinois 60601